Medical Disorders in Pregnancy

Editors

ERIKA PETERSON
JUDITH U. HIBBARD

OBSTETRICS AND GYNECOLOGY CLINICS OF NORTH AMERICA

www.obgyn.theclinics.com

Consulting Editor
WILLIAM F. RAYBURN

June 2018 • Volume 45 • Number 2

ELSEVIER

1600 John F. Kennedy Boulevard • Suite 1800 • Philadelphia, Pennsylvania, 19103-2899

http://www.theclinics.com

OBSTETRICS AND GYNECOLOGY CLINICS OF NORTH AMERICA Volume 45, Number 2
June 2018 ISSN 0889-8545, ISBN-13: 978-0-323-58407-4

Editor: Kerry Holland
Developmental Editor: Kristen Helm

Obstetrics and Gynecology Clinics (ISSN 0889-8545) is published quarterly by Elsevier Inc., 360 Park Avenue South, New York, NY 10010-1710. Months of issue are March, June, September, and December. Periodicals postage paid at New York, NY, and additional mailing offices. Subscription price per year is $313.00 (US individuals), $652.00 (US institutions), $100.00 (US students), $393.00 (Canadian individuals), $823.00 (Canadian institutions), $225.00 (Canadian students), $459.00 (international individuals), $823.00 (international institutions), and $225.00 (international students). To receive student/resident rate, orders must be accompanied by name of affiliated institution, date of term, and the signature of program/residency coordinator on institution letterhead. Orders will be billed at individual rate until proof of status is received. Foreign air speed delivery is included in all *Clinics* subscription prices. All prices are subject to change without notice. POSTMASTER: Send address changes to *Obstetrics and Gynecology Clinics*, Elsevier Health Sciences Division, Subscription Customer Service, 3251 Riverport Lane, Maryland Heights, MO 63043. **Customer Service: Telephone: 1-800-654-2452 (U.S. and Canada); 314-447-8871 (outside U.S. and Canada). Fax: 314-447-8029. E-mail: journalscustomerservice-usa@elsevier.com (for print support); journalsonlinesupport-usa@elsevier. com (for online support).**

Reprints. For copies of 100 or more of articles in this publication, please contact the Commercial Reprints Department, Elsevier Inc., 360 Park Avenue South, New York, New York 10010-1710. Tel.: 212-633-3874; Fax: 212-633-3820; E-mail: reprints@elsevier.com.

Obstetrics and Gynecology Clinics of North America is also published in Spanish by McGraw-Hill Interamericana Editores S.A., P.O. Box 5-237, 06500, Mexico; in Portuguese by Reichmann and Affonso Editores, Rio de Janeiro, Brazil; and in Greek by Paschalidis Medical Publications, Athens, Greece.

Obstetrics and Gynecology Clinics of North America is covered in MEDLINE/PubMed (Index Medicus), Excerpta Medica, Current Concepts/Clinical Medicine, Science Citation Index, BIOSIS, CINAHL, and ISI/BIOMED.

Contributors

CONSULTING EDITOR

WILLIAM F. RAYBURN, MD, MBA
Associate Dean, Continuing Medical Education and Professional Development, Distinguished Professor and Emeritus Chair, Obstetrics and Gynecology, University of New Mexico School of Medicine, Albuquerque, New Mexico

EDITORS

ERIKA PETERSON, MD
Associate Professor, Department of Obstetrics and Gynecology, Director, Division of Maternal-Fetal Medicine, Co-Director Fetal Concerns Center of Wisconsin, Medical College of Wisconsin, Milwaukee, Wisconsin

JUDITH U. HIBBARD, MD
Professor Emeritus, Professor, Vice Chair, Department of Obstetrics and Gynecology, Division of Maternal-Fetal Medicine, Medical College of Wisconsin, Milwaukee, Wisconsin

AUTHORS

KASSIE J. BOLLIG, MD
Resident Physician, Department of Obstetrics, Gynecology and Women's Health, University of Missouri School of Medicine, Columbia, Missouri

JOAN BRILLER, MD
Professor of Medicine, Director of the Heart Disease in Women Program, Division of Cardiology, Professor, Department of Obstetrics and Gynecology, University of Illinois at Chicago, Chicago, Illinois

SABRINA CRAIGO, MD
Professor of Obstetrics and Gynecology, Director of Maternal-Fetal Medicine, Tufts University School of Medicine, Tufts Medical Center, Boston, Massachusetts

MEREDITH O. CRUZ, MD, MPH, MBA
Assistant Professor, Department of Obstetrics and Gynecology, Division of Maternal-Fetal Medicine, Medical College of Wisconsin, Milwaukee, Wisconsin

JEFFREY M. DENNEY, MD, MS, FACOG
Assistant Professor, Department of Obstetrics and Gynecology, Section of Maternal-Fetal Medicine, Wake Forest University School of Medicine, Winston-Salem, North Carolina

CARA D. DOLIN, MD
Division of Maternal-Fetal Medicine, Department of Obstetrics and Gynecology, New York University Langone Health, New York, New York

JENNIFER E. DOMINGUEZ, MD, MHS
Assistant Professor, Department of Anesthesiology, Division of Women's Anesthesia, Duke University Medical Center, Durham, North Carolina

MAURICE DRUZIN, MD
Professor of Obstetrics, Obstetrics and Gynecology, Stanford University, Stanford Hospital, Stanford, California

MEGAN E. FOELLER, MD
Maternal-Fetal Medicine Fellow, Obstetrics and Gynecology, Stanford University, Stanford Hospital, Stanford, California

TIMOTHY M. FOELLER, MD
Clinical Instructor, Internal Medicine, Stanford Health Care–Valleycare, Pleasanton, California

KIMBERLY B. FORTNER, MD
Associate Professor, Department of Obstetrics and Gynecology, Division Director, Maternal-Fetal Medicine, The University of Tennessee Medical Center, Knoxville, Tennessee

LORIE M. HARPER, MD, MSCI
Associate Professor, Department of Obstetrics and Gynecology, Division of Maternal-Fetal Medicine, The University of Alabama at Birmingham, Women and Infants Center, Birmingham, Alabama

SARAH HARRIS, MS
University of North Carolina at Chapel Hill School of Medicine, Chapel Hill, North Carolina

JUDITH U. HIBBARD, MD
Professor Emeritus, Professor, Vice Chair, Department of Obstetrics and Gynecology, Division of Maternal-Fetal Medicine, Medical College of Wisconsin, Milwaukee, Wisconsin

DANIEL L. JACKSON, MD, MS
Assistant Professor, Department of Obstetrics, Gynecology and Women's Health, University of Missouri School of Medicine, Columbia, Missouri

AMANDA J. JOHNSON, MD
Department of Obstetrics and Gynecology, Division of Maternal-Fetal Medicine, Medical College of Wisconsin, Milwaukee, Wisconsin

CRESTA W. JONES, MD
Department of Obstetrics, Gynecology and Women's Health, Division of Maternal-Fetal Medicine, University of Minnesota Medical School, Minneapolis, Minnesota

SARAH J. KILPATRICK, MD, PhD
Chair, Department of Obstetrics and Gynecology, Division of Maternal-Fetal Medicine, Cedars-Sinai Medical Center, Los Angeles, California

DIANA KOLETTIS, MD
Maternal-Fetal Medicine Fellow, Tufts Medical Center, Boston, Massachusetts

MICHELLE A. KOMINIAREK, MD, MS
Division of Maternal-Fetal Medicine, Department of Obstetrics and Gynecology, Northwestern University, Chicago, Illinois

JUDETTE LOUIS, MD, MPH
Associate Professor, Department of Obstetrics and Gynecology, Division of Maternal-Fetal Medicine, MFM Division Chief, Fellowship Director, University of South Florida, Tampa, Florida

ANNA McCORMICK, DO
Department of Obstetrics and Gynecology, Medical College of Wisconsin, Milwaukee, Wisconsin

CLAUDIA NIEUWOUDT, MD
Resident Physician, Department of Obstetrics and Gynecology, The University of Tennessee Medical Center, Knoxville, Tennessee

JOHN A. OZIMEK, DO, MS
Staff Physician I, Department of Obstetrics and Gynecology, Division of Maternal-Fetal Medicine, Cedars-Sinai Medical Center, Los Angeles, California

ERIKA PETERSON, MD
Associate Professor, Department of Obstetrics and Gynecology, Director, Division of Maternal-Fetal Medicine, Co-Director Fetal Concerns Center of Wisconsin, Medical College of Wisconsin, Milwaukee, Wisconsin

KRISTEN H. QUINN, MD, MS, FACOG
Assistant Professor, Department of Obstetrics and Gynecology, Section of Maternal-Fetal Medicine, Wake Forest University School of Medicine, Winston-Salem, North Carolina

CALLIE F. REEDER, MD
Resident Physician, Department of Obstetrics and Gynecology, The University of Tennessee Medical Center, Knoxville, Tennessee

LINDA STREET, MD
Assistant Professor, Department of Obstetrics and Gynecology, Division of Maternal-Fetal Medicine, Medical College of Georgia, Augusta University, Augusta, Georgia

RONAN SUGRUE, MD, MPH
Clinical Fellow, Department of Obstetrics and Gynecology, Brigham and Women's Hospital, Harvard Medical School, Boston, Massachusetts

AMELIA L.M. SUTTON, MD, PhD
Assistant Professor, Department of Obstetrics and Gynecology, Division of Maternal-Fetal Medicine, The University of Alabama at Birmingham, Women and Infants Center, Birmingham, Alabama

GEETA K. SWAMY, MD
Senior Associate Dean Clinical Research, Associate Professor, Department of Obstetrics and Gynecology, Director, Obstetrics Clinical Research, Duke University Medical System, Durham, North Carolina

ALAN T.N. TITA, MD, PhD
Professor, Department of Obstetrics and Gynecology, Division of Maternal-Fetal Medicine, The University of Alabama at Birmingham, Women and Infants Center, Birmingham, Alabama

NEETA L. VORA, MD
Division of Maternal-Fetal Medicine, Department of Obstetrics and Gynecology,
University of North Carolina at Chapel Hill School of Medicine, Chapel Hill, North Carolina

CHLOE ZERA, MD, MPH
Assistant Professor, Division of Maternal-Fetal Medicine, Brigham and Women's
Hospital, Harvard Medical School, Boston, Massachusetts

Contents

Maternal mortality plagues much of the world. There were 303,000 maternal deaths in 2015 representing an overall global maternal mortality ratio of 216 maternal deaths per 100,000 live births. In the United States, the maternal mortality ratio had been decreasing until 1987, remained stable until 1999, and then began to increase. Racial disparities exist in the rates of maternal mortality in the United States, with maternal death affecting a higher proportion of black women compared with white women. To reduce maternal mortality, national organizations in the United States have called for standardized review of cases of maternal morbidity and mortality.

This article reviews some of the more common types of cancer that may be encountered during pregnancy. It reviews the unique challenges with the diagnosis and treatment of breast, cervical, hematologic, and colon cancers in pregnant patients.

Opioid use disorder presents an increased risk of complications in pregnancy, particularly when untreated. To optimize outcomes, medication-assisted treatment using methadone or buprenorphine as a part of a comprehensive care model is recommended. Neonatal abstinence syndrome and poor fetal growth remain significant complications of this disorder despite maternal treatment.

Pregnancy in women with obesity is an important public health problem with short- and long-term implications for maternal and child health. Obesity complicates almost all aspects of pregnancy. Given the growing prevalence of obesity in women, obstetric providers need to understand the risks associated with obesity in pregnancy and the unique aspects of management for women with obesity. Empathic and patient-centered care, along with knowledge, can optimize outcomes for women and children.

The spectrum of sleep-disordered breathing (SDB) ranges from mild snoring to obstructive sleep apnea, the most severe form of SDB. Current recommendations are to treat these women with continuous positive airway pressure despite limited data. SDB in early and mid pregnancy is associated with preeclampsia and gestational diabetes. Pregnant women with a diagnosis of obstructive sleep apnea at delivery were at significantly increased risk of having cardiomyopathy, congestive heart failure, pulmonary embolism, and in-hospital death. These effects were exacerbated in the presence of obesity. Postpartum, these women are at risk for respiratory suppression and should be monitored.

The life expectancy and quality of life of women with genetic disorders continues to improve, resulting in more women reaching reproductive age and desiring fertility. It is becoming increasingly important that obstetricians become familiar with common genetic disorders and their associated risks in pregnancy. The authors review pregnancy in women with various genetic disorders, including review of pregnancy outcomes, management recommendations, and genetic risk assessment. Most data on pregnancies in women with genetic conditions are based on case reports and literature reviews. Additional studies, including pregnancy registries, are needed to improve our understanding and care of this patient population.

Congenital heart disease comprises most maternal cardiac diseases in pregnancy and is an important cause of maternal, fetal, and neonatal morbidity and mortality worldwide. Pregnancy is often considered a high-risk state for individuals with structural heart disease as a consequence of a limited ability to adapt to the major hemodynamic changes associated with pregnancy. Preconception counseling and evaluation are of utmost importance, as pregnancy is contraindicated in certain cardiac conditions. Pregnancy can be safely accomplished in most individuals with careful risk assessment before conception and multidisciplinary care throughout pregnancy and the postpartum period.

Significant progress in understanding the pathophysiology of peripartum cardiomyopathy, especially hormonal and genetic mechanisms, has been made. Specific criteria should be used for diagnosis, but the disease remains a diagnosis of exclusion. Both long-term and recurrent pregnancy prognoses depend on recovery of cardiac function. Data from large registries and randomized controlled trials of evidence-based therapeutics hold promise for future improved clinical outcomes.

Gestational diabetes mellitus (GDM) is carbohydrate intolerance resulting in hyperglycemia with onset during pregnancy. This article provides clinicians with a working framework to minimize maternal and neonatal morbidity. Landmark historical and recent data are reviewed and presented to provide clinicians with a quick, easy reference for recognition and management of GDM. Data presented tie in insights with underlying pathophysiologic processes leading to GDM. Screening and diagnostic thresholds are discussed along with management upon diagnosis. Good clinical practice regarding screening, diagnosis, and management of GDM effectively reduces risk and improves outcomes of women and fetuses in affected pregnancies.

Diabetes is a common chronic condition in women of reproductive age. Preconception care is crucial to reducing the risk of adverse maternal and fetal outcomes, such as hypertensive disorders, abnormal fetal growth, traumatic delivery, and stillbirth, associated with poor glycemic control. Insulin is the preferred medication to optimize glucose control in women with pregestational diabetes. Frequent dose adjustments are needed during pregnancy to achieve glycemic goals, and team-based multidisciplinary care may help. Postpartum care should include lactation support, counseling on contraceptive options, and transition to primary care.

Hypertensive disorders of pregnancy are a heterogeneous group of conditions that include chronic hypertension, gestational hypertension, preeclampsia, and preeclampsia superimposed on chronic hypertension. These disorders account for a significant proportion of perinatal morbidity and mortality and nearly 10% of all maternal deaths in the United States. Given the substantial health burden of hypertensive disorders in pregnancy, there is increasing interest in optimizing management of these conditions. This article summarizes the diagnosis and management of each of the disorders in the spectrum of hypertension in pregnancy and highlights recent updates in the field.

Seizures are among the most serious neurologic complications encountered in pregnancy. This article provides a foundation for the initial

OBSTETRICS AND GYNECOLOGY CLINICS

ISSUE OF RELATED INTEREST

Rheumatic Disease Clinics of North America, May 2017 (Vol. 43, No. 2)
Reproductive Health
Lisa R. Sammaritano and Eliza F. Chakravarty, *Editors*
Available at: http://www.rheumatic.theclinics.com/

THE CLINICS ARE AVAILABLE ONLINE!
Access your subscription at:
www.theclinics.com

Foreword

Team-Based Care of Pregnant Women with Challenging Medical Disorders

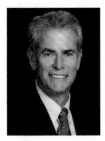

William F. Rayburn, MD, MBA
Consulting Editor

It has been nine years since our last update on medical disorders in pregnancy in the *Obstetrics and Gynecology Clinics of North America*. We appreciate Dr Judith U. Hibbard for undertaking this update again with her new coeditor Dr Erika Peterson. Both editors bring to the reader an understandable and logical approach to the evaluation and management of pregnant women who are afflicted with one or more medical conditions described in this issue. The well-regarded authors also present any updates in the diagnosis of these conditions during pregnancy.

This issue focuses on a team-based approach to patients with medical disorders that frequently antedate the pregnancy. The increased prevalence of obesity and the delay of more women in conceiving add to additional morbidity during gestation. Despite chronic illness, most reproductive-aged women are able to conceive. A patient with a newly diagnosed pregnancy and an active medical disorder is predisposed to a complexity of problems that may further complicate pregnancy. For example, obstructive sleep apnea is being encountered more often due to one-third or more of all pregnant women being obese. Many conditions discussed in this issue are associated with a greater risk of preeclampsia, fetal loss, preterm delivery, and fetal growth restriction. Thromboembolism, cardiomyopathy, and other cardiovascular diseases together account for about one-third of all maternal deaths.

Most obstetricians are familiar with the disorders described in this issue: cancer, opiate use, congenital cardiac disease, diabetes, seizures and other neurologic conditions, and hypertensive disease. However, less frequent conditions encountered in an obstetrician's practice can cause the practitioner to feel "rusty" as to what is important for continuous surveillance and treatment. While many may rely on one or many qualified subspecialists, it remains essential that the obstetrician be able to look at

Obstet Gynecol Clin N Am 45 (2018) xiii–xiv
https://doi.org/10.1016/j.ogc.2018.02.004
0889-8545/18/ **obgyn.theclinics.com**

the "big picture" and function as either a team member or a leader to provide optimal care to the mother, fetus, and family.

Each article of the issue considers the social determinants and risk factors, screening, and treatment of every medical disorder. Certain conditions, such as cardiomyopathy or cancer, are of principal concerns to the mother, while others, such as pregestational diabetes, maternal genetic disorders, and opiate use, pose a risk to the fetus, newborn, and mother. Infectious disease is perhaps the single most common medical condition encountered by the obstetrician, yet this was well covered in the December 2014 issue. Therefore, this issue provides a brief update of certain infections and emphasizes the important role of vaccines when applicable. I appreciate how preventive health is covered in many articles, especially with thromboprophylaxis, vaccines, and challenges of obesity.

Dr Hibbard and Dr Peterson selected a very capable group of accomplished maternal-fetal medicine authors. Each provided relevant information to offer contemporary strategies on their subject. Their expertise and commitment to quality care and advancement of patient safety are noteworthy. It is our hope that this single reference will aid providers in navigating these often complex and challenging issues while also understanding the most current state-of-the-science and recommendations.

William F. Rayburn, MD, MBA
Continuing Medical Education and
Professional Development
University of New Mexico School of Medicine
MSC10 5580
1 University of New Mexico
Albuquerque, NM 87131-0001, USA

E-mail address:
wrayburn@salud.unm.edu

Preface

Medical Disorders in Pregnancy

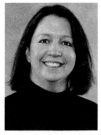
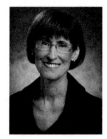

Erika Peterson, MD   Judith U. Hibbard, MD
Editors

We are both privileged to have the opportunity to edit this important issue of *Obstetrics and Gynecology Clinics of North America* on the topic of Medical Disorders in Pregnancy. Recent medical advances have led women with complex medical problems to be able to choose pregnancy and be managed successfully through an often-challenging gestation. However, the early twenty-first century has also seen an unprecedented increase in maternal mortality and morbidity in the United States. This may be due to sicker patients now being able to conceive, or a result of increased rates of obesity, advancing maternal age, and other factors leading to greater morbidity from pregnancy.

We have invited a group of eminent Maternal Fetal Medicine physicians to author articles that are both cutting edge and pertinent to changing obstetric practice. They not only review timely data on complex conditions that have become prominent in the last several decades but also address more common medical complications of pregnancy.

Our issue begins with an important article focusing on maternal mortality in the twenty-first century, an excellent starting point that puts in perspective how challenging the management of pregnancy has become. This is followed by several articles targeting an understanding of diseases that have recently come to the fore. Management of cancer in pregnancy is updated, while another article highlights the opioid epidemic and supervision of dependent women in pregnancy. We then turn our focus to obesity in pregnancy, yet another problem of epidemic proportions for which all obstetricians must be prepared, reviewing not only general complications but also weight and surgical management of the obese gravida. This is followed by a very timely review of sleep apnea in pregnancy, a problem that has risen in parallel with the obesity rate. Sleep apnea is frequently overlooked, so we are fortunate to include this appraisal of diagnosis and treatment during pregnancy.

The next several articles are all related to medical conditions that decades ago were uncommon in pregnancy, as many of these women were often not healthy enough to

Obstet Gynecol Clin N Am 45 (2018) xv–xvi
https://doi.org/10.1016/j.ogc.2018.02.003
0889-8545/18/© 2018 Published by Elsevier Inc.

obgyn.theclinics.com

reproduce. An examination of maternal genetic conditions highlights several diseases, including hereditary hemorrhagic telangiectasia and myotonic dystrophy among others. We take a fresh look at management of maternal congenital cardiac disease, now most often surgically corrected with improved outcomes.

We then shift focus to more well-known medical disorders, including a renewed assessment of peripartum cardiomyopathy, and timely reports on both gestational and pregestational diabetes highlighting recommendations on diagnosis and management. The survey on hypertensive disorders is a current, concise single reference for management of all hypertension during gestation. Comprehensive information on management of seizure disorders in pregnancy as well as recent information on antiseizure medication is included.

Our last two pieces focus on prevention of disease in pregnancy. The first targets common infections in pregnancy, including current data on Zika in pregnancy, as well as the most recent information on vaccinations in pregnancy. We finish with a review of thromboprophylaxis, including the most recent recommendations on antepartum, postpartum, and post–cesarean delivery thromboprophylaxis.

The opportunity to edit this issue of *Obstetrics and Gynecology Clinics of North America* has been challenging, rewarding, and a learning experience. We hope you will find these articles as interesting and valuable as we have.

Erika Peterson, MD
Division of Maternal Fetal Medicine
Fetal Concerns Center of Wisconsin
Medical College of Wisconsin
9200 West Wisconsin Avenue
Milwaukee, WI 53226-3522, USA

Judith U. Hibbard, MD
Medical College of Wisconsin
9200 West Wisconsin Avenue
Milwaukee, WI 53226-3522, USA

E-mail addresses:
epeterson@mcw.edu (E. Peterson)
jhibbard@mcw.edu (J.U. Hibbard)

Maternal Mortality in the Twenty-First Century

John A. Ozimek, DO, MS*, Sarah J. Kilpatrick, MD, PhD

KEYWORDS

- Maternal mortality • Severe maternal morbidity • Racial disparities
- Maternal mortality ratio • Pregnancy-related death

KEY POINTS

- Maternal mortality plagues much of the world, with 303,000 maternal deaths in 2015. This number represents a global maternal mortality ratio of 216 maternal deaths per 100,000 live births.
- The World Health Organization has created a goal to decrease the global maternal mortality ratio to 70 maternal deaths per 100,000 live births by the year 2030.
- The maternal mortality ratio is higher in the United States than in any other developed nation and has increased over the last several years.
- Significant racial disparities exist in the rates of maternal mortality in the United States.

INTRODUCTION

Maternal death was quite common in the nineteenth century with as many as 7 deaths per 100 births in some hospitals in the United States.[1] By the early twentieth century, maternal mortalities improved but plateaued at approximately 6 to 9 maternal deaths per 1000 live births.[2] Most maternal deaths during this time were secondary to poor obstetric education and delivery practices, and most of them were preventable.[2] In the 1920s, most deliveries occurred at home under the care of midwives or general practitioners. Deliveries during this time were often performed without following principles of aseptic technique, resulting in infection, with sepsis causing 40% of maternal deaths.[2] The large majority of the remaining maternal deaths were secondary to hemorrhage or preeclampsia/eclampsia.[2] In the 1930s, a link was demonstrated between poor aseptic practice, excessive operative deliveries, and high maternal mortality. These data were published in the 1933 White House Conference on Child Health Protection, Fetal, Newborn, and Maternal Mortality and Morbidity report.[2] State medical

The authors have no financial disclosures.
Department of Obstetrics and Gynecology, Division of Maternal-Fetal Medicine, Cedars-Sinai Medical Center, 8635 West 3rd Street, Suite 160-W, Los Angeles, CA 90048, USA
* Corresponding author.
E-mail address: john.ozimek@cshs.org

Obstet Gynecol Clin N Am 45 (2018) 175–186
https://doi.org/10.1016/j.ogc.2018.01.004
0889-8545/18/© 2018 Elsevier Inc. All rights reserved.

obgyn.theclinics.com

boards took note of this and previous reports, which lead to a new focus on maternal health at the state level.[2] This call to action led to the establishment of the first hospital and state maternal mortality review committees in the 1930s and 1940s. Over the following years, these committees developed institutional practice guidelines and defined minimum physician qualifications needed to gain hospital delivery privileges. Over the same period, hospital deliveries became favored over home deliveries throughout the country, increasing from 55% to 90% from 1938 to 1948.[2] Deliveries in hospitals were performed under aseptic conditions and allowed for care of the poor by state-provided services. These changes led to decreases in maternal mortality after 1930. Declines in rates of maternal mortality became even more pronounced with medical advances, including the use of antibiotics, oxytocin, improved blood transfusion technique, and better management of hypertensive conditions of pregnancy.[2] These advances and changes in practice led to a further decrease in maternal mortality of 71% over a 10-year period from 1939 to 1948.[2] From 1950 to 1973, deaths from septic abortion decreased by 89%, which is likely partially attributable to the legalization of induced abortion beginning in some states in 1967, followed by legalization in all states in 1973.[2,3]

Despite the improvements made in the twentieth century, maternal mortality continues to plague much of the world, disproportionately affecting developing nations. According to the United Nations Maternal Mortality Estimation Inter-Agency Group, there were 303,000 maternal deaths in 2015.[4] This number represents an overall global maternal mortality ratio (MMR) of 216 maternal deaths per 100,000 live births, a 44% decrease over the prior 25 years.[4] The MMR varied greatly by region ranging from 12 deaths per 100,000 live births in developed regions to 546 deaths per 100,000 live births in sub-Saharan Africa and as high as 1100 deaths per 100,000 live births in Sierra Leone.[4] Current trends in worldwide maternal mortality demonstrate a range of annual reduction from 1.8% in the Caribbean to 5.0% for Eastern Asia.[4] Although these reductions in global maternal mortality represent a trend in the right direction, this decrease fell short of the United Nations Millennium Development Goal of a reduction of 75% in the MMR between 1990 and 2015.[5] The World Health Organization (WHO) has presented new Sustainable Development Goals with the objective of reducing the global MMR to less than 70 deaths per 100,000 live births from 2015 to 2030.[6] In order to achieve this ambitious goal, countries will need to decrease their MMR at an annual rate of reduction of at least 7.5%, a far accelerated rate compared with the last 25 years.[4] Reasons cited for the decrease in maternal mortalities over the last 25 years include a decrease in the total fertility rate, increased maternal education, and increased access to skilled birth attendants among various other improvements.[7] Strategies for ongoing reduction of the global maternal mortality, as outlined in the WHO Sustainable Development Goals, include a human rights–based approach to maternal and newborn health, which includes eliminating inequities that lead to disparities in access, quality, and outcomes of care within and between countries. The need for improvements in care, including sexual and reproductive health, family planning, and newborn and child survival, are also cited as needed strategies to continue to improve maternal mortalities.[6]

Of the 171 countries studied by the United Nations Maternal-Mortality Estimation Inter-Agency Group, 158 demonstrated a reduction in maternal mortality over the 25 years studied.[4] Alarmingly, there are 13 countries that have increasing rates of maternal mortality. These countries include Bahamas, Georgia, Guyana, Jamaica, North Korea, St. Lucia, Serbia, South Africa, Suriname, Tonga, United States, Venezuela, and Zimbabwe. The United States is the ONLY developed nation with an increasing MMR, and, in fact, the current MMR in the United States is almost 2 times greater than that of the United Kingdom and more than 2 times greater than the MMR in Canada.[4,8]

MATERNAL MORTALITY IN THE UNITED STATES

To understand current maternal mortalities and trends in the United States, it is important to recognize the terminology that is used. There are several terms, each with a slightly different definition and resultant different rates of maternal mortality. The use of multiple terms often leads to differing reports of maternal mortality in both popular and scientific literature. Current frequently used terminology and definitions include the following:

- Pregnancy-Related Death (Centers for Disease Control and Prevention [CDC]): the death of a woman while pregnant or within 1 year of pregnancy termination, regardless of the duration or site of the pregnancy, from any cause related to or aggravated by the pregnancy or its management, but not from accidental or incidental causes.[9]
- Pregnancy-Related Death (WHO): the death of a woman while pregnant or with 42 days of termination of pregnancy, irrespective of the cause of death.[10]
- Maternal Death (WHO): the death of a woman while pregnant or within 42 days of termination of pregnancy, irrespective of the duration and site of the pregnancy or its management but not from accidental or incidental causes.[10]
- Pregnancy-Related Mortality Ratio (CDC): an estimate of the number of pregnancy-related deaths for every 100,000 live births. The CDC reports that there were 17.3 pregnancy-related deaths per 100,000 live births in the United States in 2014.[9]
- Maternal Mortality Ratio (WHO): the number of maternal deaths per 100,000 live births.[10] The WHO reports that the maternal mortality ratio in the United States was 14 deaths per 100,000 live births in 2015.[4]

The MMR is the most commonly used measure of maternal mortality. In the United States, the MMR had been steadily decreasing until reaching its nadir in 1987 at 6.6.[8] After 1987, the MMR remained fairly stable at between 7 and 8 maternal deaths/100,000 live births until 1999 when the MMR began to steadily increase, resulting in the most recent report of 14 deaths/100,000 live births in 2015.[4] It is postulated that some of the reported increase in the MMR in the United States is secondary to improvements in methods for identification of pregnancy-related deaths and changes in coding and classification of maternal deaths. Other factors that are thought to contribute to the increasing rate of maternal mortality include increasing maternal age, increasing maternal body mass index, and increased incidence of medical comorbidities.[11–13] A large population-level analysis, which analyzed data from the Centers for Disease Control and Prevention National Center for Health Statistics database (CDC WONDER), demonstrated that there was a significant correlation between mortality and the percentage of non-Hispanic black women in the delivery population, further illustrating known racial disparities in overall maternal outcomes in the United States.[14] The investigators also concluded that cesarean deliveries, unintended births, unmarried status, and 4 or less prenatal visits were significantly associated with increased MMR.[14]

The top 3 causes of maternal mortality in the United States have historically been hemorrhage, hypertensive disease, and thrombosis.[15] However, over time, the contribution of these causes to pregnancy-related death declined, and by 2010, deaths secondary to cardiovascular conditions and infection increased with cardiovascular conditions ranked as the leading cause.[15] Recent data from the CDC corroborate this shift in cause of death and list the top 3 causes in the United States from 2011 to 2013 as cardiovascular disease (15.5%), other medical noncardiovascular disease (14.5%), and infection/sepsis (12.7%). Hemorrhage is still listed among the top causes, ranking as the fourth leading cause at 11.4% of pregnancy-related deaths during this time (**Fig. 1**)[16] Multiple studies conducted over a similar period demonstrate a corollary trend in increased incidence of chronic heart disease,[17] hypertensive disorders,[18] obesity,[19] and diabetes,[20] among pregnant women offering additional insight into the changing trends in maternal mortality in the United States. Racial disparities in maternal mortality persist in the United States as well.[15]

An important cause of death among pregnant women is trauma. Trauma is estimated to affect 1 in 12 pregnant women and is the leading nonobstetric cause of death among reproductive-aged women in the United States.[21] The effect of trauma-related maternal mortality is not well described. Standard definitions of maternal mortality from the WHO and CDC exclude trauma-related deaths from national maternal mortality reports.[21] As trauma-related deaths are not included in national reports, this limits opportunities for further study and prevention of trauma-related deaths in pregnancy. A recent study analyzed more than 1100 trauma events among pregnant women compared with 43,600 trauma events among age-matched, nonpregnant women.[21] The investigators found that pregnant women were more likely to experience violent trauma, were 1.6 times more likely to die, and were more likely to be dead on arrival to the hospital or to die during their hospital course compared with nonpregnant women. The findings persisted despite pregnant patients having an

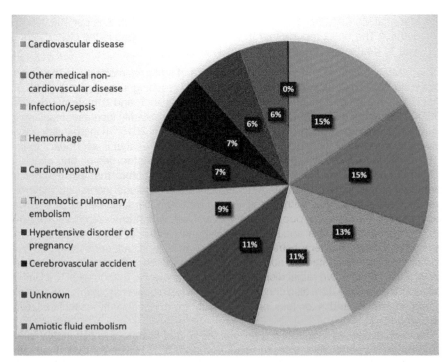

Fig. 1. Causes of pregnancy-related death in the United States: 2011 to 2013. (*Data from* Centers for Disease Control and Prevention (CDC). Pregnancy mortality surveillance system. Available at: https://www.cdc.gov/reproductivehealth/maternalinfanthealth/pmss.html.)

overall lower injury severity score. The investigators showed that pregnant trauma victims were less likely to undergo surgery and more likely to be transferred to another facility.[21] Another important finding showed that pregnant women were twice as likely to experience violent trauma and more than 3 times more likely to die of violent trauma compared with their nonpregnant counterparts.[21] These findings underscore the need for continued screening for violence in pregnancy and ongoing studies of trauma and violence among pregnant women.

RACIAL DISPARITIES AND MATERNAL MORTALITY IN THE UNITED STATES

In an analysis of pregnancy-related death in the United States from 2006 to 2010, significant racial disparities in pregnancy-related mortality ratios were demonstrated.[15] It was found that a significantly higher proportion of non-Hispanic black women experienced pregnancy-related death compared with non-Hispanic white women. Although women in all racial groups were found to be at increased risk of pregnancy-related death with increasing age, this finding was particularly pronounced among non-Hispanic black women.[15] Teenaged black women were 1.4 times more likely to die than their white counterparts; black women aged 20 to 24 years were 2.8 times more likely to die, and black women in all other age groups were more than 4 times more likely to die from pregnancy-related complications. For further perspective, the pregnancy-related mortality ratio for black women aged 40 or older in this cohort approached 150 maternal deaths per 100,000 live births versus approaching 40 deaths per 100,000 live births among white women in the same age group. The study also found that black women who died of pregnancy-related complications were younger, less educated, more likely to be unmarried, more likely to be late to prenatal care, and more likely to die of ectopic pregnancy–related complications than white women.[15]

There also appear to be location-specific disparities in the MMR across the United States, which may be secondary to the racial disparities described above.[14] In a large population-level analysis study examining data from the CDC National Center for Health Statistics database and the Detailed Mortality Underlying Cause of Death database (CDC WONDER), MMRs from 2005 to 2014 were compared at a state level.[13] The study demonstrated that there was significant variability of the MMR from state to state and that these differences tended to correlate with the percentage of non-Hispanic black women in the population. Massachusetts had the lowest MMR at 5.6 maternal deaths per 100,000 live births and ranked 25th for the percentage of non-Hispanic black births. The District of Columbia had the highest MMR at 38.8 deaths per 100,000 live births and also ranks first with the highest percentage of non-Hispanic black births and last with the lowest percentage of non-Hispanic white births. The investigators note that although the District of Columbia has the highest MMR in the United States, it also has the lowest MMR for non-Hispanic white births.[13] Although it has been postulated in the past that some of the location-specific disparities in maternal outcomes are secondary to poverty, immigration, or rural status, data from this study found no correlation between maternal mortality and any of these variables.[13] Statewide differences in medical factors, such as hypertensive disease, diabetes, tobacco use, and obesity, were analyzed as well and were not found to be significantly correlated with mortality ratios. This study demonstrated that the variation in MMR was most closely associated with social factors, such as unintended pregnancy, unmarried status, and non-Hispanic black race, further demonstrating the significant racial disparities in the United States.[14]

PREVENTABILITY

Multiple studies have demonstrated that almost half of pregnancy-related deaths in the United States are preventable.[22,23] In a retrospective study of maternal deaths in North Carolina, 108 pregnancy-related deaths were reviewed by the North Carolina Pregnancy-Related Mortality Review Committee.[22] They found that 40% of pregnancy-related deaths were potentially preventable and that preventability varied by cause. They reported that 93% of hemorrhage-related deaths, 60% of hypertension-related deaths, 43% of infection-related deaths, and 40% of cardiovascular-related deaths were potentially preventable. It was also surmised by the investigators that improved quality of medical care was the leading factor that could have led to prevention.[22] Other studies have reported similar findings with one study in Massachusetts reporting that 54% of pregnancy-associated deaths were deemed preventable.[23] Although the MMR in the United States is rising, luckily absolute numbers remain low, making it difficult to study strategies to prevent mortality. Past studies have placed maternal mortality at the end of a continuum ranging from healthy pregnancy, to maternal morbidity, to severe maternal morbidity, to death.[22,24–26] It has been suggested that, given severe maternal morbidity is a far more common occurrence than maternal death, strategies should be developed to recognize and prevent severe maternal morbidity, thereby interrupting the continuum leading to and decreasing rates of maternal mortality.

SEVERE MATERNAL MORBIDITY

Like maternal mortality, severe maternal morbidity is increasing in the United States.[11,27,28] It is currently estimated to affect at least 50,000 women per year with an occurrence of 0.5% to 1.3% of pregnancies in the United States.[27,28] Because severe maternal morbidity lies within a continuum ranging from healthy pregnancy to death, efforts to identify and prevent causes of severe maternal morbidity are thought to ultimately decrease morbidity and, hence, maternal mortality.[22,24–26] National organizations have recognized that severe maternal morbidity is increasing and have advocated for a process in which cases of severe maternal morbidity are reviewed at a hospital level.[29,30] Similar to maternal death review committees, the goal is to find where opportunities for improvement in care of such patients could have prevented morbidity from occurring, or progressing to a severe event, hence reducing both morbidity and mortality.

Identifying specific cases of severe maternal morbidity for review has been challenging because the concept is difficult to define in absolute terms. However, published guidelines have been set forth and validated to allow for sensitive methods to screen for severe maternal morbidity.[30–32] Although several methods of screening for severe maternal morbidity have been used, recent reports recommend using the following 2 screening criteria: pregnant or postpartum patients who have been admitted to the intensive care unit and/or have received ≥4 units of packed red blood cells because of their high sensitivity and specificity for identification of cases of severe maternal morbidity.[30–32] Definitive "gold-standard" guidelines to select cases of true severe maternal morbidity from those that screened positive for possible morbidity have also been established.[33] These guidelines are listed in an extensive and detailed systems-based format to help providers determine if true severe maternal morbidity has occurred.[33] Following identification of true cases of severe maternal morbidity, it has been recommended that cases in all hospitals that provide obstetric care be reviewed and presented to a multidisciplinary committee in a standardized fashion to identify where opportunities for improvement in care may have existed that could have averted severe morbidity.[28,30]

A recent, large, retrospective cohort study used the recommended screening methods, gold-standard guidelines to identify true cases of severe maternal morbidity and recommended multidisciplinary review committee approach to determine the incidence of and characterize opportunities for improvement in maternal care at a large, academic medical center.[34] The investigators found that opportunities for improvement in care existed in 44% of women who experienced severe maternal morbidity. These findings are concordant with previous studies on preventable maternal mortality, which report that nearly half of the maternal deaths in the United States are preventable and underscored the need for continued provider education to reduce morbidity and mortality.[22,23] This study also demonstrated the feasibility of the recommended review process of severe maternal morbidity.

STRATEGIES FOR REDUCTION OF MATERNAL MORTALITY

The CDC established the pregnancy mortality surveillance system in 1986, which collects data from 52 reporting areas (50 states, New York City, and Washington, DC).[9] The CDC requests that these areas voluntarily submit copies of death certificates for all women who died during pregnancy or within 1 year of pregnancy along with copies of the matching birth or fetal death certificates.[9] This information yields valuable epidemiologic data regarding causes and risk factors associated with maternal deaths. Although this information is valuable in terms of a "big picture" of maternal mortality in the United States, many states still lack standardized committees to review individual maternal deaths, which would allow for an opportunity to identify preventable causes and strategies for improvement in care.[35] Per the most recent statistics listed in a document provided by the American College of Obstetrics and Gynecology, only 28 states currently have or are forming a maternal mortality review committee.[35]

The United States lags in its system of standardized maternal mortality review compared with other developed nations with lower maternal mortalities. For example, the United Kingdom has used a national system, Confidential Enquiries into Maternal Deaths, to review maternal deaths for more than 60 years.[36] In this system, all maternal deaths in the United Kingdom are reported to the Mothers and Babies: Reducing Risk through Audits and Confidential Enquiries across the United Kingdom database.[37] These reported deaths are then cross-checked for verification and confirmed. Full medical records are obtained and made anonymous before undergoing confidential review. The record is first reviewed by a pathologist and an obstetrician to determine a cause of death. Each woman's care is then reviewed by a multidisciplinary panel of 10 to 15 expert reviewers, including obstetricians, anesthesiologists, midwives, pathologists, and other specialists as determined to be appropriate. The summary of care is then examined by a multidisciplinary writing group to elucidate the main themes for learning to be highlighted in the report.[37] This system is credited with decreasing the already low maternal mortality in the United Kingdom via implementation of recommended clinical guidelines. More recently, the system has also been credited with narrowing the gap related to pregnancy outcomes and racial disparities, significantly lowering the maternal mortality among black African women. These positive changes occurred while the maternal population in the United Kingdom faces similar health challenges that face the United States, including an older and less healthy maternal population.[36]

Although the United States may be lagging in terms of standardized review, efforts are underway to develop strategies to reduce maternal morbidity and mortality.[38–40] For example, in response to the steadily increasing maternal mortality, the California Department of Public Health, in collaboration with the California Maternal Quality Care Collaborative (CMQCC), developed the California Pregnancy-Associated Mortality Review project in 2006.[38,39] The goal of this undertaking was to identify pregnancy-related deaths, causation, and contributing factors at a state level and subsequently make recommendations on quality improvements to maternity care. Since that time, the state of California has reduced its MMR by 55% from 16.9 in 2006 to 7.3 in 2013, well below the national maternal mortality, which continued to increase over the same period.[38,39] The CMQCC (https://www.cmqcc.org) was established in 2006 in response to rising maternal mortality and morbidity rates with the goal of ending preventable morbidity, mortality, and racial disparities in California.[39] In addition to decreasing the maternal mortality, the CMQCC has succeeded in decreasing the preterm birth rate and reducing maternal morbidity by 21% among the 126 hospitals that participated in projects to reduce hemorrhage and preeclampsia.[39] The CMQCC reports these successes are secondary to multiple factors, including the following:

- The establishment of a maternal data center making real-time data available from more than 200 hospitals representing 90% of births in California.
- Creating quality improvement initiatives, including toolkits regarding early elective delivery, hemorrhage, preeclampsia, and reducing primary cesareans.
- Research collaboration with the state of California to publish the California Pregnancy-Associated Mortality review to identify quality improvement opportunities in maternity care.

The example and successes of the efforts the California Department of Public Health and the CMQCC can serve as models for other states to emulate in an effort to lower maternal mortality in the United States. Resources such as toolkits and patient safety bundles like those implemented by the CMQCC offer standardized approaches to patient management and have been shown to reduce maternal morbidity and presumably mortality.[41] There are various resources available that offer patient safety bundles free to the public. One of the most comprehensive resources for maternal patient safety bundles can be found at the Web site for the Council on Patient Safety in Women's Healthcare (https://www.safehealthcareforeverywoman.org).[41] The Council on Patient Safety in Women's Health Care is a multidisciplinary collaboration composed of several professional organizations, including the American Board of Obstetrics and Gynecology, Society for Maternal Fetal Medicine, Society for Obstetric Anesthesia and Perinatology, and approximately 20 other professional organizations.

A selection of available bundles include the following:

- Obstetric hemorrhage
- Maternal venous thromboembolism
- Reduction of peripartum racial/ethnic disparities
- Severe hypertension in pregnancy

In terms of national efforts, The American College of Obstetricians and Gynecologists and The Society for Maternal-Fetal Medicine published a consensus document calling for the creation of a system of uniform designations for levels of maternal care in an effort to reduce maternal morbidity and mortality (**Table 1**).[42] This document highlights the successes of improved neonatal outcomes following the regionalization

Table 1 Levels of maternal care	
Birth center	Peripartum care of low-risk women with uncomplicated singleton term pregnancies with a vertex presentation who are expected to have an uncomplicated birth
Level I (basic care)	Care of uncomplicated pregnancies with the ability to detect, stabilize, and initiate management of unanticipated maternal-fetal or neonatal problems that occur until the patient can be transferred to a facility at which specialty maternal care is available
Level II (specialty care)	Level I facility plus care of appropriate high-risk conditions, both directly admitted and transferred from another facility
Level III (subspecialty care)	Level II facility plus care of more complex maternal medical conditions, obstetric complications, and fetal conditions
Level IV (regional perinatal health care centers)	Level III facility plus on-site medical and surgical care of the most complex maternal conditions and critically ill pregnant women and fetuses

Adapted from American College of Obstetricians and Gynecologists and Society for Maternal–Fetal Medicine, Menard MK, Kilpatrick S, Saade G, et al. Levels of maternal care. Am J Obstet Gynecol 2015;212(3):259–71; with permission.

of neonatal care via risk-appropriate maternal transport networks, but reviews that this system focuses almost entirely on the needs of the newborn and not necessarily the mother. The investigators have created 4 objectives including creation of uniform designations for levels of maternal care available at facilities, to develop standardized definitions for facilities that provide each level of maternal care, to provide consistent guidelines per level of maternal care for use in quality improvement and health promotion, and to foster the development and equitable geographic distribution of full service maternal care facilities.[42] Through these efforts, it is hoped that maternal care can be improved and national rates of morbidity and mortality are decreased and brought in line with other developed nations.

SUMMARY

Despite improvements in rates of global maternal mortality over the last century, it remains a problem that continues to plague much of the world. Rates of maternal mortality are increasing in the United States with significant racial disparities that disproportionately affect non-Hispanic black women. Up to half of pregnancy-related deaths in the United States have been found to be preventable.[14,21,22] There are strategies that have been shown to reduce the rates of severe maternal morbidity and maternal mortality in regions of the United States.[36,38] It is imperative that these efforts are adopted on a national level to decrease the rates of maternal mortality.

REFERENCES

1. Loudon I. Death in childbirth: an international study of maternal care and maternal mortality, 1800–1950. Oxford: Clarendon Press; 1992.
2. Centers for Disease Control and Prevention (CDC). Healthier mothers and babies. MMWR Morb Mortal Wkly Rep 1999;48(38):849–58 [Erratum appears in MMWR Morb Mortal Wkly Rep 1999;48(39):892].
3. Cates W Jr, Grimes DA, Schulz KF. Abortion surveillance at CDC: creating public health light out of political heat. Am J Prev Med 2000;19(1S):12–7.

4. Alkema L, Chou D, Hogan D, et al, United Nations Maternal Mortality Estimation Inter-Agency Group Collaborators and Technical Advisory Group. Global, regional, and national levels and trends in maternal mortality between 1990 and 2015, with scenario-based projections to 2030: a systematic analysis by the UN Maternal Mortality Estimation Inter-Agency Group. Lancet 2016; 387(10017):462–74.

5. UN General Assembly. United Nations Millennium Declaration, Resolution Adopted by the General Assembly; 2000; A/RES/55/2.

6. Strategies toward ending preventable maternal mortality (EPMM). Geneva (Switzerland): World Health Organization; 2015.

7. Hogan MC, Foreman KJ, Naghavi M, et al. Maternal mortality for 181 countries, 1980-2008: a systematic analysis of progress towards Millennium Development Goal 5. Lancet 2010;375(9726):1609–23.

8. Organisation for economic co-operation and development. Available at: http://stats.oecd.org/index.aspx?DataSetCode=HEALTH_STAT#. Accessed June 5, 2017.

9. Centers for Disease Control and Prevention. Available at: www.cdc.gov/reproductivehealth/maternalinfanthealth/pmss.html. Accessed June 5, 2017.

10. World Health Organization, Health statistics and information systems. Available at: www.who.int/healthinfo/statistics/indmaternalmortality/en/. Accessed June 5, 2017.

11. Kassebaum NJ, Bertozzi-Villa A, Coggeshall MS, et al. Global, regional, and national levels and causes of maternal mortality during 1990-2013: a systematic analysis for the Global Burden of Disease Study 2013. Lancet 2014;384(9947): 980–1004.

12. Berg CJ, Chang J, Callaghan WM, et al. Pregnancy-related mortality in the United States, 1991-1997. Obstet Gynecol 2003;101(2):289–96.

13. MacKAy AP, Berg CJ, Liu X, et al. Changes in pregnancy mortality ascertainment: United States, 1999-2005. Obstet Gynecol 2011;118(1):104–10.

14. Moaddab A, Dildy GA, Brown HL, et al. Health care disparity and state-specific pregnancy-related mortality in the United States, 2005-2014. Obstet Gynecol 2016;128(4):869–75.

15. Creanga AA, Berg CJ, Syverson C, et al. Pregnancy-related mortality in the United States, 2006-2010. Obstet Gynecol 2015;125(1):5–12.

16. Centers for Disease Control and Prevention, Pregnancy Mortality Surveillance System. Available at: https://www.cdc.gov/reproductivehealth/maternalinfanthealth/pmss.html. Accessed June 5, 2017.

17. Kuklina E, Callaghan W. Chronic heart disease and severe obstetric morbidity among hospitalisations for pregnancy in the USA: 1995-2006. BJOG 2011; 118(3):345–52.

18. Kuklina EV, Ayala C, Callaghan WM. Hypertensive disorders and severe obstetric morbidity in the United States. Obstet Gynecol 2009;113(6):1299–306.

19. Hinkle SN, Sharma AJ, Kim SY, et al. Prepregnancy obesity trends among low-income women, United States, 1999-2008. Matern Child Health J 2012;16(7): 1339–48.

20. Albrecht SS, Kuklina EV, Bansil P, et al. Diabetes trends among delivery hospitalizations in the U.S., 1994-2004. Diabetes Care 2010;33(4):768–73.

21. Deshpande NA, Kucirka LM, Smith RN, et al. Pregnant trauma victims experience nearly 2-fold higher mortality compared to their nonpregnant counterparts. Am J Obstet Gynecol 2017;217(5):590.e1–9.

22. Berg CJ, Harper MA, Atkinson SM, et al. Preventability of pregnancy-related deaths: results of a state-wide review. Obstet Gynecol 2005;106(6):1228–34.

23. Nannini A, Weiss J, Goldstein R, et al. Pregnancy-associated mortality at the end of the twentieth century: Massachusetts, 1990-1999. J Am Med Womens Assoc (1972) 2002;57(3):140–3.
24. Geller SE, Rosenberg D, Cox SM, et al. The continuum of maternal morbidity and mortality: factors associated with severity. Am J Obstet Gynecol 2004;191(3): 939–44.
25. Geller SE, Cox SM, Kilpatrick SJ. A descriptive model of preventability in maternal morbidity and mortality. J Perinatol 2006;26(2):79–84.
26. Geller SE, Rosenberg D, Cox S, et al. A scoring system identified near-miss maternal morbidity during pregnancy. J Clin Epidemiol 2004;57(7):716–20.
27. Callaghan WM, Creanga AA, Kuklina EV. Severe maternal morbidity among delivery and postpartum hospitalizations in the United States. Obstet Gynecol 2012; 120(5):1029–36.
28. Callaghan WM, Mackay AP, Berg CJ. Identification of severe maternal morbidity during delivery hospitalizations, United States, 1991-2003. Am J Obstet Gynecol 2008;199(2):133.e1–8.
29. D'Alton ME, Bonanno CA, Berkowitz RL, et al. Putting the "M" back in maternal-fetal medicine. Am J Obstet Gynecol 2013;208(6):442–8.
30. Kilpatrick SJ, Berg C, Bernstein P, et al. Standardized severe maternal morbidity review: rationale and process. Obstet Gynecol 2014;124(2 Pt 1):361–6.
31. Callaghan WM, Grobman WA, Kilpatrick SJ, et al. Facility-based identification of women with severe maternal morbidity: it is time to start. Obstet Gynecol 2014; 123(5):978–81.
32. You WB, Chandrasekaran S, Sullivan J, et al. Validation of a scoring system to identify women with near-miss maternal morbidity. Am J Perinatol 2013;30(1): 21–4.
33. Main EK, Abreo A, McNulty J, et al. Measuring severe maternal morbidity: validation of potential measures. Am J Obstet Gynecol 2016;214(5):643.e1–10.
34. Ozimek JA, Eddins RM, Greene N, et al. Opportunities for improvement in care among women with severe maternal morbidity. Am J Obstet Gynecol 2016; 215(4):509.e1–6.
35. Building U.S capacity to review and prevent maternal deaths. Available at: https://www.acog.org/-/media/Departments/Government-Relations-and-Outreach/ 2017-CLC/2017-CLC-Recommended-Readings/Ask-1-Maternal-Mortality/2017Bldg CapacityforMMROverview.pdf?dmc=1&ts=20170309T1458108720. Accessed June 5, 2017.
36. Cantwell R, Clutton-Brock T, Cooper G, et al. Saving mothers' lives: reviewing maternal deaths to make motherhood safer: 2006-2008. The Eighth Report of the Confidential Enquiries into Maternal Deaths in the United Kingdom. BJOG 2011;118(Suppl 1):1–203.
37. On behalf of MBRRACE-UK, Knight M, Nair M, Tuffnell D, et al, editors. Saving lives, improving mothers' care - Surveillance of maternal deaths in the UK 2012-14 and lessons learned to inform maternity care from the UK and Ireland Confidential Enquiries into Maternal Deaths and Morbidity 2009-14. Oxford: National Perinatal Epidemiology Unit, University of Oxford; 2016.
38. State of California, Department of Public Health, California Birth and Death Statistical Master Files, 1999-2013. Available at: https://archive.cdph.ca.gov/data/ statistics/Documents/2013MaternalMortalityRates-SlideSet%20for%20MCAH%20 Website.pdf. Accessed June 5, 2017.
39. California Maternal Quality Care Collaborative. Available at: www.cmqcc.org/ research/ca-pamr-maternal-mortality-review. Accessed June 5, 2017.

40. Shields LE, Wiesner S, Fulton J, et al. Comprehensive maternal hemorrhage protocols reduce the use of blood products and improve patient safety. Am J Obstet Gynecol 2015;212(3):272–80.
41. Council on Patient Safety in Women's Healthcare. Available at: https://www.safehealthcareforeverywoman.org. Accessed June 5, 2017.
42. American College of Obstetricians and Gynecologists and Society for Maternal–Fetal Medicine, Menard MK, Kilpatrick S, et al. Levels of maternal care. Am J Obstet Gynecol 2015;212(3):259–71.

Cancer in Pregnancy

Anna McCormick, DO*, Erika Peterson, MD

KEYWORDS

- Gestational breast cancer • Cervical cancer in pregnancy
- Colon cancer in pregnancy • Hematologic cancers in pregnancy
- Lymphoma in pregnancy • Leukemia in pregnancy

KEY POINTS

- The diagnosis of cancer in the gestational period poses many difficult decisions for which multiple clinical, personal, and ethical factors need to be considered for treatment planning.
- The incidence of most gestational cancers is increasing owing to the fact that many women are deciding to delay childbearing.
- In general, most chemotherapy treatments should be delayed until the second and third trimesters to avoid fetal toxicity.
- Pregnancy should not be a reason to delay a diagnostic workup for symptoms concerning for cancer.

INTRODUCTION

Because more women are waiting to have children until later in life, cancer diagnoses in pregnancy are becoming more common. Gestational cancer is defined as a new cancer diagnosis during pregnancy or in the first year postpartum.[1] The most common cancers in reproductive aged women are breast, melanoma, thyroid, cervical, and lymphomas, listed in order of decreasing frequency.[2] The diagnosis of cancer in the gestational period poses many difficult decisions for which multiple clinical, personal, and ethical factors need to be considered for treatment planning. We review the pertinent information for some of the more common gestational cancers, as well as some less common, but with increasing prevalence in the United States.

BREAST CANCER

Gestational breast cancer is considered any breast cancer occurring either during pregnancy, in the year after delivery, or anytime during lactation. Breast cancer is

The authors have no commercial or financial conflicts of interest to disclose.
Department of Obstetrics and Gynecology, Medical College of Wisconsin, 8701 W Watertown Plank Road, Milwaukee, WI 53226, USA
* Corresponding author.
E-mail address: amccormick@mcw.edu

one of the most common pregnancy-associated cancers. Pregnancy-associated breast cancer occurs in 20% of breast cancer patients younger than 30 years of age.[3] The incidence is only 0.4% of all breast cancers diagnosed in women aged 16 to 49, however the rate is increasing.[1] This increase is most likely secondary to delaying the age at which women begin childbearing.

The majority of gestational breast cancer is infiltrating ductal carcinoma. Gestational breast cancer is more likely to be poorly differentiated and have metastases at the time of diagnosis when compared with nonpregnant women.[4] There is typically a lower incidence of estrogen receptor–positive, progesterone receptor–positive breast cancer diagnosed during pregnancy and the postpartum period, whereas human epidermal growth factor 2–positive tumors seem to be equal in incidence to that of nonpregnant women.[5]

A diagnosis of breast cancer during pregnancy or lactation is often more challenging given the normal physiologic changes in the breast during these periods.[6] For example, rapid enlargement and hypertrophy during pregnancy and the postpartum period can distort the anatomy of the breast. Often the diagnosis is delayed by pregnancy and lactation; hence, the diagnosis is made at more advanced stages during pregnancy.[7] Interestingly, a breast cancer diagnosis during lactation can be detected by the milk rejection sign, in which the nursing infant will refuse to nurse from the cancerous side.[2] Any breast mass persisting for more than 2 weeks during pregnancy or lactation needs to be evaluated. Even though 80% of breast biopsies during pregnancy are benign, delayed diagnosis because of pregnancy or lactation is critical to prognosis.[8]

If a breast mass is identified in pregnancy, it should be evaluated with imaging, typically a diagnostic mammogram. This imaging modality is considered safe during pregnancy and poses little known threat to the developing fetus.[9] An abdominal shield can be used, although the data supporting the added safety of this technique are minimal.[10–12] The standard dose of radiation of a mammogram (200–400 mrads) is negligible to the developing fetus.[9] A biopsy should be performed of any suspicious mass in pregnancy or lactation, regardless of mammogram results. Evaluation for advanced stage disease with imaging of the chest, liver, bone, and brain should also be performed. To image the chest during pregnancy a chest radiograph may be performed. The gravid uterus can make it difficult to rule out metastasis at the diaphragm or inferior lung lobes, in which case an MRI of the chest may be performed without contrast.[13] MRI without contrast has documented safety in pregnancy and can also be used to evaluate the abdomen, pelvis, and brain. There is limited information on the safety of PET scans during pregnancy and these generally should be avoided.[14] If there is suspicion for bone metastasis, a radionuclide (technetium-99M) bone scan can be obtained and also has a negligible radiation dose to the fetus.[9]

The treatment for pregnancy-associated breast cancer is challenging and should be managed by a maternal–fetal medicine specialist, breast surgeon, and oncologist. The data on treatment of gestational breast cancer are limited to retrospective reviews and case series.[15–18] In the past, it was thought that termination of pregnancy would improve prognosis and survival; however, this supposition has not been supported by evidence.[19] Elective termination of pregnancy can be considered in the instance of very advanced stage disease as a personal choice for the mother. In contrast, there is some evidence to suggest termination of pregnancy actually worsens the prognosis of breast cancer. However, these studies are retrospective and the data are likely skewed by the fact that more women with advanced disease choose termination of pregnancy.[19,20]

A key to breast cancer surgical staging is axillary lymph node dissection. This procedure can be undertaken in the pregnant patient with little if any additional risk to the fetus.[21,22] Less is known about the technique of sentinel lymph node dissection, using radiation, and its safety during pregnancy. Some authors conclude that the minimal dose of radiation used in this procedure is well below the 50-mGy threshold for fetal effects.[22] However, it is not known if the lymphatic drainage channels are altered by pregnancy and, therefore, the efficacy of this procedure is unknown in the pregnant patient.[17] There is 1 case series that documents the safety of sentinel lymph node biopsy and mapping in 12 pregnant patients.[21]

In general, the surgical treatment of breast cancer during pregnancy should be undertaken much like that in the nonpregnant population. Depending on the stage of cancer, the patient may undergo a local excision or lumpectomy versus a mastectomy.[23] For early stage treatment, a nonpregnant patient may opt for breast-conserving treatment along with radiation therapy. In a pregnant patient, a mastectomy is recommended for those patients who would like to continue their pregnancies because radiation therapy would be necessary with conservative treatment and is to be avoided during pregnancy.[24] Mastectomy can be performed with very little risk to the fetus in any trimester. Breast reconstruction surgery should be postponed until the completion of pregnancy because there is no urgency to this procedure, and it is typically postponed until completion of adjuvant treatments.

Radiation therapy, in contrast, has potential risk to the fetus.[9] Depending on gestational age, these risks include pregnancy loss and fetal anomalies if exposed in the first trimester and growth restriction and potential carcinogenic risks in childhood if exposed in the second or third trimesters.[25] The typical therapeutic radiation dose given for breast cancer is 46 to 60 Gy.[25] This translates into a fetal dose of 0.04 to 0.15 Gy. For fetuses less than 16 weeks of gestation, this is above the threshold of 0.10 to 0.2 Gy, where effects may be seen. After 16 weeks of gestation, a much higher dose is likely tolerated by the fetus, 0.50 to 0.70 Gy.[26] In most cases, radiation therapy can be avoided or delayed until after pregnancy. However, in some situations it may be beneficial to proceed with radiation therapy during pregnancy and the risks and benefits should be discussed in each unique clinical scenario.

There are supportive data to show that chemotherapy in the pregnant patient is well-tolerated by the fetus.[27,28] The most common and well-studied regimens in pregnancy are doxorubicin plus cyclophosphamide or fluorouracil, doxorubicin, and cyclophosphamide. These treatments vary slightly from the typical chemotherapy regimens in the nonpregnant patient (**Box 1**).[27] All of these agents were previously considered pregnancy risk factor category D. The most critical time period in gestation to avoid systemic chemotherapy is organogenesis, from week 5 to week 10 of gestation after the last menstrual period. This time period poses the greatest risk for fetal congenital anomalies and pregnancy loss. This risk has been estimated to be as high as 15% to 20%.[28–30] The most significant risk of chemotherapy in the second or third trimesters is not for congenital anomalies, but intrauterine growth restriction and preterm delivery.[27,28] Multiple case reports have supported the safety of anthracyclines when used in the second and third trimesters of pregnancy.[31,32] Doxirubicin is preferred to idarubicin and epirubicin during pregnancy because of reports of intrauterine demise with idarubicin and epirubicin.[31,33–36]

The use of taxanes as a chemotherapy agent is generally considered safe in the second and third trimesters of pregnancy as well.[15] The use of trastuzumab for human epidermal growth factor 2–positive breast cancers during pregnancy is considered contraindicated secondary to reported oligohydramnios and pulmonary hypoplasia.[37]

Box 1
Common chemotherapy regimens for breast cancer

Nonpregnant patients with HER2-negative breast cancer

Docetaxel and cyclophosphamide

Doxorubicin and cyclophosphamide followed by paclitaxel

Doxorubicin and cyclophosphamide

Doxorubicin and cyclophosphamide followed by paclitaxel

Docetaxel, doxorubicin, and cyclophosphamide

Cyclophosphamide, methotrexate, and fluorouracil

Fluorouracil, epirubicin, and cyclophosphamide

Fluorouracil, epirubicin, and cyclophosphamide with paclitaxel

Fluorouracil, epirubicin, and cyclophosphamide with docetaxel

Nonpregnant patients with HER2-positive breast cancer

Pertuzumab, trastuzumab, and docetaxel followed by fluorouracil, epirubicin, and cyclophosphamide

Trastuzumab, pertuzumab, carboplatin, and docetaxel

Fluorouracil, epirubicin, and cyclophosphamide followed by docetaxel, pertuzumab, and trastuzumab

Docorubicin and cyclophosphamide followed by paclitaxel and trastuzumab

Pertuzumab, trastuzumab, and docetaxel

Pregnant patients (HER2-positive/negative)

Doxorubicin and cyclophosphamide

Fluorouracil, doxorubicin, and cyclophosphamide

Abbreviation: HER2, human epidermal growth factor 2.
   Data from Giacalone PL, Laffargue F, Benos P. Chemotherapy for breast carcinoma during pregnancy: a French national survey. Cancer 1999;86(11):2266–72.

Although requested by many pregnant patients, a delay in treatment with systemic chemotherapy should be avoided. The risk of metastasis increases with every few months of delayed treatment by 5% to 10%.[7]

Tamoxifen, a selective estrogen receptor modulator, is often used as treatment and for the prevention of recurrence of breast cancer for estrogen receptor–positive cancers. Its use during pregnancy is generally avoided. The long-term effects on the neonate are not known and it has been associated with miscarriage and congenital malformations, specifically genitourinary malformations.[38,39] There have also been case reports of patients who have taken tamoxifen during pregnancy and their infants were born without anomalies.[38,40] More information is needed on the safety of this medication during pregnancy.

Tamoxifen likely inhibits the ability to breastfeed by suppressing prolactin.[41] Therefore, the potential benefits of tamoxifen in protecting the patient from recurrence must be weighed with the benefits of breastfeeding and a decision to discontinue nursing should tamoxifen therapy be desired.

The common anthracyclines and cyclophosphamide agents used for breast cancer are excreted into breast milk and should be avoided while nursing.[31,33–36] For trastuzumab, it is recommended by the manufacturer to wait at least 6 months after the last dose to begin breastfeeding owing to the 7-month wash out period for the drug concentrations to be eliminated from the body.[42]

Delivery timing should take into account nadirs in cell counts from chemotherapy. Delivery should be avoided within 3 to 4 weeks of the last chemotherapy treatment to avoid increased risks of maternal sepsis and bleeding, as well as any transient myelosuppressive effect of the chemotherapy on the fetus.[43] The optimal timing of delivery has been studied and a decision analysis model taking into account stage and hormone status concluded that for stage I and II cancers, delivery at 36 weeks results in the greatest number of overall quality-adjusted life years.[44] Route of delivery is generally not affected by breast cancer diagnosis and should be determined by normal obstetric indications.

Although studies evaluating the prognosis of pregnancy-associated breast cancer have had mixed results, in general it is thought that the survival of pregnancy-associated breast cancer is similar to that of the nonpregnant patient.[45] The diagnosis of breast cancer in the postpartum period has been postulated to be a particularly high-risk scenario, with some studies estimating increased mortality if diagnosed 4 to 6 months after delivery.[46] More epidemiologic studies need to be done to determine if this risk is actually increased because of diagnosis in the postpartum period or if it is because disease was present during pregnancy and there was a delay in diagnosis.

CERVICAL CANCER

Cervical cancer is one of the most common gynecologic cancers associated with pregnancy, but in actuality occurs rarely, 1 per 1200 to 10,000 pregnancies.[47] Depending on the stage of cervical cancer, its implications during pregnancy and future fertility range from very little impact to greatly impacting a woman's life and childbearing ability.[48] In general, the prognosis for cervical cancer is unchanged by pregnancy. However, depending on tumor size and location, cervical cancer may dictate the route of delivery.[49] As with other gestational cancers, there are no large randomized prospective studies guiding treatment. Therefore, we must rely on studies from nonpregnant patients and case series.

Women with abnormal cervical cytology who are pregnant should undergo evaluation as indicated. Colposcopy with biopsies should be performed if there is suspicion for cervical intraepithelial neoplasia II/III.[50] Colposcopy can be challenging in pregnancy given the normal physiologic changes of the cervix, including increased vascularity and ectropion that occur during pregnancy.[51] Staging of cervical cancer is typically done clinically (**Table 1**).[52] The imaging studies suggested for cervical cancer staging in pregnancy are chest radiograph with abdominal shield or computed tomography scan of the chest for suspected lung metastases.[53,54] For suspected higher stage cancers, the urinary tract, abdomen, and pelvis can be imaged with MRI to evaluate tumor size, as well as vaginal, stromal, parametrial, and lymph node involvement.[54] Cystoscopy and proctoscopy for cervical cancer staging can be performed if needed for accurate staging. Cervical cancer has not been known to metastasize to the placenta or fetus.

The management of invasive cervical cancer in pregnancy is challenging and each individual patient requires thoughtful, multidisciplinary planning. In general, definitive treatment for invasive cervical cancer in the pregnant patient should be undertaken if the patient desires termination of pregnancy in the first and early second trimesters, has positive lymph nodes, or shows progression of disease during pregnancy.[55] For desired pregnancies less than 22 weeks of gestation at the time of diagnosis, patients

Table 1
International Federation of Gynecology and Obstetrics cervical cancer staging system

Stage	Criteria
I	Carcinoma is strictly confined to the cervix.
IA	Microscopic invasion. Invasion is limited to measured stromal invasion with a maximum depth of 5 mm and no wider than 7 mm.
IA1	Measured invasion of stroma <3 mm in depth and <7 mm width.
IA2	Measured invasion of stroma >3 mm and <5 mm in depth and 7 mm width.
IB	Clinical lesions confined to the cervix of preclinical lesions greater than stage IA.
IB1	Clinical lesions no greater than 4 cm in size.
IB2	Clinical lesions >4 cm in size.
II	Carcinoma invades beyond the uterus but not to the pelvic wall or lower one-third of the vagina.
IIA	Tumor without parametrial invasion or involvement of the lower one-third of the vagina.
IIA1	Clinically visible lesion 4 cm or less in greatest dimension with involvement of less than the upper two-thirds of the vagina.
IIA2	Clinically visible lesion >4 cm in greatest dimension with involvement of less than the upper two-thirds of the vagina.
IIB	Tumor with parametrial invasion.
III	Tumor extends to pelvic wall and/or involves the lower one-third of vagina and/or causes hydronephrosis or a nonfunctioning kidney.
IIIA	Tumor involves the lower one-third of vagina, no extension to the pelvic sidewall.
IIIB	Tumor extends to the pelvic sidewall and/or causes hydronephrosis or a nonfunctioning kidney.
IVA	Tumor invades the mucosa of the bladder or rectum, and/or extends beyond the true pelvis.

Adapted from Pecorelli S. Revised FIGO staging for carcinoma of the vulva, cervix, and endometrium. Int J Gynaecol Obstet 2009;105(2):103–4; with permission.

should undergo lymphadenectomy to determine node status. This procedure can be performed laparoscopically, with little harm to the fetus based on limited data.[56]

For microinvasive disease, a cold knife cone can be performed during pregnancy.[57] There are substantial risks of bleeding as well as miscarriage with cone procedures during pregnancy and these risks increase as gestational age increases.[58]

For stage IA2 to IB1 cancers, a large conization can be performed if pregnancy continuation is desired with a reported risk of parametrial extension of less than 1%.[59,60] There is an option to place a cervical cerclage at the time of conservative surgery, although there is no evidence to support this technique; it might be extrapolated from data on trachelectomies.[61] For higher stage cervical cancers and desired pregnancy, the options include neoadjuvant chemotherapy with or without early delivery.[62] The standard chemotherapy of cisplatin and paclitaxel is generally well-tolerated by the fetus if given in the second and third trimesters, although no long-term data exist.[63] Delivery timing is optimal if the last dose of chemotherapy is given at 34 to 35 weeks of gestation with delivery at term.[53,62]

For pregnancies greater than 22 weeks of gestation at the time of diagnosis, lymphadenectomy becomes too technically challenging to be beneficial. For lower stage disease, IA to IB1, treatment can be deferred until after delivery with very little known risk of metastases.[64,65] For higher stage cancers in pregnancies greater than 22 weeks of gestation, treatment is individualized, but should include a discussion of risks of delay in treatment and the possibility of early delivery.[66,67] Often it is decided by the patient and her family to undergo chemotherapy with definitive treatment status after delivery.

The route of delivery in patients with cervical cancer also needs to be considered. With a general lack of data on this topic, it is prudent to allow for vaginal delivery in early stage cervical cancers; however, episiotomy should be avoided, because there have been case series documenting recurrence at the site of episiotomy.[67–69] The limited data support unchanged maternal outcomes for patients with lower stage disease (IA1 and 1A2) who have had vaginal deliveries.[47] For higher stages, limited case report evidence suggests cesarean delivery results in improved maternal outcomes.[70] For higher stage or bulky tumor, cesarean delivery should be performed to avoid hemorrhagic risk.

The prognosis of cervical cancer in the pregnant patient is likely not different from that of the nonpregnant patient.[62,71] The risks for the fetus include preterm delivery and growth restriction if the patient is given systemic chemotherapy.[65] A diagnosis of cervical cancer in the pregnant patient is an ethically challenging situation and each patient's care plan should be handled individually.

HEMATOLOGIC CANCERS

Of the hematologic cancers, the most common is Hodgkin lymphoma. It is the fourth most common malignancy to be diagnosed during pregnancy, likely because of the younger age of onset of this cancer.[72] The incidence of Hodgkin lymphoma in pregnancy is 1 in 1000 to 1 in 6000 pregnancies.[73] The leukemias are more rare, effecting 1 in 75,000 pregnancies.[74,75] Although more rare, there are some important perinatal risks to consider with the diagnosis of leukemia during pregnancy. Because leukemias are so rare, there is little to guide management during pregnancy.[76]

The most common type of leukemia is acute myeloid leukemia, with a typical age of onset in the reproductive years.[76] The presenting symptoms are associated with pancytopenia; the most common symptom is fatigue. The diagnosis is typically made with abnormal screening complete blood count that occurs at the first prenatal visit. Confirmation of the diagnosis is made with a bone marrow biopsy.

If diagnosed in the first trimester, consideration for termination should be given because a delay in systemic chemotherapy likely adds significant risk to the mother.[76] With the standard systemic therapy of anthracycline and cytarabine given in the second or third trimesters, the complete response rate is 87% and is similar to that of nonpregnant females.[75] Because of the underlying risk of thrombocytopenia and disseminated intravascular coagulopathy in these patients, special caution and consideration to timing of delivery should be undertaken.[77]

More is known about Hodgkin lymphoma during pregnancy. It occurs in 1 in 1000 to 1 in 6000 pregnancies and makes up 3% of all Hodgkin diagnoses.[73] Hodgkin lymphoma usually presents with symptoms of painless lymphadenopathy, fatigue, shortness of breath, anemia, or thrombocytopenia, some of which can be difficult to discern from other common pregnancy symptoms.[73] The diagnosis of Hodgkin lymphoma in pregnancy should be handled no differently than in the nonpregnant patient. This process usually consists of a lymph node biopsy. It is typically performed under local anesthesia, but can also be done under general anesthesia with little known risk to the fetus, although the effects of prolonged exposure to general anesthetic agents on the developing fetus are not known.[78] Staging evaluation typically requires chest radiograph with abdominal shielding, laboratory evaluation including a sedimentation rate (which can be elevated in pregnancy), and an MRI of the abdomen.[72]

The standard systemic chemotherapy regimen for Hodgkin lymphoma is doxorubicin, bleomycin, vinblastine, and dacarbazine. Depending on gestational age at diagnosis and the stage of the disease, this same regimen is recommended in the pregnant patient.[29] Another option often undertaken during pregnancy is maintenance therapy with vincristine alone.

There is evidence to support the safety of the doxorubicin, bleomycin, vinblastine, and dacarbazine chemotherapy regimen in pregnancy.[79] An observational study showed that there was likely more risk from iatrogenic preterm delivery to the offspring of these patients than from the exposure to chemotherapy.[79]

If the patient is diagnosed in the early first trimester, treatment should be delayed until the second or third trimesters when the teratogenic effects of chemotherapy are minimal.[80] In the second and third trimesters, systemic chemotherapy does instill a risk of intrauterine growth restriction, preterm delivery, and perhaps a long-term risk of the childhood cancer, although this finding has not been well-documented.[81] If the diagnosis is made in the third trimester of pregnancy, it is feasible for the woman to defer treatment until after delivery unless disease burden is high or progression is thought to be imminent.[80] The optimal patients for whom deferral of treatment is considered are those with early stage disease (IA to IIA) or stable disease presenting later in gestation. Although there have been no prospective trials considering deferral of treatment, there have been 2 case series supporting this approach.[82–84] Chemotherapy should be timed to avoid nadir of cell counts close to term and the goal for delivery timing should be at least 34 weeks or after, when the risks from prematurity are lower.

Pregnancy seems to have little effect on the course of disease in women with Hodgkin lymphoma.[73] One case series followed 48 pregnant women with Hodgkin lymphoma and compared outcomes with matched nonpregnant women; the 20-year survival rate was no different.[73] There have been other case series with similar results.[73,83–85] The overall survival rate for the pregnant patient with Hodgkin lymphoma is estimated to be 71% and is similar to that of the nonpregnant patient.[86]

COLON CANCER

Colon cancer is one of the less common malignancies to encounter during pregnancy; however, the age at which colon cancer is diagnosed in women is decreasing, with a median age at diagnosis of 32 years in pregnant women.[87] It is also important to consider, because many of the symptoms of colon cancer are similar to those related to pregnancy: nausea, vomiting, change in bowel habits, or rectal bleeding. The symptom of rectal bleeding is often overlooked in the pregnant patient and misdiagnosed as bleeding from hemorrhoids.[87] Any of these symptoms should prompt investigation without delay.

There is little evidence that establishes a different normal carcinoembryonic antigen level in pregnancy; therefore, any increase should be evaluated. These tests are typically drawn in the patient presenting with the symptoms listed above. Once colorectal cancer is suspected, the next step in a nonpregnant patient is a colonoscopy, barium enema, or a computed tomography scan. A colonoscopy, if needed, can be done safely during pregnancy.[87] MRI rather than a computed tomography scan is ideal for staging purposes as well as evaluation of tumor burden.[87] A systematic review of the current literature and cases of colon cancer in pregnancy concludes that survival is similar to that of nonpregnant patients; however, stage at diagnosis tends to be more advanced for pregnant women.[87] Interestingly, metastasis to the ovary is more common in pregnancy-associated colon cancer, occurring in 23% versus 8% of pregnant and nonpregnant women, respectively.[88,89] Placental metastasis is extremely rare.

If diagnosed early in pregnancy, the patient has to consider excision of tumor while pregnant versus termination of pregnancy followed by surgical excision. If diagnosed later in pregnancy, the patient will undergo surgical resection versus delivery if at a gestational age with acceptable prematurity outcomes. Chemotherapy is to be avoided during the first trimester, but can be given in the second or third trimester with little risk to the fetus.[53] The typical adjuvant chemotherapy regimen for colon cancer is Folfox (5-flurouracil, leucovorin, and oxaliplatin).[90] It is generally tolerated by the fetus later in gestation, although little is known in terms of the long-term effects.[91–96] There is especially little evidence to guide the use of oxaliplatin. There are 7 documented pregnancies exposed to this drug, 5 of which underwent treatment after the first trimester.[91–96] Only hypothyroidism was reported in one of the infants, but no birth defects were noted.[96] Two of the infants were born preterm and were noted to be small for gestational age.[96] There is more known about 5-flurouracil and leucovorin, which have some long-term follow-up information and are generally considered low risk if given in the second and third trimesters.[97]

In general, pregnancy outcomes are favorable for pregnant patients with colon cancer.[98] Patients should be counseled on the increased risk for cesarean delivery if there is large abdominal or pelvic tumors, preterm birth and small for gestational age/intrauterine growth restriction for those being treated with systemic chemotherapy.[98] Delivery timing depends on gestational age at diagnosis and the treatment plan, and should be determined with the aid of multidisciplinary teams. Delivery can generally be achieved vaginally; however, some expert opinion recommendations include cesarean section if there is an anterior rectal tumor present given the increased risks of bleeding from the tumor site during delivery.[97]

In general, the prognosis for the pregnant patient diagnosed with colon cancer is considered to be poor, but stage for stage the prognosis is similar to that of nonpregnant patients.[97] Typically, more advanced stages are being diagnosed in the pregnant patient given the risk for delay in diagnosis in this population.

SUMMARY

Cancer in pregnancy marks an emotional and devastating diagnosis that requires a multidisciplinary approach to management. Each case needs to be considered individually; there are no consensus guidelines and few prospective studies to guide treatment.

REFERENCES

1. Shachar SS, Gallagher K, McGuire K, et al. Multidisciplinary management of breast cancer during pregnancy. Oncologist 2017;22(3):324–34.
2. Saber A, Dardik H, Ibrahim IM, et al. The milk rejection sign: a natural tumor marker. Am Surg 1996;62(12):998–9.
3. Anderson BO, Petrek JA, Byrd DR, et al. Pregnancy influences breast cancer stage at diagnosis in women 30 years of age and younger. Ann Surg Oncol 1996;3(2):204–11.
4. Stensheim H, Moller B, van Dijk T, et al. Cause-specific survival for women diagnosed with cancer during pregnancy or lactation: a registry-based cohort study. J Clin Oncol 2009;27(1):45–51.

5. Elledge RM, Ciocca DR, Langone G, et al. Estrogen receptor, progesterone receptor, and HER-2/neu protein in breast cancers from pregnant patients. Cancer 1993;71(8):2499–506.

6. Sasidharan R, Harvey V. Pregnancy and breast cancer. Obstet Med 2010;3(2): 54–8.

7. Nettleton J, Long J, Kuban D, et al. Breast cancer during pregnancy: quantifying the risk of treatment delay. Obstet Gynecol 1996;87(3):414–8.

8. Collins JC, Liao S, Wile AG. Surgical management of breast masses in pregnant women. J Reprod Med 1995;40(11):785–8.

9. ACOG Committee on Obstetric Practice. ACOG Committee Opinion. Number 299, September 2004 (replaces No. 158, September 1995). Guidelines for diagnostic imaging during pregnancy. Obstet Gynecol 2004;104(3):647–51.

10. Amant F, Loibl S, Neven P, et al. Breast cancer in pregnancy. Lancet 2012; 379(9815):570–9.

11. Litton JK, Theriault RL. Breast cancer and pregnancy: current concepts in diagnosis and treatment. Oncologist 2010;15(12):1238–47.

12. Rimawi BH, Green V, Lindsay M. Fetal implications of diagnostic radiation exposure during pregnancy: evidence-based recommendations. Clin Obstet Gynecol 2016;59(2):412–8.

13. Shellock FG, Crues JV. MR procedures: biologic effects, safety, and patient care. Radiology 2004;232(3):635–52.

14. Hsieh TC, Wu YC, Sun SS, et al. FDG PET/CT of a late-term pregnant woman with breast cancer. Clin Nucl Med 2012;37(5):489–91.

15. Zagouri F, Sergentanis TN, Chrysikos D, et al. Taxanes for breast cancer during pregnancy: a systematic review. Clin Breast Cancer 2013;13(1):16–23.

16. Loibl S, Han SN, von Minckwitz G, et al. Treatment of breast cancer during pregnancy: an observational study. Lancet Oncol 2012;13(9):887–96.

17. Rovera F, Chiappa C, Coglitore A, et al. Management of breast cancer during pregnancy. Int J Surg 2013;11(Suppl 1):S64–8.

18. Krontiras H, Bland KI. When is sentinel node biopsy for breast cancer contraindicated? Surg Oncol 2003;12(3):207–10.

19. Nugent P, O'Connell TX. Breast cancer and pregnancy. Arch Surg 1985;120(11): 1221–4.

20. Clark RM, Chua T. Breast cancer and pregnancy: the ultimate challenge. Clin Oncol 1989;1(1):11–8.

21. Gentilini O, Cremonesi M, Toesca A, et al. Sentinel lymph node biopsy in pregnant patients with breast cancer. Eur J Nucl Med Mol Imaging 2010;37(1):78–83.

22. Gentilini O, Cremonesi M, Trifiro G, et al. Safety of sentinel node biopsy in pregnant patients with breast cancer. Ann Oncol 2004;15(9):1348–51.

23. Veronesi U, Cascinelli N, Mariani L, et al. Twenty-year follow-up of a randomized study comparing breast-conserving surgery with radical mastectomy for early breast cancer. N Engl J Med 2002;347(16):1227–32.

24. Woo JC, Yu T, Hurd TC. Breast cancer in pregnancy: a literature review. Arch Surg 2003;138(1):91–8 [discussion: 99].

25. Mazonakis M, Damilakis J. Estimation and reduction of the radiation dose to the fetus from external-beam radiotherapy. Phys Med 2017;43:148–52.

26. Antypas C, Sandilos P, Kouvaris J, et al. Fetal dose evaluation during breast cancer radiotherapy. Int J Radiat Oncol Biol Phys 1998;40(4):995–9.

27. Giacalone PL, Laffargue F, Benos P. Chemotherapy for breast carcinoma during pregnancy: a French national survey. Cancer 1999;86(11):2266–72.

28. Ring AE, Smith IE, Jones A, et al. Chemotherapy for breast cancer during pregnancy: an 18-year experience from five London teaching hospitals. J Clin Oncol 2005;23(18):4192–7.
29. Doll DC, Ringenberg QS, Yarbro JW. Antineoplastic agents and pregnancy. Semin Oncol 1989;16(5):337–46.
30. Ebert U, Loffler H, Kirch W. Cytotoxic therapy and pregnancy. Pharmacol Ther 1997;74(2):207–20.
31. Murthy RK, Theriault RL, Barnett CM, et al. Outcomes of children exposed in utero to chemotherapy for breast cancer. Breast Cancer Res 2014;16(6):500.
32. Turchi JJ, Villasis C. Anthracyclines in the treatment of malignancy in pregnancy. Cancer 1988;61(3):435–40.
33. Achtari C, Hohlfeld P. Cardiotoxic transplacental effect of idarubicin administered during the second trimester of pregnancy. Am J Obstet Gynecol 2000;183(2):511–2.
34. Germann N, Goffinet F, Goldwasser F. Anthracyclines during pregnancy: embryo-fetal outcome in 160 patients. Ann Oncol 2004;15(1):146–50.
35. Reynoso EE, Huerta F. Acute leukemia and pregnancy–fatal fetal outcome after exposure to idarubicin during the second trimester. Acta Oncol 1994;33(6):709–10.
36. Siu BL, Alonzo MR, Vargo TA, et al. Transient dilated cardiomyopathy in a newborn exposed to idarubicin and all-trans-retinoic acid (ATRA) early in the second trimester of pregnancy. Int J Gynecol Cancer 2002;12(4):399–402.
37. Zagouri F, Sergentanis TN, Chrysikos D, et al. Trastuzumab administration during pregnancy: a systematic review and meta-analysis. Breast Cancer Res Treat 2013;137(2):349–57.
38. Isaacs RJ, Hunter W, Clark K. Tamoxifen as systemic treatment of advanced breast cancer during pregnancy–case report and literature review. Gynecol Oncol 2001;80(3):405–8.
39. Tewari K, Bonebrake RG, Asrat T, et al. Ambiguous genitalia in infant exposed to tamoxifen in utero. Lancet 1997;350(9072):183.
40. Koca E, Kuzan TY, Babacan T, et al. Safety of tamoxifen during pregnancy: 3 case reports and review of the literature. Breast Care (Basel) 2013;8(6):453–4.
41. Shaaban MM. Suppression of lactation by an antiestrogen, tamoxifen. Eur J Obstet Gynecol Reprod Biol 1975;4(5):167–9.
42. Lactmed. Available at: https://toxnet.nlm.nih.gov/cgi-bin/sis/search2/r?dbs+lactmed:@term+@DOCNO+1017.
43. Koren G, Carey N, Gagnon R, et al. Cancer chemotherapy and pregnancy. J Obstet Gynaecol Can 2013;35(3):263–78.
44. Kuo K, Caughey AB. Optimal timing of delivery for women with breast cancer, according to cancer stage and hormone status: a decision-analytic model. J Matern Fetal Neonatal Med 2017;1–10 [Epub ahead of print].
45. Lee GE, Mayer EL, Partridge A. Prognosis of pregnancy-associated breast cancer. Breast Cancer Res Treat 2017;163(3):417–21.
46. Schedin P. Pregnancy-associated breast cancer and metastasis. Nat Rev Cancer 2006;6(4):281–91.
47. Nguyen C, Montz FJ, Bristow RE. Management of stage I cervical cancer in pregnancy. Obstet Gynecol Surv 2000;55(10):633–43.
48. Bruinsma FJ, Quinn MA. The risk of preterm birth following treatment for precancerous changes in the cervix: a systematic review and meta-analysis. BJOG 2011;118(9):1031–41.

49. Kyrgiou M, Athanasiou A, Kalliala IEJ, et al. Obstetric outcomes after conservative treatment for cervical intraepithelial lesions and early invasive disease. Cochrane Database Syst Rev 2017;(11):CD012847.

50. Guidelines N. https://www.tri-kobe.org/nccn/guideline/gynecological/english/cervical.pdf.

51. Baldauf JJ, Dreyfus M, Ritter J, et al. Colposcopy and directed biopsy reliability during pregnancy: a cohort study. Eur J Obstet Gynecol Reprod Biol 1995;62(1):31–6.

52. Pecorelli S, Zigliani L, Odicino F. Revised FIGO staging for carcinoma of the cervix. Int J Gynaecol Obstet 2009;105(2):107–8.

53. Cordeiro CN, Gemignani ML. Gynecologic malignancies in pregnancy: balancing fetal risks with oncologic safety. Obstet Gynecol Surv 2017;72(3):184–93.

54. Reznek RH, Sahdev A. MR imaging in cervical cancer: seeing is believing. The 2004 Mackenzie Davidson Memorial Lecture. Br J Radiol 2005;78(Spec No 2):S73–85.

55. Amant F, Halaska MJ, Fumagalli M, et al. Gynecologic cancers in pregnancy: guidelines of a second international consensus meeting. Int J Gynecol Cancer 2014;24(3):394–403.

56. Vercellino GF, Koehler C, Erdemoglu E, et al. Laparoscopic pelvic lymphadenectomy in 32 pregnant patients with cervical cancer: rationale, description of the technique, and outcome. Int J Gynecol Cancer 2014;24(2):364–71.

57. Yahata T, Numata M, Kashima K, et al. Conservative treatment of stage IA1 adenocarcinoma of the cervix during pregnancy. Gynecol Oncol 2008;109(1):49–52.

58. Connor JP. Noninvasive cervical cancer complicating pregnancy. Obstet Gynecol Clin North Am 1998;25(2):331–42.

59. Takushi M, Moromizato H, Sakumoto K, et al. Management of invasive carcinoma of the uterine cervix associated with pregnancy: outcome of intentional delay in treatment. Gynecol Oncol 2002;87(2):185–9.

60. Herod JJ, Decruze SB, Patel RD. A report of two cases of the management of cervical cancer in pregnancy by cone biopsy and laparoscopic pelvic node dissection. BJOG 2010;117(12):1558–61.

61. Ishioka S, Endo T, Baba T, et al. Successful delivery after transabdominal cerclage of uterine cervix for cervical incompetence after radical trachelectomy. J Obstet Gynaecol Res 2015;41(8):1295–9.

62. Hopkins MP, Morley GW. The prognosis and management of cervical cancer associated with pregnancy. Obstet Gynecol 1992;80(1):9–13.

63. Cardonick E, Bhat A, Gilmandyar D, et al. Maternal and fetal outcomes of taxane chemotherapy in breast and ovarian cancer during pregnancy: case series and review of the literature. Ann Oncol 2012;23(12):3016–23.

64. van der Vange N, Weverling GJ, Ketting BW, et al. The prognosis of cervical cancer associated with pregnancy: a matched cohort study. Obstet Gynecol 1995;85(6):1022–6.

65. Karam A, Feldman N, Holschneider CH. Neoadjuvant cisplatin and radical cesarean hysterectomy for cervical cancer in pregnancy. Nat Clin Pract Oncol 2007;4(6):375–80.

66. Germann N, Haie-Meder C, Morice P, et al. Management and clinical outcomes of pregnant patients with invasive cervical cancer. Ann Oncol 2005;16(3):397–402.

67. Iavazzo C, Karachalios C, Iavazzo PE, et al. The implantation of cervical neoplasia at postpartum episiotomy scar: the clinical evidence. Ir J Med Sci 2015;184(1):113–8.

68. Van den Broek NR, Lopes AD, Ansink A, et al. "Microinvasive" adenocarcinoma of the cervix implanting in an episiotomy scar. Gynecol Oncol 1995;59(2):297–9.
69. Neumann G, Rasmussen KL, Petersen LK. Cervical adenosquamous carcinoma: tumor implantation in an episiotomy scar. Obstet Gynecol 2007;110(2 Pt 2):467–9.
70. Baloglu A, Uysal D, Aslan N, et al. Advanced stage of cervical carcinoma undiagnosed during antenatal period in term pregnancy and concomitant metastasis on episiotomy scar during delivery: a case report and review of the literature. Int J Gynecol Cancer 2007;17(5):1155–9.
71. Zemlickis D, Lishner M, Degendorfer P, et al. Maternal and fetal outcome after invasive cervical cancer in pregnancy. J Clin Oncol 1991;9(11):1956–61.
72. Moshe Y, Bentur OS, Lishner M, et al. The management of Hodgkin lymphomas in pregnancies. Eur J Haematol 2017;99(5):385–91.
73. Lishner M, Zemlickis D, Degendorfer P, et al. Maternal and foetal outcome following Hodgkin's disease in pregnancy. Br J Cancer 1992;65(1):114–7.
74. Pavlidis NA. Coexistence of pregnancy and malignancy. Oncologist 2002;7(4): 279–87.
75. Horowitz NA, Henig I, Henig O, et al. Acute myeloid leukemia during pregnancy: a systematic review and meta-analysis. Leuk Lymphoma 2018;59(3):610–6.
76. Ali S, Jones GL, Culligan DJ, et al. Guidelines for the diagnosis and management of acute myeloid leukaemia in pregnancy. Br J Haematol 2015;170(4):487–95.
77. Consoli U, Figuera A, Milone G, et al. Acute promyelocytic leukemia during pregnancy: report of 3 cases. Int J Hematol 2004;79(1):31–6.
78. Olutoye OA, Baker BW, Belfort MA, et al. Food and Drug Administration warning on anesthesia and brain development: implications for obstetric and fetal surgery. Am J Obstet Gynecol 2018;218(1):98–102.
79. Amant F, Van Calsteren K, Halaska MJ, et al. Long-term cognitive and cardiac outcomes after prenatal exposure to chemotherapy in children aged 18 months or older: an observational study. Lancet Oncol 2012;13(3):256–64.
80. Bachanova V, Connors JM. How is Hodgkin lymphoma in pregnancy best treated? ASH evidence-based review 2008. Hematology Am Soc Hematol Educ Program 2008;33–4.
81. Ngu SF, Ngan HY. Chemotherapy in pregnancy. Best Pract Res Clin Obstet Gynaecol 2016;33:86–101.
82. Connors JM. Challenging problems: coincident pregnancy, HIV infection, and older age. Hematology Am Soc Hematol Educ Program 2008;334–9.
83. Jacobs C, Donaldson SS, Rosenberg SA, et al. Management of the pregnant patient with Hodgkin's disease. Ann Intern Med 1981;95(6):669–75.
84. Gelb AB, van de Rijn M, Warnke RA, et al. Pregnancy-associated lymphomas. A clinicopathologic study. Cancer 1996;78(2):304–10.
85. Yahalom J. Treatment options for Hodgkin's disease during pregnancy. Leuk Lymphoma 1990;2(3–4):151–61.
86. Woo SY, Fuller LM, Cundiff JH, et al. Radiotherapy during pregnancy for clinical stages IA-IIA Hodgkin's disease. Int J Radiat Oncol Biol Phys 1992;23(2):407–12.
87. Pellino G, Simillis C, Kontovounisios C, et al. Colorectal cancer diagnosed during pregnancy: systematic review and treatment pathways. Eur J Gastroenterol Hepatol 2017;29(7):743–53.
88. Mason MH 3rd, Kovalcik PJ. Ovarian metastases from colon carcinoma. J Surg Oncol 1981;17(1):33–8.
89. Tsukamoto N, Uchino H, Matsukuma K, et al. Carcinoma of the colon presenting as bilateral ovarian tumors during pregnancy. Gynecol Oncol 1986;24(3):386–91.

90. National Comprehensive Cancer Network (NCCN). Homepage on the Internet/ Available: https://www.nccn.org.

91. Makoshi Z, Perrott C, Al-Khatani K, et al. Chemotherapeutic treatment of colorectal cancer in pregnancy: case report. J Med Case Rep 2015;9:140.

92. Kanate AS, Auber ML, Higa GM. Priorities and uncertainties of administering chemotherapy in a pregnant woman with newly diagnosed colorectal cancer. J Oncol Pharm Pract 2009;15(1):5–8.

93. Jeppesen JB, Osterlind K. Successful twin pregnancy outcome after in utero exposure to FOLFOX for metastatic colon cancer: a case report and review of the literature. Clin Colorectal Cancer 2011;10(4):348–52.

94. Gensheimer M, Jones CA, Graves CR, et al. Administration of oxaliplatin to a pregnant woman with rectal cancer. Cancer Chemother Pharmacol 2009;63(2): 371–3.

95. Dogan NU, Tastekin D, Kerimoglu OS, et al. Rectal cancer in pregnancy: a case report and review of the literature. J Gastrointest Cancer 2013;44(3):354–6.

96. Rogers JE, Dasari A, Eng C. The treatment of colorectal cancer during pregnancy: cytotoxic chemotherapy and targeted therapy challenges. Oncologist 2016;21(5):563–70.

97. Nesbitt JC, Moise KJ, Sawyers JL. Colorectal carcinoma in pregnancy. Arch Surg 1985;120(5):636–40.

98. Dahling MT, Xing G, Cress R, et al. Pregnancy-associated colon and rectal cancer: perinatal and cancer outcomes. J Matern Fetal Neonatal Med 2009;22(3): 204–11.

Opioid Use Disorders and Pregnancy

Amanda J. Johnson, MD[a], Cresta W. Jones, MD[b],*

KEYWORDS

- Opioid use disorder • Methadone • Buprenorphine • Pregnancy
- Neonatal abstinence syndrome

KEY POINTS

- Opioid use disorder is associated with an increased risk of pregnancy complications.
- Recommended treatment of opioid use disorder in pregnancy includes medication-assisted therapy using methadone or buprenorphine.
- Medically assisted withdrawal may be considered for women for whom medication-assisted therapy is not a current treatment option, but has a higher risk of maternal relapse.
- Both opioid use disorder and medication assisted therapy are associated with neonatal withdrawal, or neonatal abstinence syndrome.
- A comprehensive care approach is recommended for optimal outcomes with opioid use disorder in pregnancy.

INTRODUCTION

Over the last several decades, the United States has suffered from an increasing epidemic of opioid misuse and dependence, with opioid related overdoses among US adults increasing by 200%.[1] This crisis spans across demographics, including women of childbearing age and who are pregnant.[2,3] As the crisis has intensified, so have the costs of opioid use disorder (OUD) and its sequelae increased. The care of pregnant women affected by opioid use is associated with a substantial economic burden to the health care system, with mean hospital charges for infants affected by opioid withdrawal, or neonatal abstinence syndrome (NAS), at

Disclosure Statement: Neither author has any relationship with a commercial company that has a direct financial interest in subject matter or materials discussed in article or with a company making a competing product.
[a] Department of Obstetrics and Gynecology, Division of Maternal-Fetal Medicine, Medical College of Wisconsin, 9200 West Wisconsin Avenue, Milwaukee, WI 53226, USA; [b] Department of Obstetrics, Gynecology and Women's Health, Division of Maternal-Fetal Medicine, University of Minnesota Medical School, 606 24th Avenue S, Suite 400, Minneapolis, MN 55455, USA
* Corresponding author.
E-mail address: jonesc@umn.edu

approximately 19 times the costs of non-NAS infants.[4,5] This article provides an overview of significant issues associated with OUDs that are of importance to providers of obstetric care.

Defining Opioid Use Disorder

An OUD is currently defined as the repeated occurrence, over a 1-year time period, of 2 or more specific criteria related to opioid use. These criteria include giving up important life events to use more opioids, excessive time spent obtaining and using opioids, and withdrawal when opioid use is stopped abruptly.[6] It is important to note that women on chronic opioids for medically indicated treatment may have opioid withdrawal when medications are abruptly stopped, but withdrawal alone does not identify a patient as suffering from an OUD.

ISSUES IN PREGNANCY
Screening

The identification of opioid misuse and dependence is key to optimizing patient outcomes. Because the misuse of opioids crosses societal boundaries, and risk factor-based screening may lead to missed cases,[7] it is essential that substance use screening be universal.[8] Screening for substance use should, therefore, be considered a routine component of initial prenatal care.[9] Multiple screening tools for substance use and abuse are available, although few have been validated for opioid misuse in pregnancy.[10] Most tools can be administered in written or verbal fashion during the history component of a clinical visit, by any trained health care provider. Urine drug testing as a primary screening tool cannot be recommended at this time, owing to ongoing concerns about the ability to accurately identify patients with substance use disorders. Urine drug screening only assesses recent use, it may miss many substances of abuse, and it is associated with a high false-positive rate.[8,11,12] The Screening, Brief Intervention, and Referral for Treatment technique is recommended for use in pregnancy as a helpful tool for identifying patients with substance use disorders and for providing the first steps to initiating treatment.[13] Because of societal stereotypes and stigmas associated with substance use disorders, health care providers should screen patients in a caring and nonjudgmental manner, and should assure patients that screening is undertaken to allow for optimal maternal care and outcomes during pregnancy and beyond. It is important for all providers to educate themselves on state and federal laws surrounding substance use screening and reporting, before implementing any universal screening protocols, owing to the potential for mandatory reporting of use in some states.

Complications of Opioid Use Disorder

Untreated OUD has been associated with significant complications during pregnancy for the mother, fetus, and neonate (**Table 1**).[14,15] Women experiencing OUD in pregnancy without treatment often have limited prenatal care and are exposed to at-risk behaviors, which increases the risk of sexually transmitted infections, violence, and adverse legal consequences, as well as to a significant risk of overdose and death. The fetus is at an increased risk of intrauterine growth restriction, placental abruption, preterm birth, and fetal death. Many of these complications are significantly reduced or improved with maternal treatment,[16,17] although some complications may persist, such as suboptimal fetal growth and risk of neonatal opioid withdrawal syndrome (also known as NAS). NAS is characterized by disturbances in the gastrointestinal, autonomic, and central nervous systems, and can be associated with extended

Table 1 Complications of untreated opioid use disorder in pregnancy	
Maternal	• Limited prenatal care • Infectious exposure • Miscarriage • Preterm labor and delivery • Opioid overdose and death
Fetal	• Intrauterine growth restriction • Preterm birth • Congenital anomalies (uncertain)
Neonatal	• Small for gestational age • Neonatal abstinence syndrome • Long-term developmental effects (uncertain)

newborn hospitalizations to treat withdrawal symptoms. Infants exposed to chronic opioids in utero are typically observed for a minimum of 4 to 7 days for signs or symptoms of NAS. If NAS is identified, it is often treated with oral morphine or methadone at a dose that alleviates the signs and symptoms of withdrawal, with the dose weaned over days to weeks.[12]

Although NAS is the most common term used to represent the pattern of findings typically associated with opioid withdrawal in the newborn, it is important to note that the US Food and Drug Administration now embraces the term "neonatal opioid withdrawal syndrome," which more accurately identifies the constellation of symptoms specifically associated with prenatal exposure to opioids.[18]

NAS was described initially in infants of mothers with illicit opioid use, but its development can be associated with any chronic maternal opioid use in pregnancy, including for treatment of OUD as well as of chronic pain. Rates of development of NAS have varied widely, from 30% to 80%,[12,19] and the incidence cannot be predicted by the amount of opioids used by the mother before delivery.[20,21] The incidence of NAS in the United States has increased approximately 400% in recent years.[4] In addition, NAS risk seems to be doubled in infants of mothers with coexposure to antidepressants, benzodiazepines, and gabapentin.[22] Patient should be counseled to limit exposure to these medications if not medically indicated.

Treatment

Although not approved for use in pregnancy by the US Food and Drug Administration, several therapies are currently considered standard of care for maternal treatment, and several others require additional data on outcomes before recommendations can be made (**Table 2**).[12,15]

Table 2 Treatment options for opioid use disorder in pregnancy	
Preferred treatment	• Methadone • Buprenorphine
Treatment reported, not preferred	• Buprenorphine/naloxone combination therapy • Medically supervised withdrawal
Limited data in pregnancy	• Naltrexone

Medication-assisted therapy

The preferred treatment options for OUD in pregnancy include 2 forms of medication-assisted treatment (MAT): methadone or buprenorphine.[12,23,24] The rationale for treatment with MAT includes the prevention of opioid withdrawal, the prevention of complications owing to nonmedical opioid use and relapse to use, improved compliance with prenatal care and comprehensive addiction treatment, and a reduced risk of obstetric complications.[8]

It is recommended that all obstetric providers be familiar with the federal guideline on emergency narcotic addiction treatment, 21 CFR 1306.07(b).[25] This exception, known as the "3-day rule" allows a practitioner who is not separately registered as a narcotic treatment provider to administer (but not prescribe) narcotic drugs to relieve acute withdrawal while arranging for a patient's referral for treatment. Treatment can be provided for no more than 72 hours, and should be performed in consultation or collaboration with a specialist comfortable with initiating treatment for OUD. This provision may be useful when a pregnant patient presents in withdrawal at a time of day when access to immediate OUD treatment is not available, such as evenings and weekends.

Methadone Methadone is a pure opioid receptor agonist that binds to and activates μ-opioid receptors. It is provided through federally regulated opiate treatment programs that dispense daily medication doses as a component of comprehensive addiction care. The dose is increased slowly over several weeks to reach a therapeutic level while minimizing the increased risk of overdose during treatment initiation. Methadone has long been used as a treatment for OUD in pregnancy, with clear evidence of improvement in obstetric outcomes.[26] Because treatment with methadone can only be continued through a federally regulated opiate treatment program, open communication between the opioid treatment program and the obstetric team is necessary for optimal care. However, this communication must be done while following special guidelines for disclosure of information regarding addiction and substance use treatment.[27]

Although long considered the standard of care for OUD in pregnancy, methadone treatment is not without its adverse effects. These effects include respiratory depression and risk of overdose, QTc interval prolongation, as well as interaction with other drugs, including antiretroviral agents.[23] In addition, as with all currently used MAT options for OUD in pregnancy, it is also associated with the risk of NAS.

Buprenorphine Buprenorphine is a partial μ-receptor agonist that binds with a high affinity to the μ-opioid receptor, but does not activate the receptor completely when bound. The partial agonistic activity makes overdose less likely when use is compared with other opioids.[28] However, owing to its high affinity for the opioid receptor, patients must demonstrate withdrawal symptoms before initiating treatment, to avoid precipitated withdrawal, which can be very difficult to treat.[23]

Buprenorphine is accessible through office-based maintenance therapy, which can be undertaken by a licensed provider who has obtained a DATA-2000 waiver from the US Drug Enforcement Agency. This process requires additional provider training, which can be obtained by several routes, the simplest of which is a full-day training program available on-line or in person. Buprenorphine has many advantages that allow for patient discretion and accessibility outside of areas where daily methadone treatment is an option. Buprenorphine treatment can be incorporated into a comprehensive obstetric treatment program if a waivered physician is available.

Most buprenorphine treatment programs outside of pregnancy use primarily a buprenorphine/naloxone combination medication.[23] Naloxone is added to help deter alternative administration of buprenorphine in an abuse/diversion setting. Although naloxone does not seem to have systemic absorption when taken correctly in a combination sublingual treatment, buprenorphine monotherapy is currently recommended in pregnancy.[8,12,15] However, recent data suggest that buprenorphine/naloxone combination therapy may be an additional option during pregnancy. At this time, no maternal, fetal, or neonatal adverse effects have been identified with the combination product.[29–31] It is expected that the use of this treatment in pregnancy will increase as more data become available.

If a patient maintained on combination therapy becomes pregnant, and she is unwilling or unable to change to monotherapy, informed consent on limited outcomes is recommended before continuing treatment.

A recently available buprenorphine implant is being used in addiction treatment,[32,33] as opposed to conventional sublingual therapy. However, there are currently no data on the use of this treatment in a pregnant population.

Methadone versus buprenorphine: initiating therapy in pregnancy Both methadone and buprenorphine are appropriate choices for initiating treatment in pregnancy. A personalized approach to treatment is required, because there are benefits and downfalls to both therapies (**Table 3**).[8,12,15] Data do indicate less severe manifestations of

Table 3
Medication specific issues: medication-assisted therapy in pregnancy

Treatment	Pros	Cons
Methadone	• Demonstrated safety and efficacy in pregnancy • Decreased medication diversion • More structured program • More effective for polysubstance abuse • Effective if failed buprenorphine treatment • Safe for breastfeeding	• Daily clinic treatment required • Higher risk of overdose • Interactions with other medication • Prolongation of QT interval • Neonatal abstinence syndrome
Buprenorphine	• Does not require proximity for daily clinic visits • Decreased overdose risk • Decreased interactions with other medications • Less severe, shorter neonatal abstinence • More discreet • Safe for breastfeeding	• Risk of precipitated withdrawal during initiation • Lack of long-term data on child outcomes • Increased diversion risk • Lower retention in treatment • Less effective if buprenorphine drug of abuse • Requires mild withdrawal to start treatment
Buprenorphine + naloxone	• Decreased diversion risk • Similar outcomes to buprenorphine alone • Limited breastfeeding data	• Severe withdrawal if used incorrectly (ie, injected) • Lack of long-term data on child outcomes
Naltrexone	• Requires completed opioid withdrawal to initiate • Limits overdose risk • No maternal withdrawal if treatment stopped • Minimal breastfeeding data	• Limited effectiveness of opioid treatment if required (eg, after a cesarean section) • Lack of long-term data on infant and child outcomes • Minimal data on pregnancy and breastfeeding • Minimal data on long-term maternal outcomes

NAS with maternal treatment using buprenorphine,[19] and a recent systematic review and metaanalysis suggested that buprenorphine treatment was associated with a lower risk of preterm birth, greater birth weight, and larger neonatal head circumference, with no increase in adverse events.[34] However, methadone has been associated with a higher treatment retention rate[35] and individual patient characteristics must be considered when choosing the best treatment to minimize relapse risk.

It is important to note that, owing to physiologic and metabolic changes of pregnancy, dosages of methadone and buprenorphine often require multiple dose changes during pregnancy.[36–38] Patients can be reassured by their obstetricians that such changes are common in pregnancy and should be considered when patients report a return of or an increase in withdrawal symptoms. The decision for a dosage increase is determined by the opioid- agonist therapy provider, based on the presence of withdrawal symptoms or patient reported urges for illicit use, often in collaboration with the obstetric providers. Changes may include increasing the overall dose and/or increasing the frequency of dosing to control withdrawal symptoms.[39,40] It is of note that methadone and buprenorphine doses do not seem to have a consistent effect on the incidence and severity of NAS[41,42]; therefore, maternal treatment goals must be to manage withdrawal symptoms and prevent relapse and illicit use, rather than to minimize daily treatment dosages.

Patient often express concern about the long-term implications of prenatal exposure to MAT. Studies are complicated by substantial difficulties in isolating the effects of opioid treatment from other confounders often seen in women experiencing OUD.[43] However, limited data suggest the possibility of potential vision, motor, behavioral, and cognitive problems, as well as an increased rate of otitis media.[44,45] It is important that these families be identified early and be provided with additional support to optimize long-term outcomes.

Alternative treatment options Although methadone and buprenorphine are both recommended as first-line therapy for treatment of OUD in pregnancy, they may not be acceptable treatments for some patients for a variety of reasons, including financial, geographic, or stigma. Therefore, it is important that obstetric providers be familiar with alternative treatments that may be provided to their patients.[12,15]

Medically assisted withdrawal Although opioid withdrawal has historically been associated with a higher risk of miscarriage and fetal demise,[46] available recent data do not support a significantly increased risk of fetal complications with medically assisted withdrawal during pregnancy.[47,48] MAT is currently considered as the first-line treatment of OUD in pregnancy, but medically supervised withdrawal may be considered in situations in which a woman will not accept MAT, or MAT is not available.[8,12] Although recent studies have described successful outcomes after medically supervised withdrawal in pregnancy,[48,49] there remains a high risk of maternal relapse as well as NAS, likely related to relapse.[50] Significant ancillary services are often required, such as intensive outpatient therapy, for the successful maintenance of abstinence. In addition, there are no studies addressing the long-term outcomes for patients treated with medically supervised withdrawal during pregnancy.[51]

Owing to concerns and guilt related to the risk of NAS, women may request self-wean from MAT and abstinence from all treatment. It is important to educate patients that success is low with self-wean, and most patients end up maintaining or increasing their current dose.[52] In addition, with a clinical focus based on treatment of a chronic maternal disease, goals must be directed toward long-term success in recovery for the patient. Owing to the high relapse rate associated with maternal withdrawal and abstinence (90%), medically assisted withdrawal cannot currently be considered a recommended form of treatment.

Naltrexone Naltrexone therapy, in oral, injectable, and implant forms, has been gaining more attention as an alternative to opioid-based treatments.[53] Naltrexone is a pure opioid antagonist, similar to naloxone, and it seems to block most opioid receptors. Naltrexone has been shown to reduce the risk of relapse in nonpregnant populations.[23,54] Management of acute pain while using this medication has been found to be challenging, which would certainly complicate analgesia surrounding childbirth.[55] In addition, currently available data on use in pregnancy are limited, although no significant adverse outcomes have been noted when compared with other MAT.[56] Initiating naltrexone requires complete withdrawal from opioids, making the initiation of therapy difficult even outside of pregnancy. Data are currently limited on both the safety and effectiveness of naltrexone in pregnancy. If a pregnancy is identified in a woman currently undergoing naltrexone treatment, a significant discussion of possible benefits and unknown risks will need to be undertaken.[53]

COMPREHENSIVE OBSTETRIC CARE AND OPIOID USE DISORDERS

To best provide obstetric care for women experiencing OUD, a "whole-women" approach must be taken.[15] This means comprehensive management of the other medical and social issues often associated with OUD in pregnancy. A modified care schedule may include flexible appointments, grouping prenatal visits with ultrasound and social services, and offering convenient consultations with lactation specialists and pediatrics.[11,12] Even in women who are not engaged in treatment of substance use disorders, participation in prenatal care has been associated with significant reductions in prematurity and low birth weight infants.[57]

Antepartum Care

Communication
A vital component of obstetric care is adequate collaboration among all care providers. It is important for providers to obtain written permission from the patient to coordinate care and follow up with her substance use disorder and psychiatric providers, as well as with social services, as is required by federal law for patients undergoing addiction treatment.[27] Pregnant women with ongoing active substance use must be encouraged to continue to engage in prenatal care and legal action to address perinatal OUDs is strongly discouraged.[58] Supportive obstetric care without criminal ramifications for the mother with substance use will allow for the best outcomes for both mother and infant.

Owing to the ongoing risk of maternal relapse to illicit use, which carries an increased risk of overdose and death, prescription of naloxone, the opioid antagonist administered to rapidly reverse the effects of an opioid overdose, for emergency administration should be considered. A patient's family and caregivers should be instructed on use, with the fetal risks of acute maternal withdrawal clearly outweighed by the risk of maternal death from overdose.

Psychiatric disorders
Just fewer than one-half of individuals suffering from OUD have coexisting mental health concerns,[59] many of which are underdiagnosed and undertreated, and may be associated with increased psychological, social, and medical impairments.[60,61] The most common codiagnoses include depression and anxiety. It is important to take a thorough mental health history and to refer patients for additional services as

indicated. This step also includes an assessment for the impact of victimization and trauma in the patient's life to best guide health care delivery, a principle termed trauma-informed care.[62] Patients should be scheduled for a follow-up phone call or visit before the routine postpartum visit, to assess for the risk of postpartum depression and psychosis.

Tobacco use disorders

Tobacco use in pregnancy has been associated with an increased risk of adverse pregnancy outcomes including poor fetal growth, placental abruption, preterm birth, and stillbirth.[63] Tobacco use disorders are much more prevalent in pregnant women experiencing OUD (95%) than in pregnant women without substance use concerns (15%).[64,65] This population also has much more limited success in quitting smoking during pregnancy. Recent studies suggest some success with incentive-based treatment programs.[66] Even a decrease in the amount of daily tobacco use, if cessation is unachievable, is associated with improved neonatal outcomes.[67] Tobacco use has also been shown to increase the duration and medication required for infants suffering from NAS.[68,69]

Infectious complications

Infectious disease is more common in women suffering from OUD.[70] In particular, 1 study suggested a rate of hepatitis C exposure of 53% and chronic infection of 37%.[71] Thus, women with identified OUD should be screened for hepatitis C at prenatal intake. In addition, testing for infections such as sexually transmitted infections, hepatitis B, and tuberculosis should be considered, and repeated in later pregnancy for women considered to be at ongoing risk of new exposure. Women not previously immunized should also be offered hepatitis A and B vaccination.[8,23]

Constipation

Patients using opioids including MAT for OUD are at significant risk of opioid-induced constipation and bowel dysfunction. Constipation-related issues should be addressed with patients at each visit. Medications including bisacodyl, Senna, and polyethylene glycol have been shown to be effective for opioid-induced constipation in nonpregnant patients,[72] although no data are currently available regarding the treatment of opioid-induced constipation in pregnancy.

Fetal surveillance

Although opioids are consistently associated with the risk of NAS, studies have demonstrated uncertainty regarding the association of opioid exposure and an increased risk of fetal anomalies.[73] A targeted anatomic survey should be considered to evaluate for possible fetal anomalies, which can be present in up to 2% to 3% of normal pregnancies. Given the increased risk of fetal growth abnormalities with OUDs,[74,75] fetal growth assessments may be considered, either through close clinical examination or via fetal ultrasound examination. For women who are stable in treatment, consideration should be given to sonographic evaluation of fetal growth in the third trimester. In the absence of fetal growth restriction or any additional maternal complications, there are no current recommendations for additional fetal surveillance during the pregnancy. For women with ongoing illicit substance use, more frequent evaluation, including antepartum surveillance, may be considered. No late preterm or early term delivery is currently recommended for maternal OUD, and delivery should be facilitated as obstetrically indicated.[8,12]

It is important to note that antepartum surveillance, if indicated, may demonstrate such abnormalities as decreased fetal heart rate baseline, decreased variability, and fewer accelerations, likely owing to suppressed motor activity in the fetus.[76,77] Surveillance performed immediately before or immediately after medication is administered, thus avoiding peak effects, is recommended when possible.

Patient expectations

It is important to establish clear expectations for the patient to best optimize the patient–provider relationship. This process includes guidelines for best partnership for prenatal care, what to expect during labor and delivery, and how to best partner to prevent an increased risk of relapse after delivery. Prenatal consultations are suggested with anesthesia, pediatrics/neonatology, and lactation support, and delivery unit tours should be considered. In addition, it is recommended to discuss with the patient how her pain will be managed during labor as well as upon discharge.

Patients with OUD may experience substantial barriers to routine prenatal care, including an inability to attend consistent prenatal appointments owing to transportation or childcare issues. There remains an ongoing need for focused programming that allows for opportunities to overcome these issues.[78]

Peripartum Care

Intrapartum

Patients should be continued on MAT throughout labor and delivery to avoid withdrawal symptoms.[8,12] Although theoretic concerns about precipitated withdrawal have been raised with using buprenorphine in conjunction with pure opioid antagonists (which may be used for labor analgesia), buprenorphine can be safely continued without interruption through labor and delivery, as well as through the postpartum period.[79] Because patients may have hyperalgesia as a result of treatment, it is important to consider early epidural and to remember that MAT will not cover the pain associated with the childbirth process. Alternative pain management protocols such as transverse abduminus plane blocks or nitrous oxide may also be beneficial.[80] Finally, it is very important to avoid treatment with partial opioid antagonists such as nalbuphine and butorphanol during labor and delivery, because these agents can precipitate withdrawal symptoms.

Birthing center staff should be counseled on intrapartum fetal heart rate tracings for patients on methadone, including the potential for reduced variability and accelerations, and a lower baseline.[81] No data are currently available on the potential changes in intrapartum fetal monitoring with buprenorphine therapy.

Postpartum

Limited studies indicate that women with OUD on MAT who undergo cesarean section may require up to 70% more opioid analgesia than women without OUD to adequately treat their pain.[82,83] After delivery, women should continue with a pregnancy-level dosing of MAT, because most studies suggest that medication does not need to be reduced to prepregnancy levels for several weeks.[84] Patients may require a short course of narcotics at discharge after cesarean delivery, and this has not been shown to be a risk factor for relapse for postsurgical patients on methadone or buprenorphine therapy.[85] Higher nonopioid medication use may also be required.[86]

The importance of parental participation in reducing the sequelae of NAS for the infant and for the mother cannot be underestimated.[87] It is important to encourage women who are stable in treatment to consider breastfeeding, which has been shown to improve maternal bonding and potentially decrease the severity of NAS.[88] Contraindications to breastfeeding include active relapse to illicit drug use and infectious complications such as with human immunodeficiency virus.[89] In addition, rooming-in, skin-to-skin care, and parenting education and support may further improve outcomes for the family unit. The addition of parenting support groups exclusively for women in MAT has also been found to be beneficial.[90]

It is important to address contraception during prenatal care and again at the time of discharge, because the majority of pregnancies are unplanned and women in MAT have lower use of contraception. In addition, they often lack information about effective long-acting reversible contraception.[91,92]

RESPONSIBLE OPIOID PRESCRIBING

Health care providers play an important role in reducing opioid overprescribing, which is an important contributor to the opioid epidemic.[2,3] This role includes limited prescriptions for opioids during pregnancy and at hospital discharge,[93,94] as well as adequate patient education at the time of postdelivery discharge.[95] When prescribing opioids outside of pregnancy to women of childbearing age, discussion of plans for pregnancy, use of reliable contraception, and risks of ongoing opiate use must be considered as primary prevention of both OUD and NAS.[96] Regular use of state-established prescription drug monitoring programs will also help to avoid duplicate prescriptions and doctor shopping, and may also facilitate the identification of women experiencing OUD. Outside of pregnancy, guidelines and best practice statements now exist to help limit the overuse of opioids for chronic pain disorders.[97,98]

Although women with chronic pain may experience physical opioid dependence, they often represent a subset of patients at risk of NAS, but without the other clinical issues associated with OUD. There are few data available on the effects of medically indicated chronic opioid use on pregnancy outcomes, other than the risk of NAS. Although new data and guidelines do not support the use of long-term opioids for chronic pain, many women have already been placed on long-term therapy before achieving pregnancy. There are currently limited data on this population and specific obstetric risks, including the incidence of NAS, that might be encountered. Best practice should include a discussion of limiting opioid use to the minimum required, supporting the use of alternative and complementary pain treatment, and consultations with anesthesia and pediatrics before delivery.[99,100]

SUMMARY

OUDs have significant implications in pregnancy, and outcomes are improved when patients are cared for in an environment that addresses both the treatment of OUD and focused obstetric care tailored to the unique issues that may arise. A personalized approach will identify the best treatment for each patient, with current recommendations focusing on MAT using methadone or buprenorphine. Focused obstetric care allows for appropriate and supportive pregnancy care during the pregnancy and after delivery, with special attention paid to contraception and postpartum depression. Providers must also take steps to minimize ongoing opioid prescribing, using currently accepted guidelines to limit excessive prescriptions.

REFERENCES

1. Rudd RA, Aleshire N, Zibbell JE, et al. Increases in drug and opioid overdose deaths – United States, 2000-2014. MMWR Morb Mortal Wkly Rep 2016;64(50–51):1378–82.
2. Kozhimannil KB, Graves AJ, Jarlenski M, et al. Non-medical opioid use and sources of opioids among pregnant and non-pregnant reproductive-aged women. Drug Alcohol Depend 2017;174:201–8.

3. Kozhimannil KB, Graves AJ, Levy R, et al. Nonmedical use of prescription opioids among pregnant U.S. women. Womens Health Issues 2017;27(3):308–15.

4. Patrick SW, Davis MM, Lehman CU, et al. Increasing incidence and geographic distribution of neonatal abstinence syndrome: United States 2009 to 2012. J Perinatol 2015;35(8):650–5.

5. Corr TE, Hollenbeak CS. The economic burden of neonatal abstinence syndrome in the United States. Addiction 2017;112(9):1590–9.

6. American Psychiatric Association (APA). Diagnostic and statistical manual of mental disorders. 5th edition. Arlington (VA): APA; 2013.

7. Schauberger CW, Newbury EJ, Coburn JM, et al. Prevalence of illicit drug use in pregnant women in a Wisconsin private practice setting. Am J Obstet Gynecol 2014;211(3):255.e1-4.

8. American College of Obstetrics and Gynecology (ACOG) Committee on Obstetric Practice. ACOG practice bulletin no. 711. Opioid use and opioid use disorder in pregnancy. Obstet Gynecol 2017;130(2):e81–94.

9. American College of Obstetrics and Gynecology (ACOG) Committee on Ethics. ACOG committee opinion no. 633. Alcohol abuse and other substance use disorders: ethical issues in obstetric and gynecologic practice. Obstet Gynecol 2015;125(6):1529–37.

10. Chasnoff IJ, Wells AM, McGourty RF, et al. Validation of the 4Ps plus screen for substance use in pregnancy validation of the 4Ps plus. J Perinatol 2007;27(12): 744–8.

11. Jones HE, Deppen K, Hudak ML, et al. Clinical care for opioid-using pregnant and postpartum women: the role of obstetric providers. Am J Obstet Gynecol 2014;210(4):302–10.

12. Reddy UM, Davis JM, Ren X, et al. Opioid use in pregnancy, neonatal abstinence syndrome, and childhood outcomes: executive summary of a joint workshop by the Eunice Kennedy Shriver National Institute of Child Health and Human Development, American College of Obstetricians and Gynecologists, American Academy of Pediatrics, Society for Maternal-Fetal Medicine, Centers for Disease Control and Prevention, and the March of Dimes Foundation. Obstet Gynecol 2017;130(1):10–28.

13. Wright TE, Terplan M, Ondersma SJ, et al. The role of screening, brief intervention, and referral to treatment in the perinatal period. Am J Obstet Gynecol 2016; 215(5):539–47.

14. Mozurkewich EL, Rayburn WF. Buprenorphine and methadone for opioid addiction during pregnancy. Obstet Gynecol Clin North Am 2014;41(2):241–53.

15. Substance Abuse and Mental Health Services Administration (SAMHSA). A collaborative approach to the treatment of pregnant women with opioid use disorders. HHS Publication No. (SMA)16-4978. Rockville (MD): SAMHSA; 2016. Available at: https://ncsacw.samsha.gov/files/Collaborative_Approach_508.pdf. Accessed August 10, 2017.

16. Fullerton CA, Kim M, Thomas CP, et al. Medication-assisted treatment with methadone: assessing the evidence. Psychiatr Serv 2014;65(2):146–57.

17. Thomas CP, Fullerton CA, Kim M, et al. Medication-assisted treatment with buprenorphine: assessing the evidence. Psychiatr Serv 2014;65(2):158–70.

18. US Food and Drug Administration (FDA). What is the federal government doing to combat the opioid abuse epidemic? U.S. Food and Drug Administration; 2015. Available at: http://www.fda.gov/newsevents/testimony/ucm446076.htm. Accessed September 8, 2017.

19. Jones HE, Kaltenbach K, Heil SH, et al. Neonatal abstinence syndrome after methadone or buprenorphine exposure. N Engl J Med 2010;363(24): 2320–31.

20. Jones HE, Dengler E, Garrison A, et al. Neonatal outcomes and their relationship to maternal buprenorphine dose during pregnancy. Drug Alcohol Depend 2014; 334:414–7.

21. Bakstad B, Sarfi M, Welle-Strand GK, et al. Opioid maintenance treatment during pregnancy: occurrence and severity of neonatal abstinence syndrome. A national prospective study. Eur Addict Res 2009;15(3):128–34.

22. Huybrechts KF, Bateman BT, Desai RJ, et al. Risk of neonatal withdrawal after intrauterine co-exposure to opioids and psychotropic medications: cohort study. BMJ 2017;358:j3326.

23. Kampman K, Jarvis M. American Society of Addiction Medicine (ASAM) national practice guideline for the use of medications in the treatment of addiction involving opioid use. J Addict Med 2015;9(5):358–67.

24. World Health Organization (WHO). Guidelines for identification and management of substance use and substance use disorders in pregnancy. Geneva (Switzerland): World Health Organization; 2014.

25. Title 21 code of federal regulations. US Drug Enforcement Administration Web site. Available at: http://deadiversion.usdoj.gov/21cfr/cfr/1306/1306_07.htm. Accessed September 8, 2017.

26. Harper RG, Solish GI, Purow HM, et al. The effect of a methadone treatment program upon pregnant heroin addicts and their newborn infants. Pediatrics 1974; 54:300–5.

27. Substance abuse confidentiality regulations. Substance Abuse and Mental Health Services Administration Web. 2016. Available at: http://www.samhsa.gov/about-us/who-we-are/laws/confidentiality-regulations-faqs. Accessed August 10, 2017.

28. Bell JR, Butler B, Lawrance A, et al. Comparing overdose mortality associated with methadone and buprenorphine treatment. Drug Alcohol Depend 2009; 104(1–2):73–7.

29. Wiegand SL, Stringer EM, Stuebe AM, et al. Buprenorphine and naloxone compared with methadone treatment in pregnancy. Obstet Gynecol 2015; 125(2):363–8.

30. Lund IO, Fischer G, Welle-Strand GK, et al. A comparison of buprenorphine + naloxone to buprenorphine and methadone in the treatment of opioid dependence during pregnancy: maternal and neonatal outcomes. Subst Abuse 2013;6:61–74.

31. Debelak K, Morrone WR, O'Grady KE, et al. Buprenorphine + naloxone compared with methadone treatment during pregnancy – initial patient care and outcome data. Am J Addict 2013;22(3):252–4.

32. Chavoustie S, Frost M, Snyder O, et al. Buprenorphine implants in medical treatment of opioid addiction. Expert Rev Clin Pharmacol 2017;10(8):799–807.

33. Rosenthal RN, Lofwall MR, Kim S, et al. Effect of buprenorphine implants on illicit opioid use among abstinent adults with opioid dependence treated with sublingual buprenorphine: a randomized clinical trial. JAMA 2016;316(3):282–90.

34. Zedler BK, Mann AL, Kim MM, et al. Buprenorphine compared with methadone to treat pregnant women with opioid use disorder: a systematic review and meta-analysis of safety in the mother, fetus and child. Addiction 2016;111(12): 2115–28.

35. Minozzi S, Amato L, Bellisario C, et al. Maintenance agonist treatments for opiate-dependent pregnant women. Cochrane Database Syst Rev 2013;(12):CD0006318.

36. Albright B, de la Torre L, Skipper B, et al. Changes in methadone maintenance therapy during and after pregnancy. J Subst Abuse Treat 2011;41(4):347–53.
37. Wolff K, Boys A, Rostami-Hodjegan A, et al. Changes to methadone clearance during pregnancy. Eur J Clin Pharmacol 2005;61(10):763–8.
38. Bastian JR, Chen H, Zhang H, et al. Dose-adjusted plasma concentrations of sublingual buprenorphine are lower during than after pregnancy. Am J Obstet Gynecol 2017;216(1):64.e1-7.
39. Caritis SN, Bastian JR, Zhang H, et al. An evidence-based recommendation to increase the dosing frequency of buprenorphine during pregnancy. Am J Obstet Gynecol 2017. https://doi.org/10.1016/j.ajog.2017.06.029.
40. McCarthy JJ, Leamon MH, Willits HN, et al. The effect of methadone dose regimen on neonatal abstinence syndrome. J Addict Med 2015;9(2):105–10.
41. Cleary BJ, Donnelly J, Strawbridge J, et al. Methadone dose and neonatal abstinence syndrome – systematic review and meta-analysis. Addiction 2010; 105(12):2071–84.
42. O'Connor AB, O'Brien L, Alto WA. Maternal buprenorphine dose at delivery and its relationship to neonatal outcomes. Eur Addict Res 2016;22(3):127–30.
43. Logan BA, Brown MS, Hayes MJ. Neonatal abstinence syndrome: treatment and pediatric outcomes. Clin Obstet Gynecol 2013;56(1):186–92.
44. Maguire DJ, Taylor S, Armstrong K, et al. Long-term outcomes of infants with neonatal abstinence syndrome. Neonatal Netw 2016;35(5):277–86.
45. Oei JL, Melhuish E, Uebel H, et al. Neonatal abstinence syndrome and high school performance. Pediatrics 2017;139(2). https://doi.org/10.1542/peds. 2016-2651.
46. Rementeria JL, Nunag NN. Narcotic withdrawal in pregnancy: stillbirth incidence with a case report. Am J Obstet Gynecol 1973;116:1152–6.
47. Luty J, Nikolaou V, Bearn J. Is opiate detoxification unsafe in pregnancy? J Subst Abuse Treat 2003;24(4):363–7.
48. Bell J, Towers CV, Hennessy MD, et al. Detoxification from opiate drugs during pregnancy. Am J Obstet Gynecol 2016;215(3):374.e1-6.
49. Stewart RD, Nelson DB, Adjikari EH, et al. The obstetrical and neonatal impact of maternal opioid detoxification in pregnancy. Am J Obstet Gynecol 2013; 209(3):267.e1-5.
50. Jones HE, O'Grady KE, Malfi D, et al. Methadone maintenance vs. methadone taper during pregnancy: maternal and neonatal outcomes. Am J Addict 2008; 17(5):372–86.
51. Jones HE, Terplan M, Meyer M. Medically assisted withdrawal (detoxification): considering the mother-infant dyad. J Addict Med 2017;11(2):90–2.
52. Welle-Strand GK, Skurtveit S, Tanum L, et al. Tapering from methadone or buprenorphine during pregnancy: maternal and neonatal outcomes in Norway 1996-2009. Eur Addict Res 2015;21(5):253–61.
53. Jones HE, Chisolm MS, Jansson LM, et al. Naltrexone in the treatment of opioid-dependent pregnant women: the case for a considered and measured approach to research. Addiction 2013;108(2):233–47.
54. Rea F, Bell JR, Young MR, et al. A randomised, controlled trial of low dose naltrexone for the treatment of opioid dependence. Drug Alcohol Depend 2004;75(1):79–88.
55. Vickers BP, Jolly A. Naltrexone and problems in pain management. BMJ 2006; 332(7534):132–3.
56. Kelty E, Hulse G. A retrospective cohort study of obstetric outcomes in opioid-dependent women treated with implant naltrexone, oral methadone

or sublingual buprenorphine, and non-dependent controls. Drugs 2017; 77(11):1199–210.

57. El-Mohandes A, Herman AA, Nabil El-Khorazaty M, et al. Prenatal care reduces the impact of illicit drug use on perinatal outcomes. J Perinatol 2003;23(5): 354–60.

58. ACOG Committee on Health Care for Underserved Women. ACOG committee opinion no. 473. Substance abuse reporting and pregnancy: the role of the obstetrician-gynecologist. Obstet Gynecol 2011;117(1):200–1.

59. Zhang C, Brook JS, Leukefeld CG, et al. Associations between compulsive buying and substance dependence/abuse, major depressive episodes, and generalized anxiety disorder among men and women. J Addict Dis 2016; 35(4):298–304.

60. Benningfield MM, Arria AM, Kaltenbach K, et al. Co-occurring psychiatric symptoms are associated with increased psychological, social, and medical impairment in opioid dependent pregnant women. Am J Addict 2010;19(5):416–21.

61. Holbrook A, Kaltenbach K. Co-occurring psychiatric symptoms in opioid-dependent women: the prevalence of antenatal and postnatal depression. Am J Drug Alcohol Abuse 2012;38(6):575–9.

62. Torchalla I, Linden IA, Strehlau V, et al. "Like a lots happened in my whole childhood": violence, trauma and addiction in pregnant and postpartum women from Vancouver's Downtown Eastside. Harm Reduct J 2015;12:1.

63. Salihu HM, Wilson RE. Epidemiology of prenatal smoking and perinatal outcomes. Early Hum Dev 2007;83(11):713–20.

64. Chisolm MS, Fitzsimons H, Leoutsakos JM, et al. A comparison of cigarette smoking profiles in opioid-dependent pregnant patients receiving methadone or buprenorphine. Nicotine Tob Res 2013;15(7):1297–304.

65. Substance Abuse and Mental Health Services Administration (SAMHSA). Results from the 2012 National survey on drug use and health. Summary of national findings. NSDUH series H-46, HHS. Publication No. (SMA) 13-4795. Rockville (MD): SAMHSA; 2013.

66. Akerman SC, Brunette MF, Green AI, et al. Treating tobacco use disorder in pregnant women in medication-assisted treatment for an opioid use disorder: a systematic review. J Subst Abuse Treat 2015;52:40–7.

67. Winklbaur B, Baewert A, Jagsch R, et al. Association between prenatal tobacco exposure and outcomes of neonates born to opioid-maintained mothers. Implications for treatment. Eur Addict Res 2009;15(3):150–6.

68. Choo RE, Huestis MA, Schroeder JR, et al. Neonatal abstinence syndrome in methadone-exposed infants is altered by level of prenatal tobacco exposure. Drug Alcohol Depend 2004;75(3):253–60.

69. Jones HE, Heil SH, Tuten M, et al. Cigarette smoking in opioid-dependent pregnant women: neonatal and maternal outcomes. Drug Alcohol Depend 2013; 131(3):271–7.

70. Holbrook AM, Baxter JK, Jones HE, et al. Infections and obstetric outcomes in opioid-dependent pregnant women maintained on methadone or buprenorphine. Addiction 2012;107(S1):83–90.

71. Page K, Leeman L, Bishop S, et al. Hepatitis C cascade of care among pregnant women on opioid agonist pharmacotherapy attending a comprehensive prenatal program. Matern Child Health J 2017. https://doi.org/10.1007/s10995-017-2316-x.

72. Muller-Lissner S, Bassotti G, Coffin B, et al. Opioid-induced constipation and bowel dysfunction: a clinical guideline. Pain Med 2016. https://doi.org/10.1093/pm/pnw255.

73. Lind JN, Interrante JD, Ailes EC, et al. Maternal use of opioids during pregnancy and congenital malformations: a systematic review. Pediatrics 2017;139(6). https://doi.org/10.1542/peds.2016-4131.

74. Mactier H, Shipton D, Dryden C, et al. Reduced fetal growth in methadone-maintained pregnancies is not fully explained by smoking or socio-economic depravation. Addiction 2014;109(3):482–8.

75. Liu AJ, Sithamparanathan S, Jones MP, et al. Growth restriction in pregnancies of opioid-dependent mothers. Arch Dis Child Fetal Neonatal Ed 2010;95(4):F258–62.

76. Jansson LM, Velez M, McConnell K, et al. Maternal buprenorphine treatment and fetal neurobehavioral development. Am J Obstet Gynecol 2017;216(5):529.e1-8.

77. Jansson LM, Dipietro J, Elko A. Fetal response to maternal methadone administration. Am J Obstet Gynecol 2005;193(3 Pt 1):611–7.

78. Terplan M, Longinaker N, Appel L. Women-centered drug treatment services and need in the United States, 2002-2009. Am J Public Health 2015;105(11):e50–4.

79. Jones HE, Johnson RE, Milio L. Post-cesarean pain management of patients maintained on methadone or buprenorphine. Am J Addict 2006;15(3):528–9.

80. Pan A, Zakowski M. Peripartum anesthetic management of the opioid-tolerant of buprenorphine/suboxone-dependent patient. Clin Obstet Gynecol 2017;60(2):447–58.

81. Ramirez-Cacho WA, Flores S, Schrader RM, et al. Effect of chronic methadone therapy on intrapartum fetal heart rate patterns. J Soc Gynecol Investig 2006;13(2):108–11.

82. Meyer M, Wagner K, Benvenuto A, et al. Intrapartum and postpartum analgesia for women maintained on buprenorphine during pregnancy. Obstet Gynecol 2007;110(2Pt1):261–6.

83. Meyer M, Paranya G, Keefer Norris A, et al. Intrapartum and postpartum analgesia for women maintained on buprenorphine during pregnancy. Eur J Pain 2010;14(9):939–43.

84. Jones HE, Johnson RE, O'Grady KE, et al. Dosing adjustments in postpartum patients maintained on buprenorphine or methadone. J Addict Med 2008;2(2):103–7.

85. Alford DP, Compton P, Samet JH. Acute pain management for patients receiving maintenance methadone or buprenorphine therapy. Ann Intern Med 2006;144(2):127–34.

86. Jones HE, O'Grady K, Dahne J, et al. Management of acute postpartum pain in patients maintained on methadone or buprenorphine during pregnancy. Am J Drug Alcohol Abuse 2009;35(3):151–6.

87. Bagley SM, Wachman EM, Holland E, et al. Review of the assessment and management of neonatal abstinence syndrome. Addict Sci Clin Pract 2014;9(1):19.

88. O'Conner AB, Collett A, Alto WA, et al. Breastfeeding rates and the relationship between breastfeeding and neonatal abstinence syndrome in women being maintained on buprenorphine during pregnancy. J Midwifery Womens Health 2013;58(4):383–8.

89. American Academy of Pediatrics (AAP) Committee on Drugs. Transfer of drugs and other chemicals into human milk. Pediatrics 2001;108(3):776–89.

90. Kahn LS, Mendel WE, Fallin KL, et al. A parenting education program for women in treatment for opioid-use disorder at an outpatient medical practice. Soc Work Health Care 2017;56(7):649–65.

91. Terplan M, Hand DJ, Hutchinson M, et al. Contraceptive use and method choice among women with opioid and other substance use disorders: a systematic review. Prev Med 2015;80:23–31.

92. Matusiewicz AK, Melbostad HS, Heil SH. Knowledge of and concerns about long-acting reversible contraception among women in medication–assisted treatment for opioid use disorder. Contraception 2017. https://doi.org/10.1016/j.contraception.2017.07.167.

93. Bateman BT, Cole NM, Maeda A, et al. Patterns of opioid prescription and use after cesarean delivery. Obstet Gynecol 2017;130(1):29–35.

94. Osmundson SS, Schornack LA, Grasch JL, et al. Postdischarge opioid use after cesarean delivery. Obstet Gynecol 2017;130(1):36–41.

95. Prabhu M, McQuaid-Hanson E, Hopp S, et al. A shared decision-making intervention to guide opioid prescribing after cesarean delivery. Obstet Gynecol 2017;130(1):42–6.

96. Ko JY, Wolicki S, Barfield WD, et al. CDC grand rounds: public health strategies to prevent neonatal abstinence syndrome. MMWR Morb Mortal Wkly Rep 2017; 66(9):242–5.

97. Wisconsin Medical Examining Board Opioid Prescribing Guideline – November 16, 2016. 2016. State of Wisconsin Department of Safety and Professional Services. Available at: www.dsps.wi.gov/Documents/Board%20Services/Other%20Resources/MEB/20161116_MEB_Guidelines_v4.pdf. Accessed August 11, 2017.

98. Centers for Disease Control and Prevention (CDC). CDC guidelines for prescribing opioids for chronic pain – United States, 2016. Centers for Disease Control and Prevention. 2016. Available at: www.cdc.gov/mmwr/volumes/65/rr/rr6501e1.htm. Accessed September 8, 2017.

99. Kallen B, Reis M. Ongoing pharmacological management of chronic pain in pregnancy. Drugs 2016;76(9):915–24.

100. Pritham UA, McKay L. Safe management of chronic pain in the pregnancy in an era of opioid misuse and abuse. J Obstet Gynecol Neonatal Nurs 2014;43(5): 554–67.

Pregnancy in Women with Obesity

Cara D. Dolin, MD[a],*, Michelle A. Kominiarek, MD, MS[b]

KEYWORDS

- Pregnancy • Maternal obesity • Morbid obesity • Complications

KEY POINTS

- Obesity complicates almost all aspects of pregnancy.
- Antepartum management of women with obesity is complicated by limitations of screening tools, increased risks to the fetus, and underlying maternal medical comorbidities.
- Obesity increases risk of abnormal labor, cesarean delivery, and postpartum complications.
- Care of women with obesity should include an empathic and patient-centered approach.

INTRODUCTION

Pregnancy in women with obesity is an important public health problem with short- and long-term implications for maternal and child health. During pregnancy, weight status is assessed using a woman's prepregnancy body mass index (BMI) whereby a BMI greater than or equal to 30 kg/m^2 is considered obese. There is an increasing prevalence of obesity among women in the United States. Notably, 37% of reproductive-age women are obese and 10% have morbid obesity (BMI $\geq$40 kg/m^2).[1] There is a significant racial disparity in the prevalence of obesity. More than half of reproductive-age black women are obese compared with one-third of reproductive-age white women (**Fig. 1**).[1] Given the growing prevalence of obesity in women, obstetric providers need to understand the risks associated with obesity in pregnancy and the unique aspects of antepartum and intrapartum management for women with obesity.

The authors report no conflicts of interest.
There was no financial support of this study.
[a] Division of Maternal-Fetal Medicine, Department of Obstetrics and Gynecology, New York University Langone Health, 550 1st Avenue, New York, NY 10016, USA; [b] Division of Maternal-Fetal Medicine, Department of Obstetrics and Gynecology, Northwestern University, 250 East Superior Street Suite 05-2175, Chicago, IL 60611, USA
* Corresponding author.
E-mail address: Cara.Dolin@nyumc.org

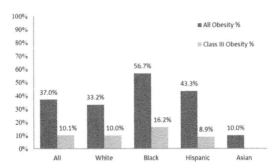

Fig. 1. Prevalence of obesity and class III obesity in women 20 to 39 years old in the United States by race, 2013 to 2014. Data not shown for class III obesity and Asian race because it only included two participants. (*Data from* Flegal KM, Kruszon-Moran D, Carroll MD, et al. Trends in obesity among adults in the United States, 2005 to 2014. JAMA 2016;315(21):2284–91.)

ANTEPARTUM MANAGEMENT OF PREGNANCY IN WOMEN WITH OBESITY
Counseling Women with Obesity

Ideally, women should achieve a normal weight before pregnancy to optimize maternal and neonatal outcomes.[2] Pregnancy is not a time for medical or surgical weight loss because of the potential negative consequences on the developing fetus. Women with obesity before pregnancy should be offered interventions aimed at assisting in long-term weight loss, as recommended by the US Preventative Task Force.[3] However, currently there is little evidence on the effectiveness of preconception interventions for women with obesity.[4]

During pregnancy, counseling on nutrition, exercise, and weight gain should occur at each prenatal visit.[5] In counseling women with obesity, it is important not to stigmatize obesity and instead treat it as a medical condition.[6] Be aware of any personal bias, such as thinking of these women as "lazy" or "noncompliant," which may influence the care provided to women with obesity.[7] Women should never feel judged, because this can harm the physician-patient relationship.[6] Motivational interviewing is a counseling style that has been shown to have an impact on behavior modification, including diet and physical activity.[8] Through reflective listening, providers impart empathy while personalizing feedback and promoting self-efficacy and self-motivation within the woman.[9]

Social factors that contribute to unhealthy lifestyle choices for pregnant women with obesity should be considered when counseling women. Low socioeconomic status is a risk factor for obesity, particularly in women.[10] Women with low socioeconomic status may be unable to access or afford healthy food. Furthermore, the neighborhood and environment may limit the ability to engage in regular physical activity,[5] which has been shown to decrease the risk of pregnancy complications, including gestational diabetes and excess gestational weight gain (GWG).[11–13] If a woman with obesity is otherwise healthy and without any contraindications to exercise, it is recommended that she spend at least 150 minutes per week engaging in low- to moderate-intensity physical activity.[11]

Gestational Weight Gain

Prepregnancy BMI should be calculated at the initial prenatal visit for all women using reported prepregnancy weight or measured first trimester weight. Currently, GWG recommendations are based on the 2009 Institute of Medicine (IOM) guidelines

(**Table 1**).[14] These recommendations are limited in that there is a single recommendation for all women with BMI greater than or equal to 30 kg/m^2. Among women with obesity, 57% have excessive GWG, whereas 13% have inadequate GWG and 6% lose weight during pregnancy.[15]

Studies published after the release of the IOM guidelines have demonstrated improved maternal outcomes in women with obesity who gain less than the recommended GWG.[15,16] However, there are also data that low GWG and even weight loss during pregnancy may be associated with small-for-gestational-age infants.[15,16] Until further evidence is available all women with obesity should be counseled to gain between 11 and 20 pounds during pregnancy according to the IOM guidelines.

Ultrasound Limitations

Antenatal ultrasound in the obese population is challenging. Abdominal adiposity limits visualization because of the increased depth of insonation required and increased absorption of ultrasound energy by surrounding tissue.[17] Techniques to improve visualization include reducing the transducer frequency for better penetration, use of ultrasound settings that increase the signal-to-background noise ratio, and approaching the fetus during transabdominal ultrasound from areas with less adipose tissue (**Box 1**).[17] Importantly, the impaired visualization of the fetus in women with obesity is associated with up to a 30% lower detection rate of fetal anomalies.[18,19] An early second-trimester anatomy ultrasound and use of transvaginal ultrasound has been found to increase the rate of complete anatomy scans in women with obesity, especially women with morbid obesity.[17,20,21]

Genetic Screening and Testing

Accuracy of genetic screening is influenced by maternal obesity. Failure to visualize the nasal bone and obtain a nuchal translucency measurement increases with increasing maternal BMI.[22,23] The interpretation of traditional serum screening tests, such as the quadruple marker test, is affected by obesity.[24,25] Maternal weight is reported with serum samples; however, most laboratories use a standard weight correction to a maximum weight of approximately 270 lbs. This correction standard is used for all women who weigh more than the cutoff, increasing the risk of false-positive screening results in women with morbid obesity.[26]

Noninvasive prenatal testing (NIPT) through maternal serum cell-free DNA testing is also affected by obesity. Fetal fraction decreases with increasing maternal weight.[27] Furthermore, the proportion of women with NIPT failure (fetal fraction <4%) significantly increases with increased maternal weight. At a maternal weight of 160 kg,

Table 1
Recommended gestational weight gain by prepregnancy weight category

Prepregnancy Weight Category	BMI	Recommended GWG
Underweight	<18.5	28–40 lb (12.5–18 kg)
Normal weight	18.5–24.9	25–35 lb (11.5–16 kg)
Overweight	25–29.9	15–25 lb (7–11.5 kg)
Obese	≥30	11–20 lb (5–9 kg)

Modified from Institute of Medicine (US) and National Research Council (US) Committee to Reexamine IOM Pregnancy Weight Guidelines, Rasmussen KM, Yaktine AL, editors. Weight gain during pregnancy: reexamining the guidelines. Washington, DC: National Academies Press (US); 2009; with permission.

Box 1
Techniques to improve obstetric ultrasound visualization in women with obesity

Ultrasound settings
  Reduce frequency
  Speckle reduction filter
  Harmonic imaging
  Compound imaging

Approach fetus during transabdominal ultrasound from areas with less adipose tissue
  Suprapubic
  Periumbilical
  Right or left iliac fossae

Consider early anatomy ultrasound (13–16 weeks)

Use color Doppler for cardiac assessment

Consider transvaginal ultrasound for central nervous system assessment if fetus cephalic

Adapted from Paladini D. Sonography in obese and overweight pregnant women: clinical, medicolegal and technical issues. Ultrasound Obstet Gynecol 2009;33(6):726; with permission.

---

more than half of women have NIPT failure (**Table 2**).[27] The cause of a high NIPT failure rate in women with obesity is unknown. It may be secondary to a dilutional effect of obesity or increased adipocyte death contributing to higher levels of maternal cell-free DNA in the circulation.[27,28] Given that a low fetal fraction is also associated with fetal aneuploidy, counseling obese women with NIPT failure is challenging and the limitations of the screening test should be discussed.

Invasive diagnostic procedures are more technically challenging in women with obesity. Because of excess adipose tissue, visualization of the needle may be limited and the longer distance from entry to the uterus increases the need for multiple attempts.[29] However, in a large retrospective study of more than 15,000 women, 25% of whom had obesity, there was no difference in the risk of fetal loss before 24 weeks after amniocentesis or chorionic villus sampling in women with obesity compared with those without obesity.[29] However, there was a significantly higher risk for fetal loss after amniocentesis for those with a BMI greater than or equal to 40 kg/m^2 when compared with women with a BMI less than 25 kg/m^2 (adjusted odds ratio [aOR], 2.2; 95% confidence interval [CI], 1.2–3.9).[29]

Fetal Anomalies

The association between obesity and congenital anomalies has been shown in numerous studies.[30–32] An analysis of a cohort from Sweden including 1.2 million

---

Table 2
Estimated median fetal fraction in maternal plasma cell-free DNA and proportion of women with low fetal fraction by maternal weight

Maternal Weight, kg	Median Fetal Fraction, %	Proportion Low Fetal Fraction, % (<4%)
60	11.7	0.7
100	8.1	7.1
160	3.9	51.1

Modified from Ashoor G, Syngelaki A, Poon LC, et al. Fetal fraction in maternal plasma cell-free DNA at 11-13 weeks' gestation: relation to maternal and fetal characteristics. Ultrasound Obstet Gynecol 2013;41(1):30; with permission.

singletons found a progressive increase in the risk of congenital anomalies with increasing BMI (adjusted relative risk [aRR], 1.37; 95% CI, 1.26–1.49; with BMI ≥40 kg/m²).[31] Risk of fetal cardiac, central nervous system, and limb anomalies increased with increasing BMI. The largest risk was seen in central nervous system anomalies (aRR, 1.88; 95% CI, 1.20–2.94; with BMI ≥40 kg/m²).[31] In a meta-analysis, maternal obesity was associated with an increased risk of a range of fetal anomalies, including neural tube defects, cardiac anomalies, cleft lip and palate, ano-rectal atresia, hydrocephaly, and limb reduction anomalies **(Table 3)**.[30]

The exact cause of fetal anomalies in women with obesity is unknown. Metabolic abnormalities, including elevated levels of insulin, triglycerides, uric acid, and estrogen, or chronic hypoxia and hypercapnia, may have a teratogenic effect on the fetus.[17] Nutritional deficiency, as a result of poor diet, prior bariatric surgery, or inadequate doses of supplementation, may contribute to anomalies.[17]

Spontaneous Abortion

Women with obesity have higher odds of spontaneous abortion than women with a normal weight (odds ratio [OR], 1.2; 95% CI, 1.01–1.46).[33] Additionally, the risk of recurrent early pregnancy loss is significantly higher in women with obesity (OR, 3.5; 95% CI, 1.02–12.01).[33,34] The cause of spontaneous abortion in women with obesity is not fully understood. Obesity has known adverse effects on the oocyte; however, women with obesity continue to experience higher odds of pregnancy loss even with oocyte donation.[35,36] Obesity impairs endometrial decidualization and receptivity, potentially leading to higher rates of spontaneous abortion.[36]

Medical Complications

Pre-existing medical problems, including cardiovascular disease, diabetes, arthritis, sleep disorders, and liver and gallbladder disease, are more common in women with obesity.[5] Ideally, management of these conditions should be optimized before conception, including discontinuing potentially teratogenic medications.[37] Management of nonobstetric medical conditions during pregnancy should include a multidisciplinary approach.

Obstructive sleep apnea in pregnancy has been associated with adverse maternal and neonatal outcomes. Up to 15% of reproductive-age women have obstructive sleep apnea; however, most are undiagnosed. Because obesity is an important risk factor for obstructive sleep apnea, pregnant women with obesity should be asked about a history of snoring and excessive daytime sleepiness and referred to a sleep specialist for further evaluation as needed[38] (See Jennifer E. Dominguez and

Table 3		
Odds ratio of congenital anomalies in women with obesity		
Congenital Anomaly	OR	95% CI
Neural tube defects	1.87	1.62–2.15
Cardiovascular defects	1.30	1.12–1.51
Cleft lip and palate	1.20	1.03–1.40
Anorectal atresia	1.48	1.12–1.97
Hydrocephaly	1.68	1.19–2.36
Limb reduction anomalies	1.34	1.03–1.73

Data from Stothard KJ, Tennant PW, Bell R, et al. Maternal overweight and obesity and the risk of congenital anomalies: a systematic review and meta-analysis. JAMA 2009;301(6):636–50.

colleagues' article, "Management of Obstructive Sleep Apnea in Pregnancy," in this issue).

Given the increased risk of undiagnosed pregestational diabetes, all women with obesity should be screened for diabetes at their initial prenatal visit[39] (See Ronan Sugrue and Chloe Zera's article, "Pregestational Diabetes in Pregnancy," in this issue). Even if early screening is negative, second-trimester screening for gestational diabetes mellitus should still be performed[39] (See Jeffrey M. Denney and Kristen H. Quinn's article, "Gestational Diabetes: Underpinning Principles, Surveillance and Management," in this issue). Not only are women with obesity more likely to have chronic hypertension, they have a higher risk of developing hypertensive disorders of pregnancy. The risk of preeclampsia in women with obesity is almost three-fold higher than women with normal BMI (aOR, 2.9; 95% CI, 1.6–5.3).[40] The US Preventive Services Task Force recommends low-dose aspirin during pregnancy for women at risk of preeclampsia. Obesity is considered a moderate risk factor and aspirin to prevent preeclampsia should be considered in the setting of other moderate risk factors, such as nulliparity, advanced maternal age, low socioeconomic status, and family or personal history[41] (See Amelia L.M. Sutton and colleagues' article, "Hypertensive Disorders in Pregnancy," in this issue).

Stillbirth

Obesity is an important risk factor for stillbirth.[42–45] The risk of stillbirth increases with increasing BMI (**Table 4**).[42,46] There are many theories as to why maternal obesity puts fetuses at risk of intrauterine demise including medical comorbidities and fetal anomalies. Underlying metabolic disorders, lipid metabolism, inflammation, and vascular dysfunction have all been proposed as potential mechanisms.[46] Although there is a higher risk of stillbirth in women with obesity, there is no evidence to support routine antepartum surveillance.[47]

Fetal Growth

Obesity is an independent risk factor for large-for-gestational age, even after controlling for diabetes (aOR, 1.5; 95% CI, 1.4–1.9).[48] This risk increases with increasing BMI. In a meta-analysis, women with class III obesity were found to have a significantly higher risk of large-for-gestational age as compared with those with class I or II obesity.[49] Women with obesity are also at risk of intrauterine growth restriction, because conditions that predispose to growth restriction, such as hypertensive disorders and history of prior bariatric surgery, are seen more commonly in these women. Given the limitations of fundal height

Table 4		
Adjusted hazard ratio of stillbirth by obesity class compared with normal BMI		
Obesity Class (BMI)	**Adjusted HR**	**95% CI**
Overweight (25–29.9)	1.36	1.29–1.43
Class I obesity (30–34.9)	1.71	1.62–1.83
Class II obesity (35–39.9)	2.04	1.89–2.21
Class III obesity (40–40.9)	2.50	2.28–2.74
Superobesity (≥50)	3.11	2.54–3.81

Abbreviation: HR, hazard ratio.

Modified from Yao R, Ananth CV, Park BY, et al. Obesity and the risk of stillbirth: a population-based cohort study. Am J Obstet Gynecol 2014;210(5):457.e6; with permission.

measurement in women with obesity, fetal growth assessment should be performed by ultrasound.[50]

Prior Bariatric Surgery

Bariatric surgery is a proven method for weight loss that is increasingly being used. Importantly for the obstetrician, 80% of bariatric procedures are performed on women, many of whom are reproductive age, and weight loss after bariatric surgery has been shown to increase fertility.[51,52] Weight loss is achieved through caloric restriction and malabsorption, and neurohormonal changes that influence metabolism and hunger.[53]

The ideal timing of pregnancy after bariatric surgery to optimize maternal and neonatal outcomes is unknown. Most weight loss occurs during the first 12 months after surgery.[54] Some experts advise to delay pregnancy for 12 to 24 months after surgery.[52] The rate of gestational diabetes is significantly lower in women after bariatric surgery compared with women with obesity who have not undergone bariatric surgery (OR, 0.25; 95% CI, 0.13–0.47).[55] Bariatric surgery has been associated with neonatal outcomes, including a decreased risk for large-for-gestational-age infants, an increased risk for small-for-gestational-age infants, neonatal intensive care unit admissions, and preterm births (**Table 5**).[55,56] Fetal growth should be monitored by serial ultrasound assessment in women who become pregnant within 12 months of bariatric surgery.[52]

Women are at risk of malnutrition after bariatric surgery. Evaluation for micronutrient deficiencies should take place during the initial prenatal evaluation and be re-evaluated each trimester.[52] In addition to a standard prenatal vitamin, women with a history of bariatric surgery should receive additional supplementation as needed based on their laboratory testing results. There are no specific recommendations for GWG in these women; as such the IOM guidelines for GWG are appropriate.[14] When evaluating women with a history of prior bariatric surgery who present during pregnancy with abdominal pain, nausea, or vomiting, it is important to consider bariatric surgical complications. Women with prior bariatric surgery have an increased risk of abdominal surgery for nonobstetric indications during pregnancy (OR, 11.3; 95% CI, 6.9–18.5).[57]

INTRAPARTUM MANAGEMENT OF PREGNANCY IN WOMEN WITH OBESITY
Resource and Equipment Considerations

Caring for women with obesity during pregnancy requires additional resources. Appropriate equipment must be available, including large speculums, long

Table 5		
Adjusted relative risk of obstetric and neonatal outcomes in pregnancies after bariatric surgery		
Outcome	**aRR**	**95% CI**
Preterm birth	1.57	1.33–1.85
NICU admission	1.25	1.08–1.44
SGA	1.93	1.65–2.26
LGA	0.53	0.44–0.65
Cesarean delivery	1.21	1.12–1.31

Abbreviations: LGA, large-for-gestational age; NICU, neonatal intensive care unit; SGA, small-for-gestational age.

Data from Parent B, Martopullo I, Weiss NS, et al. Bariatric surgery in women of childbearing age, timing between an operation and birth, and associated perinatal complications. JAMA Surg 2017;152(2):1–8.

instruments, and wide examination and operating room tables that can accommodate higher weights (**Box 2**).[6] Providers should be familiar with the equipment at their institution. Most standard operating tables can accommodate up to 500 lbs. Bariatric tables can typically accommodate 600 to 1000 lbs. All staff should take care when transferring a woman with obesity. A slide board or air mattress should be used and additional personnel available to ensure the safety of the medical staff and the woman.

It is important to ensure the appropriate-sized arm cuff is used to measure blood pressure in women with obesity. If a correctly fitting upper arm cuff is not available, blood pressure should be taken using an arm cuff on the wrist held at the level of the patient's heart. A wrist blood pressure has a higher sensitivity and specificity (92% sensitivity, 92% specificity) than using the wrong size cuff on the upper arm (73% sensitivity, 76% specificity) or taking the measurement on the forearm (84% sensitivity, 75% specificity).[58]

Labor Abnormalities

Women with obesity have lower rates of spontaneous labor and higher rates of post-term pregnancies compared with women with normal weight.[45,59,60] A large study of 11,752 women found that at each week of gestation after 37 weeks, women with obesity are significantly less likely to go into spontaneous labor.[59] The odds of presenting in spontaneous labor decreases as BMI increases.[45,59] Obesity is associated with pregnancy progressing past 40 weeks (aOR, 1.63; 95% CI, 1.39–1.92), 41 weeks (aOR, 1.81; 95% CI, 1.50–2.18), and 42 weeks (aOR, 1.69; 95% CI, 1.23–2.31).[60] The reason for prolonged pregnancies in women with obesity in unknown but may involve metabolic and endocrine dysfunction affecting initiation of labor.[45,60,61] Women with obesity have higher concentrations of estrogen in adipose tissue, which may disrupt hormonal balance and mechanisms that regulate labor.[61]

Women with obesity are more likely to undergo an induction of labor compared with normal-weight women.[62] The odds of induction failure are higher (aOR, 2.16; 95% CI, 2.07–2.27) for women with obesity compared with normal-weight women. The rate of induction failure increases with increasing BMI. In a large, retrospective study of 80,887 women undergoing induction of labor, 13% of women with normal weight had a failed induction, whereas the rate was more than twice that (29%) for women with a BMI greater than or equal to 40 kg/m^2.[62] It is not completely understood how maternal obesity leads to abnormal labor and risk for arrest disorders. One theory is that myometrial contractility is somehow impaired in these women.[63,64]

Box 2
Equipment to care for women with obesity during pregnancy

Large blood pressure cuffs or normal-size cuff on wrist

Large speculum

Wide examination table or table extenders

Large labor beds that can accommodate weight

Long instruments

Bariatric operating table

Self-retaining retractor

Panniculus retractor

Slide board or air mattress for transfer

Cesarean Delivery

Increasing maternal weight is associated with an increasing risk of cesarean delivery. For each additional 1 kg/m^2 in BMI the risk of cesarean delivery increases by 4%.[65] The cesarean delivery rate in women with BMI greater than or equal to 50 kg/m^2 is almost 50% and one in three of these procedures are accompanied by wound complications.[66,67] Obesity is a risk factor for failed trial of labor after cesarean delivery in women with obesity (OR, 1.99; 95% CI, 1.20–3.30) and morbid obesity (OR, 2.22; 95% CI, 1.11–4.44).[68] In a large study of 13,529 women, the rate of successful vaginal birth after cesarean delivery was 68.4% in women with obesity compared with 79.6% in women without obesity.[69]

Labor and Delivery Anesthesia

Physiologic changes in women with obesity put them at higher risk of complications related to anesthesia during labor and delivery. In the supine position, the increased weight of the chest wall leads to decreased expiratory reserve volume, residual volume, and functional residual capacity.[70] These physiologic changes combined with the increased oxygen demand associated with obesity puts the pregnant woman with obesity at higher risk of hypoxemia.[70] The body habitus of women with obesity has been shown to change the epidural space, decreasing the epidural space volume while increasing the epidural space pressure.[71] This can lead to larger cephalad spread of medications administered during regional anesthesia.[71] Women with morbid obesity have been found to have higher rates of hypotension and fetal heart rate decelerations after epidural placement compared with normal-weight women.[72]

The rate of labor epidural failure is 17% in women with morbid obesity compared with only 3% in matched control subjects.[73] It is recommended that an epidural catheter be placed in early labor in women with obesity given their increased risk of failed epidural anesthesia.[47] Confirmation of a working epidural early in pregnancy is thought to decrease time to delivery and need for general anesthesia in event of an emergency cesarean delivery.[70] General anesthesia poses additional risks in the pregnant woman with obesity. At baseline, the anatomic changes in pregnancy make intubation challenging. In the woman with obesity, increased adipose tissue in the back and neck increase the risk of failed intubation, which has deadly consequences.[70] Antenatal anesthesiology consultation may be considered, particularly for women with BMI greater than or equal to 50 kg/m^2.[74]

Prevention of Venous Thromboembolism

Venous thromboembolism is an important cause of maternal mortality.[75] Pregnant women with obesity are at even higher risk for venous thromboembolism (aOR, 5.3; 95% CI, 2.1–13.5) and specifically pulmonary embolism (aOR, 14.9; 95% CI, 3.0–74.8) than pregnant women without obesity.[76] Although it is recommended that mechanical thromboprophylaxis be used during antepartum admissions and cesarean delivery, strong consideration should be given to pharmacologic thromboprophlaxis, especially in women with a BMI greater than or equal to 40 kg/m^2.[75] Weight-based dosing regimens as opposed to standard doses (eg, 40 mg daily) are preferable. A study of anti-Xa levels in postpartum women receiving weight-based dosing of enoxaparin compared with those receiving standard dosing found a significantly higher percentage of patients with prophylactic range anti-Xa levels in the weight-based group (86% vs 26%; $P<.001$).[77]

Prevention of Wound Complications

Obesity is an independent risk factor for surgical site infection after cesarean delivery (OR, 2.0; 95% CI, 1.6–2.5) and this risk increases with increasing BMI (BMI >35 kg/m^2; OR, 3.7; 95% CI, 2.6–5.2).[78,79] Women with obesity undergoing cesarean delivery should receive antibiotic prophylaxis with 2 g of cefazolin.[47] Although it has been suggested that women with obesity may potentially benefit from a higher dose, randomized controlled trials have demonstrated sufficient concentrations of cefazolin in maternal tissue at the 2-g dose.[80,81]

In women with greater than 2 cm of subcutaneous tissue, this tissue should be approximated to decrease risk of wound disruption (RR, 0.66; 95% CI, 0.48–0.91).[82] However, there is evidence that subcutaneous drains may increase wound complications and should not be used.[83,84] The incision should be closed with suture and not staples. In a meta-analysis, the risk of wound complications in women with obesity was almost halved when the incision was closed with sutures rather than staples (RR, 0.51; 95% CI, 0.34–0.75).[85] One randomized trial found no benefit to placing a wound vacuum after cesarean delivery in women with obesity.[86]

POSTPARTUM MANAGEMENT OF WOMEN WITH OBESITY
Breastfeeding

Women with obesity have less intentions to breastfeed, lower rates of breastfeeding initiation, and shortened duration of exclusive and any breastfeeding.[87] A large study that examined breastfeeding status at the time of postpartum discharge in more than 12,000 women found the rate of breastfeeding was inversely correlated with increasing BMI (**Fig. 2**).[88] Breastfeeding is challenging for women with obesity for several reasons. Physiologically, there is a delay in lactogenesis II, potentially because of abnormal levels of leptin and insulin.[89] Additionally, women with obesity are more likely to have complicated labors, cesarean deliveries, and be separated from the infant postpartum, all of which contribute to decreased rate of breastfeeding initiation. The size of the breast can make latching and positioning more difficult.[89] Counseling about breastfeeding should begin prenatally and additional support provided postpartum (**Box 3**).

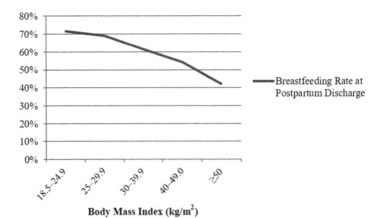

Fig. 2. Rate of breastfeeding at postpartum discharge by body mass index. (*Data from* Ramji N, Challa S, Murphy PA, et al. A comparison of breastfeeding rates by obesity class. J Matern Fetal Neonatal Med 2017:1–6. [Epub ahead of print].)

Box 3
Breastfeeding support for women with obesity

Reassurance and guidance on how to know infant is receiving enough milk

Demonstration of feeding positions
  Side-lying
  Cradle/cross-cradle hold
  Clutch/football/underarm hold

Assistance to support large breasts
  Rolled towel or breast sling to elevate breast

Assistance to better visualize latch

Demonstration of reverse pressure softening around areola to enable deeper latch

Guidance to supplement when necessary

Continued postpartum support
  Telephone support
  Breastfeeding support group
  Skilled in-person care

Adapted from Bever Babendure J, Reifsnider E, Mendias E, et al. Reduced breastfeeding rates among obese mothers: a review of contributing factors, clinical considerations and future directions. Int Breastfeed J 2015;10:21; with permission.

Contraception

Obesity should be considered when counseling about contraception choices. Postpartum tubal ligation is more technically challenging and associated with greater operative morbidity in women with obesity. Because of the changes in metabolism associated with obesity, there is concern that hormonal contraceptives may not have the same effectiveness in women with obesity; however, most studies have not shown an increased risk of pregnancy.[90] One exception is the transdermal contraceptive patch; its use should be limited to those weighing less than or equal to 90 kg.[91] Obesity is a risk factor for endometrial cancer. The levonorgestrel intrauterine device provides endometrial protection in addition to reliable contraception.[92] Because of the malabsorption associated with bariatric surgery, women should not use oral contraception after malabsorptive bariatric procedures.[52]

SUMMARY

Obesity complicates almost all aspects of pregnancy. As the proportion of women with obesity continues to rise, obstetric providers must consider the impact of obesity throughout pregnancy. Empathic and patient-centered care, along with knowledge of the complexity of a pregnancy complicated by obesity, can optimize outcomes for women and children.

REFERENCES

1. Flegal KM, Kruszon-Moran D, Carroll MD, et al. Trends in obesity among adults in the United States, 2005 to 2014. JAMA 2016;315(21):2284–91.
2. ACOG committee opinion no. 549: obesity in pregnancy. Obstet Gynecol 2013; 121(1):213–7.
3. Moyer VA. Screening for and management of obesity in adults: U.S. Preventive Services Task Force recommendation statement. Ann Intern Med 2012;157(5):373–8.

4. Opray N, Grivell RM, Deussen AR, et al. Directed preconception health programs and interventions for improving pregnancy outcomes for women who are overweight or obese. Cochrane Database Syst Rev 2015;(7):CD010932.

5. Committee opinion no. 591: challenges for overweight and obese women. Obstet Gynecol 2014;123(3):726–30.

6. ACOG committee opinion no. 600: ethical issues in the care of the obese woman. Obstet Gynecol 2014;123(6):1388–93.

7. Hebl MR, Xu J. Weighing the care: physicians' reactions to the size of a patient. Int J Obes Relat Metab Disord 2001;25(8):1246–52.

8. Rubak S, Sandbaek A, Lauritzen T, et al. Motivational interviewing: a systematic review and meta-analysis. Br J Gen Pract 2005;55(513):305–12.

9. ACOG committee opinion no. 423: motivational interviewing: a tool for behavioral change. Obstet Gynecol 2009;113(1):243–6.

10. Harvey JR, Ogden DE. Obesity treatment in disadvantaged population groups: where do we stand and what can we do? Prev Med 2014;68:71–5.

11. ACOG committee opinion no. 650: physical activity and exercise during pregnancy and the postpartum period. Obstet Gynecol 2015;126(6):e135–42.

12. Magro-Malosso ER, Saccone G, Di Mascio D, et al. Exercise during pregnancy and risk of preterm birth in overweight and obese women: a systematic review and meta-analysis of randomized controlled trials. Acta Obstet Gynecol Scand 2017;96(3):263–73.

13. Wang C, Wei Y, Zhang X, et al. A randomized clinical trial of exercise during pregnancy to prevent gestational diabetes mellitus and improve pregnancy outcome in overweight and obese pregnant women. Am J Obstet Gynecol 2017;216(4): 340–51.

14. Institute of Medicine, National Research Council Committee to Reexamine Institute of Medicine Pregnancy Weight Guidelines. The national academies collection: reports funded by National Institutes of Health. In: Rasmussen KM, Yaktine AL, editors. Weight gain during pregnancy: reexamining the guidelines. Washington, DC: National Academies Press (US) National Academy of Sciences; 2009.

15. Goldstein RF, Abell SK, Ranasinha S, et al. Association of gestational weight gain with maternal and infant outcomes: a systematic review and meta-analysis. JAMA 2017;317(21):2207–25.

16. Kominiarek MA, Peaceman AM. Gestational weight gain. Am J Obstet Gynecol 2017;217(6):642–51.

17. Paladini D. Sonography in obese and overweight pregnant women: clinical, medicolegal and technical issues. Ultrasound Obstet Gynecol 2009;33(6):720–9.

18. Dashe JS, McIntire DD, Twickler DM. Effect of maternal obesity on the ultrasound detection of anomalous fetuses. Obstet Gynecol 2009;113(5):1001–7.

19. Aagaard-Tillery KM, Flint Porter T, Malone FD, et al. Influence of maternal BMI on genetic sonography in the FaSTER trial. Prenat Diagn 2010;30(1):14–22.

20. Gupta S, Timor-Tritsch IE, Oh C, et al. Early second-trimester sonography to improve the fetal anatomic survey in obese patients. J Ultrasound Med 2014; 33(9):1579–83.

21. Romary L, Sinkovskaya E, Ali S, et al. The role of early gestation ultrasound in the assessment of fetal anatomy in maternal obesity. J Ultrasound Med 2017;36(6): 1161–8.

22. Thornburg LL, Mulconry M, Post A, et al. Fetal nuchal translucency thickness evaluation in the overweight and obese gravida. Ultrasound Obstet Gynecol 2009;33(6):665–9.

23. Gandhi M, Fox NS, Russo-Stieglitz K, et al. Effect of increased body mass index on first-trimester ultrasound examination for aneuploidy risk assessment. Obstet Gynecol 2009;114(4):856–9.

24. Neveux LM, Palomaki GE, Larrivee DA, et al. Refinements in managing maternal weight adjustment for interpreting prenatal screening results. Prenat Diagn 1996; 16(12):1115–9.

25. Spencer K, Bindra R, Nicolaides KH. Maternal weight correction of maternal serum PAPP-A and free beta-hCG MoM when screening for trisomy 21 in the first trimester of pregnancy. Prenat Diagn 2003;23(10):851–5.

26. Rose NC. Genetic screening and the obese gravida. Clin Obstet Gynecol 2016; 59(1):140–7.

27. Ashoor G, Syngelaki A, Poon LC, et al. Fetal fraction in maternal plasma cell-free DNA at 11-13 weeks' gestation: relation to maternal and fetal characteristics. Ultrasound Obstet Gynecol 2013;41(1):26–32.

28. Haghiac M, Vora NL, Basu S, et al. Increased death of adipose cells, a path to release cell-free DNA into systemic circulation of obese women. Obesity (Silver Spring) 2012;20(11):2213–9.

29. Harper LM, Cahill AG, Smith K, et al. Effect of maternal obesity on the risk of fetal loss after amniocentesis and chorionic villus sampling. Obstet Gynecol 2012; 119(4):745–51.

30. Stothard KJ, Tennant PW, Bell R, et al. Maternal overweight and obesity and the risk of congenital anomalies: a systematic review and meta-analysis. JAMA 2009; 301(6):636–50.

31. Persson M, Cnattingius S, Villamor E, et al. Risk of major congenital malformations in relation to maternal overweight and obesity severity: cohort study of 1.2 million singletons. BMJ 2017;357:j2563.

32. Huang HY, Chen HL, Feng LP. Maternal obesity and the risk of neural tube defects in offspring: a meta-analysis. Obes Res Clin Pract 2017;11(2):188–97.

33. Lashen H, Fear K, Sturdee DW. Obesity is associated with increased risk of first trimester and recurrent miscarriage: matched case-control study. Hum Reprod 2004;19(7):1644–6.

34. Boots C, Stephenson MD. Does obesity increase the risk of miscarriage in spontaneous conception: a systematic review. Semin Reprod Med 2011;29(6):507–13.

35. Metwally M, Ong KJ, Ledger WL, et al. Does high body mass index increase the risk of miscarriage after spontaneous and assisted conception? A meta-analysis of the evidence. Fertil Steril 2008;90(3):714–26.

36. Broughton DE, Moley KH. Obesity and female infertility: potential mediators of obesity's impact. Fertil Steril 2017;107(4):840–7.

37. ACOG committee opinion number 313, September 2005. The importance of preconception care in the continuum of women's health care. Obstet Gynecol 2005; 106(3):665–6.

38. Cain MA, Louis JM. Sleep disordered breathing and adverse pregnancy outcomes. Clin Lab Med 2016;36(2):435–46.

39. Practice bulletin no. 180: gestational diabetes mellitus. Obstet Gynecol 2017; 130(1):e17–37.

40. Bodnar LM, Ness RB, Markovic N, et al. The risk of preeclampsia rises with increasing prepregnancy body mass index. Ann Epidemiol 2005;15(7):475–82.

41. LeFevre ML. Low-dose aspirin use for the prevention of morbidity and mortality from preeclampsia: U.S. Preventive Services Task Force recommendation statement. Ann Intern Med 2014;161(11):819–26.

42. Yao R, Ananth CV, Park BY, et al. Obesity and the risk of stillbirth: a population-based cohort study. Am J Obstet Gynecol 2014;210(5):457.e1-9.
43. Fretts RC. Etiology and prevention of stillbirth. Am J Obstet Gynecol 2005;193(6): 1923–35.
44. Nohr EA, Bech BH, Davies MJ, et al. Prepregnancy obesity and fetal death: a study within the Danish National Birth Cohort. Obstet Gynecol 2005;106(2): 250–9.
45. Denison FC, Price J, Graham C, et al. Maternal obesity, length of gestation, risk of postdates pregnancy and spontaneous onset of labour at term. BJOG 2008; 115(6):720–5.
46. Aune D, Saugstad OD, Henriksen T, et al. Maternal body mass index and the risk of fetal death, stillbirth, and infant death: a systematic review and meta-analysis. JAMA 2014;311(15):1536–46.
47. ACOG practice bulletin no 156: obesity in pregnancy. Obstet Gynecol 2015; 126(6):e112–26.
48. Ehrenberg HM, Mercer BM, Catalano PM. The influence of obesity and diabetes on the prevalence of macrosomia. Am J Obstet Gynecol 2004;191(3):964–8.
49. Lutsiv O, Mah J, Beyene J, et al. The effects of morbid obesity on maternal and neonatal health outcomes: a systematic review and meta-analyses. Obes Rev 2015;16(7):531–46.
50. ACOG practice bulletin no. 134: fetal growth restriction. Obstet Gynecol 2013; 121(5):1122–33.
51. Kominiarek MA, Jungheim ES, Hoeger KM, et al. American Society for Metabolic and Bariatric Surgery position statement on the impact of obesity and obesity treatment on fertility and fertility therapy Endorsed by the American College of Obstetricians and Gynecologists and the Obesity Society. Surg Obes Relat Dis 2017;13(5):750–7.
52. ACOG practice bulletin no. 105: bariatric surgery and pregnancy. Obstet Gynecol 2009;113(6):1405–13.
53. Korner J, Bessler M, Cirilo LJ, et al. Effects of Roux-en-Y gastric bypass surgery on fasting and postprandial concentrations of plasma ghrelin, peptide YY, and insulin. J Clin Endocrinol Metab 2005;90(1):359–65.
54. Sjostrom L, Narbro K, Sjostrom CD, et al. Effects of bariatric surgery on mortality in Swedish obese subjects. N Engl J Med 2007;357(8):741–52.
55. Johansson K, Cnattingius S, Naslund I, et al. Outcomes of pregnancy after bariatric surgery. N Engl J Med 2015;372(9):814–24.
56. Parent B, Martopullo I, Weiss NS, et al. Bariatric surgery in women of childbearing age, timing between an operation and birth, and associated perinatal complications. JAMA Surg 2017;152(2):1–8.
57. Stuart A, Kallen K. Risk of abdominal surgery in pregnancy among women who have undergone bariatric surgery. Obstet Gynecol 2017;129(5):887–95.
58. Irving G, Holden J, Stevens R. Which cuff should I use? Indirect blood pressure measurement for the diagnosis of hypertension in patients with obesity: a diagnostic accuracy review. BMJ Open 2016;6(11):e012429.
59. Frolova AI, Wang JJ, Conner SN, et al. Spontaneous labor onset and outcomes in obese women at term. Am J Perinatol 2018;35(1):59–64.
60. Stotland NE, Washington AE, Caughey AB. Prepregnancy body mass index and the length of gestation at term. Am J Obstet Gynecol 2007;197(4):378.e1-5.
61. Smith R, Mesiano S, McGrath S. Hormone trajectories leading to human birth. Regul Pept 2002;108(2–3):159–64.

62. Wolfe KB, Rossi RA, Warshak CR. The effect of maternal obesity on the rate of failed induction of labor. Am J Obstet Gynecol 2011;205(2):128.e1-7.
63. Zhang J, Bricker L, Wray S, et al. Poor uterine contractility in obese women. BJOG 2007;114(3):343–8.
64. Chin JR, Henry E, Holmgren CM, et al. Maternal obesity and contraction strength in the first stage of labor. Am J Obstet Gynecol 2012;207(2):129.e1-6.
65. Kominiarek MA, Vanveldhuisen P, Hibbard J, et al. The maternal body mass index: a strong association with delivery route. Am J Obstet Gynecol 2010; 203(3):264.e1-7.
66. Alanis MC, Villers MS, Law TL, et al. Complications of cesarean delivery in the massively obese parturient. Am J Obstet Gynecol 2010;203(3):271.e1-7.
67. Marshall NE, Guild C, Cheng YW, et al. Maternal superobesity and perinatal outcomes. Am J Obstet Gynecol 2012;206(5):417.e1-6.
68. Goodall PT, Ahn JT, Chapa JB, et al. Obesity as a risk factor for failed trial of labor in patients with previous cesarean delivery. Am J Obstet Gynecol 2005;192(5): 1423–6.
69. Landon MB, Leindecker S, Spong CY, et al. The MFMU Cesarean Registry: factors affecting the success of trial of labor after previous cesarean delivery. Am J Obstet Gynecol 2005;193(3 Pt 2):1016–23.
70. Tan T, Sia AT. Anesthesia considerations in the obese gravida. Semin Perinatol 2011;35(6):350–5.
71. Hodgkinson R, Husain FJ. Obesity and the cephalad spread of analgesia following epidural administration of bupivacaine for cesarean section. Anesth Analg 1980;59(2):89–92.
72. Vricella LK, Louis JM, Mercer BM, et al. Impact of morbid obesity on epidural anesthesia complications in labor. Am J Obstet Gynecol 2011;205(4): 370.e1-6.
73. Tonidandel A, Booth J, D'Angelo R, et al. Anesthetic and obstetric outcomes in morbidly obese parturients: a 20-year follow-up retrospective cohort study. Int J Obstet Anesth 2014;23(4):357–64.
74. Practice bulletin no. 177: obstetric analgesia and anesthesia. Obstet Gynecol 2017;129(4):e73–89.
75. Friedman AM, D'Alton ME. Venous thromboembolism bundle: risk assessment and prophylaxis for obstetric patients. Semin Perinatol 2016;40(2):87–92.
76. Larsen TB, Sorensen HT, Gislum M, et al. Maternal smoking, obesity, and risk of venous thromboembolism during pregnancy and the puerperium: a population-based nested case-control study. Thromb Res 2007;120(4):505–9.
77. Overcash RT, Somers AT, LaCoursiere DY. Enoxaparin dosing after cesarean delivery in morbidly obese women. Obstet Gynecol 2015;125(6):1371–6.
78. Krieger Y, Walfisch A, Sheiner E. Surgical site infection following cesarean deliveries: trends and risk factors. J Matern Fetal Neonatal Med 2017;30(1):8–12.
79. Wloch C, Wilson J, Lamagni T, et al. Risk factors for surgical site infection following caesarean section in England: results from a multicentre cohort study. BJOG 2012;119(11):1324–33.
80. Young OM, Shaik IH, Twedt R, et al. Pharmacokinetics of cefazolin prophylaxis in obese gravidae at time of cesarean delivery. Am J Obstet Gynecol 2015;213(4): 541.e1-7.
81. Maggio L, Nicolau DP, DaCosta M, et al. Cefazolin prophylaxis in obese women undergoing cesarean delivery: a randomized controlled trial. Obstet Gynecol 2015;125(5):1205–10.

82. Chelmow D, Rodriguez EJ, Sabatini MM. Suture closure of subcutaneous fat and wound disruption after cesarean delivery: a meta-analysis. Obstet Gynecol 2004; 103(5 Pt 1):974–80.

83. Ramsey PS, White AM, Guinn DA, et al. Subcutaneous tissue reapproximation, alone or in combination with drain, in obese women undergoing cesarean delivery. Obstet Gynecol 2005;105(5 Pt 1):967–73.

84. Gates S, Anderson ER. Wound drainage for caesarean section. Cochrane Database Syst Rev 2013;(12):CD004549.

85. Mackeen AD, Schuster M, Berghella V. Suture versus staples for skin closure after cesarean: a metaanalysis. Am J Obstet Gynecol 2015;212(5):621.e1-10.

86. Ruhstaller K, Downes KL, Chandrasekaran S, et al. Prophylactic wound vacuum therapy after cesarean section to prevent wound complications in the obese population: a randomized controlled trial (the ProVac study). Am J Perinatol 2017; 34(11):1125–30.

87. Turcksin R, Bel S, Galjaard S, et al. Maternal obesity and breastfeeding intention, initiation, intensity and duration: a systematic review. Matern Child Nutr 2014; 10(2):166–83.

88. Ramji N, Challa S, Murphy PA, et al. A comparison of breastfeeding rates by obesity class. J Matern Fetal Neonatal Med 2017;1–6 [Epub ahead of print].

89. Bever Babendure J, Reifsnider E, Mendias E, et al. Reduced breastfeeding rates among obese mothers: a review of contributing factors, clinical considerations and future directions. Int Breastfeed J 2015;10:21.

90. Lopez LM, Bernholc A, Chen M, et al. Hormonal contraceptives for contraception in overweight or obese women. Cochrane Database Syst Rev 2016;(8):CD008452.

91. Simmons KB, Edelman AB. Hormonal contraception and obesity. Fertil Steril 2016;106(6):1282–8.

92. Practice bulletin no. 149: endometrial cancer. Obstet Gynecol 2015;125(4): 1006–26.

Management of Obstructive Sleep Apnea in Pregnancy

Jennifer E. Dominguez, MD, MHS[a], Linda Street, MD[b], Judette Louis, MD, MPH[c],*

KEYWORDS

- Obstructive sleep apnea • Obesity • Pregnancy • Diabetes • Preeclampsia
- Anesthesia • Sleep-disordered breathing • Hypoxia

KEY POINTS

- All women with known or suspected sleep apnea should undergo treatment with a goal to normalize oxygenation during sleep.
- Sleep apnea is associated with hypertensive disorders of pregnancy, gestational diabetes, severe maternal morbidities including cardiomyopathy and venous thromboembolism, and in-hospital death.
- Management of women with sleep apnea should be multidisciplinary and include specialists in sleep medicine and anesthesiology.
- After delivery, women with sleep apnea are at risk for severe respiratory suppression and medications that suppress respiration should be limited in use.

Obstetric patients have been underrecognized as a population at risk for sleep-disordered breathing (SDB). SDB is likely underappreciated in pregnancy because of several factors including limited provider education, a lack of reliable screening tools, and a need for additional studies characterizing the dynamic effects of pregnancy on SDB and perinatal outcomes.[1] In addition, several of the most common risk factors for SDB recognized by clinicians were established from studies that excluded women of reproductive age.[2] It is now recognized that SDB may present differently in women of reproductive age, which can further complicate screening and diagnosis.[3]

Disclosure Statement: Dr J.E. Dominguez's work is supported in part by the NIH 5T32GM008600-20. Devices used in our research have been loaned by ResMed and Itamar Medical, Ltd. No Disclosures (L. Street, J. Louis).
[a] Department of Anesthesiology, Obstetric Anesthesiology, Division of Women's Anesthesia, Duke University Medical Center, Mail Sort #9, DUMC Box 3094, Durham, NC 27710, USA; [b] Division of Maternal Fetal Medicine, Department of OB/GYN, Medical College of Georgia, Augusta University, 1120 15th Street, BA-7410, Augusta, GA 30912, USA; [c] Division of Maternal Fetal Medicine, Department of OB/GYN, University of South Florida, 2 Tampa General Circle Suite 6050, Tampa, FL 33606, USA
* Corresponding author.
E-mail address: Jlouis1@health.usf.edu

Studies of SDB in recent years indicate there are significant implications for pregnancy. Women affected by SDB are more likely to experience pregnancy complications and adverse pregnancy outcomes.[4–10] This article reviews SDB, the implications for pregnancy, and ways that a practicing physician can improve clinical outcomes.

WHAT IS SLEEP-DISORDERED BREATHING?

SDB is a group of disorders characterized by ventilation abnormalities during sleep. The spectrum of SDB ranges from mild snoring to obstructive sleep apnea (OSA), the most severe form of SDB.[11] OSA involves multiple episodes of apnea or hypopnea during sleep that result from diminished airflow through the upper airway during respiratory effort, caused by partial or complete upper airway tissue collapse. This phenomenon leads to sleep fragmentation, sympathetic stimulation, hypercarbia, and intermittent cycles of hypoxemia and reoxygenation.[12] These pathophysiologic perturbations in turn contribute to inflammation, endothelial dysfunction, insulin resistance, and cardiovascular disease.[12] Repeated nocturnal arousals can result in excessive daytime sleepiness, and increased risk when driving or operating machinery.[12–14] The terms SDB and sleep apnea have been used interchangeably in the obstetric literature.

GESTATIONAL OBSTRUCTIVE SLEEP APNEA

Women diagnosed with OSA during pregnancy likely represent one of two distinct clinical phenotypes: women with pre-existing OSA that become pregnant (chronic OSA), and pregnant women who develop OSA (gestational OSA). Women with gestational OSA may enter pregnancy with snoring, and develop worsening airway obstruction because of physiologic and hormonal changes of pregnancy or in association with other comorbidities developed in pregnancy (multiple gestations, hypertensive disorders of pregnancy, or gestational diabetes). Some physiologic changes of pregnancy that may predispose women to OSA include upper airway edema and respiratory-driven changes leading to larger negative upper airway pressures caused by elevated estrogen and progesterone.[15] There is some evidence that gestational OSA may improve or resolve entirely after pregnancy.[16–18] However, the term "gestational sleep apnea" has not been formally defined. To date, the progression and impact of these two phenotypes has not been well described in either the perinatal period or beyond.

EPIDEMIOLOGY AND RISK FACTORS

The risk factors for OSA are well established in the general population and include male gender, older age, obesity, African-American race, craniofacial abnormalities, and smoking.[19,20] OSA is also associated with other comorbid conditions including type II diabetes, hypertension, cardiac arrhythmias, and cardiovascular disease.[12] Women who have those risk factors before pregnancy may be at increased risk for OSA. The existing studies in pregnancy also recognize increasing gestation, increasing maternal age, obesity, chronic hypertension, and frequent snoring ($\geq$3 times per week) as risk factors.[8,10,21] In the largest prospective study to date, women with OSA were older, had higher body mass index, larger neck circumference, and were more likely to have chronic hypertension, which is consistent with prior studies.[6]

Longitudinal studies of OSA indicate an increased prevalence across gestation.[6,22] In the largest prospective study currently published, the prevalence of OSA was estimated to be 3.6% in early pregnancy and increased across gestation with rates of 8.3% in the third trimester among the 3132 nulliparous women who completed objective testing for OSA.[6] These data are congruent with the findings of Pien and colleagues,[22] which also found an increase from 10.5% women with OSA in the first trimester to 26.7% in the third trimester among a group of women who underwent overnight polysomnography (PSG) at the two time points in pregnancy. Although the first trimester prevalence likely represents women with pre-existing chronic OSA, the increase throughout gestation is evidence of impact of pregnancy on the prevalence of the disease. With increased obesity rates, OSA is expected to affect a greater proportion. Approximately 15% to 20% of obese pregnant women are estimated to have OSA.[7,10,21] With delayed childbearing, women are older at the time of their first pregnancy, further increasing the risk for OSA.

SCREENING AND DIAGNOSIS

The screening questionnaires developed and validated in the nonpregnant population (Berlin questionnaire, Epworth Sleepiness Scale, and STOP-BANG questionnaires) have not been demonstrated to be useful in the obstetric population with reported sensitivities and specificities that are 36% to 39% and 68% to 77%, respectively, in current literature.[2,7,23–26] Although they are limited, in the absence of a better screening tool, some clinicians choose to use them. As an alternative, Facco and colleagues[21] proposed that most cases of OSA can be identified using three factors: (1) age, (2) body mass index, and (3) presence of chronic hypertension. Larger scale studies are needed to identify the best approach for screening pregnant women.

The gold standard for the diagnosis of OSA is overnight, attended, in-laboratory PSG.[14] However, in many medical centers, the availability of in-laboratory PSG requires significant wait times that may not allow for treatment to occur during pregnancy. Furthermore, in-laboratory PSG is costly, and requires an overnight, inpatient stay, which may not be practical for many patients that are unable to spend a night away from children in the home. Because of these challenges, many sleep physicians and insurers are turning to home sleep testing using portable devices as a practical alternative for select populations. Home sleep apnea testing devices have been used in several studies with pregnant women and some have been validated in pregnant populations.[10,21,27] However, although home sleep testing is widely accepted, there are some limitations. Home sleep tests are unattended and do not measure sleep time with electroencephalogram, so they are prone to underestimate sleep apnea severity or provide false-negative results.[14,28] They are particularly confounded by frequent waking during sleep, such as occurs for many pregnant women who may have a more frequent need to urinate. Routine electroencephalogram offers direct clinical observation along with electrophysiologic and cardiorespiratory monitoring to measure actual sleep time; most home tests are missing that component.[29] Despite these limitations, home sleep testing is likely to detect moderate to severe OSA, especially when using mild-range apnea-hypopnea index (AHI) scores (>5/h) as the threshold for treatment or further testing.[30] Sleep apnea severity is scored based on the AHI, a measure of how many apneas (cessation of airflow for $\geq$10 seconds accompanied by an arousal or oxyhemoglobin desaturation) and hypopneas (reduction of airflow for $\geq$10 seconds accompanied by an arousal or oxyhemoglobin desaturation) are present per hour of sleep. Mild OSA is defined as five less than or equal to AHI less than 15 per hour, moderate is considered 15 less than or equal to AHI less than 30, and severe OSA is 30 or greater per hour.[31]

Some insurers prefer that their insured customers receive home sleep tests instead of in-laboratory PSG because of the cost savings as proof of diagnosis of OSA for coverage of continuous positive airway pressure (CPAP) therapy; the Centers for Medicare and Medicaid Services began covering home sleep testing in 2016.[32] At this point, because of barriers of in-laboratory studies, home sleep testing is a viable alternative in select patients. However, the results should be interpreted with caution, and if significant clinical suspicion for OSA remains, it is recommended that the patient undergo overnight, in-laboratory PSG.[14]

TREATMENT

In the general population, CPAP is the preferred treatment of mild, moderate, and severe OSA.[33] More than 15 randomized clinical trials in the general population have suggested that treatment reduces hypertension, cardiovascular morbidities, and motor vehicle crashes.[34–37] Although the data on improvement of symptoms, quality of life, and automobile crashes have been consistent, recent data have failed to demonstrate a benefit in the reduction of cardiovascular disease.[38] However, some of the difficulty in finding a difference may be caused by diminished efficacy of CPAP secondary to poor patient adherence. Customized oral mandibular repositioning devices are an alternative that keep the airway open by pulling the lower jaw forward. Although these oral devices are an effective treatment of mild to moderate OSA for individuals with good dentition, they are considered second-line treatment and only recommended if the patient cannot tolerate CPAP or desire alternative therapy.[39]

There are few data to direct the treatment of OSA in pregnancy. Small studies examined CPAP treatment using short-term intermediary outcomes, such as maternal blood pressure.[40–42] However, with such small sample sizes, they were insufficiently powered to detect treatment impact or safety. Therefore, despite a consistent body of evidence showing an increased risk of adverse pregnancy outcomes associated with OSA in pregnancy, there is no evidence that treatment in the short term of pregnancy improves maternal or neonatal outcome. Rather, the benefits demonstrated in the general populations and the existing treatment guidelines are extrapolated to pregnancy.[33]

MATERNAL MORBIDITY

The Sleep Disordered Breathing Sub-study of the Nulliparous Pregnancy Outcomes Study was a multicenter, prospective cohort study seeking to investigate whether SDB during pregnancy is a risk factor for the development of hypertensive disorders of pregnancy and gestational diabetes.[6,18] Most of these subjects who tested positive for OSA in their pregnancies had mild-moderate OSA (AHI 5–14.9/h). SDB in early and midpregnancy was associated with preeclampsia (adjusted odds ratio [aOR], 1.94 [95% confidence interval (CI), 1.07–3.51] and 1.95 [95% CI, 1.18–3.23]), and gestational diabetes (aOR, 3.47 [95% CI, 1.95–6.19] and 2.79 [95% CI, 1.63–4.77]). There was a demonstrated dose response for women with severe OSA in midpregnancy (AHI >15/h) showing an even greater risk of hypertensive diseases of pregnancy (aOR, 4.27; 95% CI, 1.74–10.45). The findings of that study confirmed the findings of other smaller retrospective and prospective cohort studies that consistently found a two-fold increased adjusted odds of preeclampsia and a nearly two-fold increased adjusted odds of gestational diabetes in association with SDB or OSA, in two meta-analyses of the existing studies.[8,43]

Another study that included a military-treatment facility cohort indicated that the association persisted even in a "healthier cohort." Women with an OSA diagnosis were more likely to have a cesarean delivery (aOR, 1.60; 95% CI, 1.06–2.40), gestational hypertension (aOR, 2.46; 95% CI, 1.30–4.68), preeclampsia (aOR, 2.42; 95% CI, 1.43–4.09), and preterm delivery (aOR, 1.90; 95% CI, 1.09–3.30).[44]

SEVERE MATERNAL MORBIDITY

Severe maternal morbidities are those clinical events that can proximally lead to maternal death. Evidence from a large, national inpatient database study showed that pregnant women with a diagnosis of OSA during their hospital admission (by diagnosis code) at delivery were at significantly increased risk of having cardiomyopathy (aOR, 9.0; 95% CI, 7.47–10.87), congestive heart failure (aOR, 8.94; 95% CI, 7.45–10.73), and pulmonary embolism (aOR, 4.5; 95% CI, 2.3–8.9). This study also showed a five-fold increase of in-hospital mortality during a pregnancy or delivery in women with OSA.[7] These effects were exacerbated in the presence of obesity. The findings seem to indicate an effect of OSA that is independent of obesity. This study has yet to be replicated with other data sets with large enough numbers to confirm these uncommon findings but suggest serious complications for pregnant women with OSA.

NEONATAL MORBIDITY

The adverse fetal and neonatal consequences of sleep apnea in pregnancy are delineated to a lesser extent than that of maternal consequences. Maternal OSA is associated with 1.5- to two-fold increased frequency of low birth weight and small for gestational age infants.[8,43,45] These findings persist after controlling for comorbid maternal conditions that predispose to growth restriction, such as hypertension.[8,43,45] However, associations with large for gestational age infants born to women with SDB have also been reported.[46] This association may be partially explained by the high rates of maternal obesity and diabetes, two risk factors for large for gestational age infants.

Infants born to women with OSA are more likely to be born preterm and admitted to the neonatal intensive care unit despite similar gestational age at delivery.[10] Definitive studies examining the relationship do not exist. However, the findings are not completely unexpected given the high rates of cesarean delivery among women with OSA (up to 50%).[10] There are no studies that indicate an increased risk of fetal death or miscarriage in association with sleep apnea.[7]

In addition to the studies on immediate infant outcomes, smaller studies indicate that there may be longer term consequences for these infants.[47,48] Seventy-four mom-baby pairs of which 24% had OSA were followed in one study. Although there was no difference in general motor scores, there was an increased frequency of low social development scores in neonates of moms with OSA (64% vs 25%; $P = .036$) at 12 months of age.[47] Another recent study showed that the infants of women at risk for SDB determined by sleep questionnaires administered at hospital admission for delivery had shorter telomere lengths in the DNA collected from their cord blood.[49] Shorter telomere length has been observed in the DNA of adults with OSA, and is associated with age-related disease.[49,50] It is difficult to draw conclusions from these small, preliminary studies, but they may inform future directions for research.

MECHANISMS OF DISEASE

To date, the mechanisms that link OSA to adverse outcomes of pregnancy have not been well defined. Sleep apnea is a state in which there is overlap of proinflammatory states, oxidative stress, and sympathetic activation.[48] This cascade of events is thought to lead to endothelial dysfunction, although the role of oxidative stress in these pathways has been questioned by the findings of recent studies in nonpregnant and pregnant cohorts.[15,51,52] Endothelial dysfunction has been implicated in nonpregnant adults to link OSA and cardiovascular disease.[53] Some of these same mechanisms have been implicated in the development of preeclampsia and adverse pregnancy outcome (**Fig. 1**).[54]

The pathophysiologic mechanisms that connect OSA with the associated cardiovascular and metabolic disease share significant overlap with known pathways involved in preeclampsia.[55,56] OSA and preeclampsia both seem to be proinflammatory states, and studies in both populations demonstrate sympathetic nervous system activation.[57–60] To our knowledge, no studies have been done investigating these pathways in women with OSA and preeclampsia. In OSA, as in preeclampsia, up-regulation of antiangiogenic proteins seems to lead to endothelial dysfunction.[61,62] This endothelial dysfunction is implicated in vasoconstriction, hypertension, and proteinuria associated with preeclampsia, and the hypertension and cardiovascular

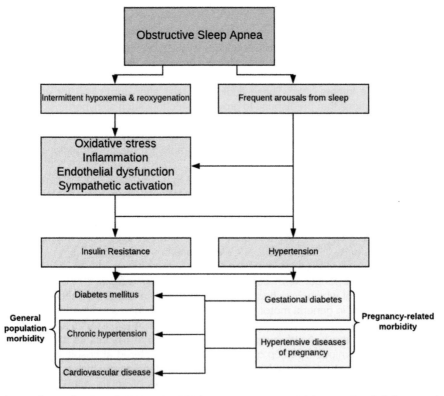

Fig. 1. The mechanisms that connect OSA in pregnant women with gestational diabetes and preeclampsia are not well-elucidated, but may share common pathways with cardiovascular and metabolic diseases associated with OSA in nonpregnant adults. OSA is associated with proinflammatory states, oxidative stress, and sympathetic activation. This cascade of events is thought to lead to endothelial dysfunction. Some of these same mechanisms have been implicated in the development of gestational diabetes and preeclampsia, but few studies have investigated these pathophysiologic mechanisms in women with OSA in pregnancy.

disease associated with OSA.[63,64] Preliminary evidence that imbalances of proangiogenic/antiangiogenic proteins are associated with a diagnosis of OSA were found in a small retrospective study of pregnant women with OSA.[55]

The explanations for the fetal growth abnormalities may differ. Pregnant women that live at high altitude have chronically low arterial oxygen partial pressures and studies have shown that they have an increased risk of hypertensive disorders of pregnancy and fetal growth restriction.[65,66] Both animal model and human studies suggest that the placenta and fetus adapt via compensatory mechanisms to the low oxygen tension.[67,68]

However, there are currently no studies in pregnant women with OSA that have specifically investigated the effects of repetitive, nocturnal exposure to hypoxemia in this disease state.[67,68] In vitro and animal studies suggest that oxygen tension plays a specific role in the early development of the placenta, and that alterations may predispose to the pathologic placental development that is subsequently seen in hypertensive disorders of pregnancy and fetal growth restriction.[69–72] Hypoxia-inducible factors 1 and 2 are transcription factors that play a vital role in the cellular response to low oxygen tension.[73] Hypoxia-inducible factors 1 and 2 are overexpressed in the placentas of women living at high altitude, women with hypertensive disorders of pregnancy, and rats with growth-restricted fetuses.[74–76] Hypoxia-inducible factors have also been studied for their role in OSA with hypertension in nonpregnant adults, as mediators of hypoxemia, sympathetic nervous system activators, oxidative stress, and endothelial dysfunction.[77] These different mechanisms can serve as targets for future interventional studies.

LONG-TERM IMPLICATIONS OF SLEEP APNEA

Untreated OSA has a bidirectional association with type II diabetes, cardiovascular disease, and hypertension.[78–80] It is also known that pregnancy is a time that most patients seek medical help, often for the first time, providing an opportunity to impact future health outcomes. Developing complications, such as preeclampsia and gestational diabetes, increases the future risk of cardiovascular disease and type II diabetes among the affected women.[81–84] Because of this relationship, it is hypothesized that SDB and OSA may further predispose these women to future cardiovascular disease. The extent to which SDB impacts the already observed relationship between preeclampsia and cardiovascular disease is unknown (**Fig. 2**).[16,85] It is also unknown if postpartum resolution of OSA has a lasting impact, or if treating OSA during pregnancy would modify these outcomes.

Future studies are needed to ascertain if treatment of OSA can impact the course of these comorbid diseases in pregnant women because their consequences are far reaching and extend beyond completion of pregnancy. Preeclampsia has been linked to a three- to 12-fold increased risk of cardiovascular events later in life and a two-fold to eight-fold increased risk of death from a cardiovascular event.[86,87] Up to 62% of women diagnosed with gestational diabetes go on to develop type II diabetes later in life.[88] This does not even begin to take into account the potential for gestational OSA to persist after pregnancy. Rates of long-term postpartum persistence of OSA or development of OSA later in life are not well defined at this time, but it is reasonable to presume that in some women gestational OSA is a precursor for life-long risks discussed previously.

CLINICAL CARE
Antepartum Care

A multidisciplinary approach should be taken when managing pregnant women with OSA, which should continue to the postpartum period.[89] Women with known OSA

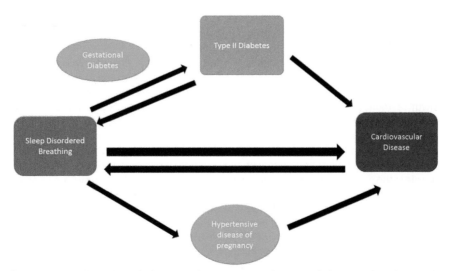

Fig. 2. Untreated SDB has a bidirectional association with type II diabetes and cardiovascular disease in nonpregnant adults. SDB has also been associated with gestational diabetes and hypertensive diseases of pregnancy in recent studies. Developing complications, such as pre-eclampsia and gestational diabetes, have been shown to increase the future risk of cardiovascular disease and type II diabetes among the affected women.

who become pregnant should be evaluated by a sleep medicine specialist to optimize CPAP settings. The goal is to achieve and maintain a normalized AHI and oxygenation throughout gestation through the consistent use of CPAP therapy. Follow-up visits or an automatically titrating CPAP machine are useful because CPAP requirements may increase with advancing gestation and worsening obstruction.[6,22,90] The patient should be counseled about the known perinatal consequences of sleep apnea and a multidisciplinary plan must be formulated. Patients with moderate to severe OSA may have comorbid cardiovascular disease or pulmonary hypertension, and echocardiography should be considered. Obstetric providers should be mindful of the risk of hypertensive disorders and diabetes and should focus on early detection or prevention of these conditions. Women who are suspected of having OSA but have not been diagnosed should be referred to a sleep medicine specialist for evaluation. Situations where a suspicion of sleep apnea may arise include but are not limited to maternal symptoms of excessive daytime sleepiness or generalized fatigue, witnessed apneas, loud and frequent snoring, headaches, and/or observed maternal hypoxia in the absence of cardiorespiratory pathology.[90] After referral, the sleep medicine provider can evaluate the patient and make recommendations regarding diagnosis and management during the pregnancy and in the postpartum period. In the absence of pregnancy-specific data to direct treatment, we currently suggest treatment of all women with OSA. Studies have not been conducted to evaluate the safety of CPAP in pregnancy, but it is widely accepted as safe in pregnancy. An individualized plan can be developed with the sleep medicine provider.

Intrapartum and Immediate Postpartum Management

Women with OSA are also more likely to have comorbid conditions that also predispose them to cesarean deliveries.[10] The American Society of Anesthesiologists guidelines advise preoperative evaluation and treatment of OSA is optimal in surgical patients.[91] There are no guidelines specifically regarding pregnant women with OSA, however, they represent a high-risk cohort and should be treated like other presurgical patients.[9]

Perioperative risks to gravid women with sleep apnea include a greater risk of difficult intubation and ventilation. When OSA is comorbid with severe obesity, neuraxial anesthesia, which is the gold standard anesthetic for cesarean delivery, is technically difficult. This can increase the need for conversion to general anesthesia.[92] A preoperative anesthesia consultation for airway assessment and evaluation for placement of neuraxial anesthesia should occur.

These women are at risk for postoperative respiratory suppression and should have continuous pulse oximetry monitoring after discharge from the recovery room; continuous oximetry should be maintained as long as patients remain at increased risk.[93] Although some institutions have implemented protocols that include monitoring for a 12- to 24-hour period of time, there are no studies to guide the effectiveness of these protocols and to determine the optimal duration of that monitoring.[89] If frequent or severe airway obstruction or hypoxemia are noted, CPAP or noninvasive positive pressure ventilation in an intensive care unit setting should be strongly considered.[93] In a case series of anesthesia-related maternal deaths in Michigan, half of the anesthesia-related deaths were determined to be caused by lapses in postoperative monitoring, either in the postanesthesia care unit or the hospital room.[94] Patients should be encouraged to maintain a 45-degree head elevation and avoid supine position because this was associated with a decrease in the number of apnea and hypopnea events in a study of postpartum women.[95] Multimodal postoperative analgesia with nonsteroidal anti-inflammatory agents and acetaminophen is recommended when possible to decrease the risk of sedation and hypoventilation associated with opioids. The use of neuraxial morphine in this population because of the theoretic risk of delayed respiratory depression is controversial.[96] Some centers avoid the use of neuraxial morphine for postcesarean delivery analgesia in women with morbid obesity and OSA. Others have argued that the parenteral opioid-sparing effect of a small dose of neuraxial morphine outweighs the small risk of respiratory depression.[97] Transversus abdominis plane block, local anesthetic wound catheters, and neuraxial techniques are options to consider for postoperative analgesia when appropriate.[98] Sedating medications, such as antiemetics, antihistamines, anxiolytics, and sleep aids should be avoided or used sparingly with extreme caution in monitored settings, particularly when used along with opioids. Standing order for narcotics and basal dosing should be avoided, and patient-controlled systemic opioids should be used cautiously.

During the postpartum period, all women with a diagnosis or suspicion of OSA during pregnancy should be evaluated by a sleep medicine provider to allow for reassessment of OSA severity and overall management/treatment strategy.

SUMMARY

OSA in pregnancy is a common and underrecognized disorder that carries implications for the mother and the fetus. These women are at a higher risk of pregnancy and anesthesia-related complications. A lack of effective screening tools and limited understanding of the dynamic effects of pregnancy on OSA throughout gestation continue to make diagnosis and management challenging. Increased awareness with appropriate diagnosis, treatment, and perioperative management could improve outcomes in these pregnancies, although data on the impact of OSA treatment on adverse pregnancy outcomes are still needed. Additionally, identifying OSA early in a woman's life may positively impact her long-term health. Because pregnancy is often the only time many young women seek health care, this may be the best opportunity for early detection in some at-risk women.

REFERENCES

1. Bourjeily G, Raker C, Paglia MJ, et al. Patient and provider perceptions of sleep disordered breathing assessment during prenatal care: a survey-based observational study. Ther Adv Respir Dis 2012;6:211–9.
2. Chung F, Subramanyam R, Liao P, et al. High STOP-bang score indicates a high probability of obstructive sleep apnoea. Br J Anaesth 2012;108:768–75.
3. Shah N, Hanna DB, Teng Y, et al. Sex-specific prediction models for sleep apnea from the Hispanic community health study/study of Latinos. Chest 2016;149: 1409–18.
4. O'Brien LM, Bullough AS, Chames MC, et al. Hypertension, snoring, and obstructive sleep apnoea during pregnancy: a cohort study. BJOG 2014;121:1685–93.
5. O'Brien LM, Bullough AS, Owusu JT, et al. Pregnancy-onset habitual snoring, gestational hypertension, and preeclampsia: prospective cohort study. Am J Obstet Gynecol 2012;207(487):e481–9.
6. Facco FL, Parker CB, Reddy UM, et al. Association between sleep-disordered breathing and hypertensive disorders of pregnancy and gestational diabetes mellitus. Obstet Gynecol 2017;129:31–41.
7. Louis JM, Mogos MF, Salemi JL, et al. Obstructive sleep apnea and severe maternal-infant morbidity/mortality in the United States, 1998-2009. Sleep 2014; 37:843–9.
8. Pamidi S, Pinto LM, Marc I, et al. Maternal sleep-disordered breathing and adverse pregnancy outcomes: a systematic review and metaanalysis. Am J Obstet Gynecol 2014;210:52.e1–14.
9. Xu T, Feng Y, Peng H, et al. Obstructive sleep apnea and the risk of perinatal outcomes: a meta-analysis of cohort studies. Sci Rep 2014;4:6982.
10. Louis J, Auckley D, Miladinovic B, et al. Perinatal outcomes associated with obstructive sleep apnea in obese pregnant women. Obstet Gynecol 2012;120: 1085–92.
11. Chervin RD, Guilleminault C. Obstructive sleep apnea and related disorders. Neurol Clin 1996;14:583–609.
12. Jordan AS, McSharry DG, Malhotra A. Adult obstructive sleep apnoea. Lancet 2014;383:736–47.
13. Alam I, Lewis K, Stephens JW, et al. Obesity, metabolic syndrome and sleep apnoea: all pro-inflammatory states. Obes Rev 2007;8:119–27.
14. Kapur VK, Auckley DH, Chowdhuri S, et al. Clinical practice guideline for diagnostic testing for adult obstructive sleep apnea: an American Academy of Sleep Medicine Clinical Practice Guideline. J Clin Sleep Med 2017;13:479–504.
15. Bourjeily G, Ankner G, Mohsenin V. Sleep-disordered breathing in pregnancy. Clin Chest Med 2011;32:175–89, x.
16. Reid J, Glew RA, Skomro R, et al. Sleep disordered breathing and gestational hypertension: postpartum follow-up study. Sleep 2013;36:717–21B.
17. Edwards N, Blyton DM, Hennessy A, et al. Severity of sleep-disordered breathing improves following parturition. Sleep 2005;28:737–41.
18. Facco FL, Parker CB, Reddy UM, et al. NuMoM2b sleep-disordered breathing study: objectives and methods. Am J Obstet Gynecol 2015;212:542.e1–127.
19. Young T, Peppard PE, Gottlieb DJ. Epidemiology of obstructive sleep apnea: a population health perspective. Am J Respir Crit Care Med 2002;165:1217–39.

20. Punjabi NM. The epidemiology of adult obstructive sleep apnea. Proc Am Thorac Soc 2008;5:136–43.
21. Facco FL, Ouyang DW, Zee PC, et al. Development of a pregnancy-specific screening tool for sleep apnea. J Clin Sleep Med 2012;8:389–94.
22. Pien GW, Pack AI, Jackson N, et al. Risk factors for sleep-disordered breathing in pregnancy. Thorax 2014;69:371–7.
23. Netzer NC, Stoohs RA, Netzer CM, et al. Using the Berlin Questionnaire to identify patients at risk for the sleep apnea syndrome. Ann Intern Med 1999;131:485–91.
24. Lockhart EM, Ben Abdallah A, Tuuli MG, et al. Obstructive sleep apnea in pregnancy: assessment of current screening tools. Obstet Gynecol 2015; 126:93–102.
25. Johns MW. A new method for measuring daytime sleepiness: the Epworth Sleepiness Scale. Sleep 1991;14:540–5.
26. Johns MW. Reliability and factor analysis of the Epworth Sleepiness Scale. Sleep 1992;15:376–81.
27. O'Brien LM, Bullough AS, Shelgikar AV, et al. Validation of Watch-PAT-200 against polysomnography during pregnancy. J Clin Sleep Med 2012;8:287–94.
28. Ghegan MD, Angelos PC, Stonebraker AC, et al. Laboratory versus portable sleep studies: a meta-analysis. Laryngoscope 2006;116:859–64.
29. Karakis I, Chiappa KH, San Luciano M, et al. The utility of routine EEG in the diagnosis of sleep disordered breathing. J Clin Neurophysiol 2012;29:333–8.
30. Chai-Coetzer CL, Antic NA, Rowland LS, et al. A simplified model of screening questionnaire and home monitoring for obstructive sleep apnoea in primary care. Thorax 2011;66:213–9.
31. Berry RB, Brooks R, Gamaldo CE, et al. The AASM manual for the scoring of sleep and associated events. Rules, terminology and technical specifications. Darien (IL): American Academy of Sleep Medicine; 2012.
32. Chiao W, Durr ML. Trends in sleep studies performed for Medicare beneficiaries. Laryngoscope 2017;127(12):2891–6.
33. Adult Obstructive Sleep Apnea Task Force of the American Academy of Sleep Medicine. Clinical guideline for the evaluation, management and long-term care of obstructive sleep apnea in adults. J Clin Sleep Med 2009;5:263–76.
34. Buchner NJ, Sanner BM, Borgel J, et al. Continuous positive airway pressure treatment of mild to moderate obstructive sleep apnea reduces cardiovascular risk. Am J Respir Crit Care Med 2007;176:1274–80.
35. Haentjens P, Van Meerhaeghe A, Moscariello A, et al. The impact of continuous positive airway pressure on blood pressure in patients with obstructive sleep apnea syndrome: evidence from a meta-analysis of placebo-controlled randomized trials. Arch Intern Med 2007;167:757–64.
36. Tregear S, Reston J, Schoelles K, et al. Continuous positive airway pressure reduces risk of motor vehicle crash among drivers with obstructive sleep apnea: systematic review and meta-analysis. Sleep 2010;33:1373–80.
37. Mehra R. Sleep apnea ABCs: airway, breathing, circulation. Cleve Clin J Med 2014;81:479–89.
38. Yu J, Zhou Z, McEvoy R, et al. Association of positive airway pressure with cardiovascular events and death in adults with sleep apnea: a systematic review and meta-analysis. JAMA 2017;318:156–66.
39. Ramar K, Dort LC, Katz SG, et al. Clinical practice guideline for the treatment of obstructive sleep apnea and snoring with oral appliance therapy: an update for 2015. J Clin Sleep Med 2015;11:773–827.

40. Blyton DM, Sullivan CE, Edwards N. Reduced nocturnal cardiac output associ-
    ated with preeclampsia is minimized with the use of nocturnal nasal CPAP. Sleep
    2004;27:79–84.
41. Guilleminault C, Palombini L, Poyares D, et al. Pre-eclampsia and nasal CPAP:
    part 1. Early intervention with nasal CPAP in pregnant women with risk-factors
    for pre-eclampsia: preliminary findings. Sleep Med 2007;9:9–14.
42. Poyares D, Guilleminault C, Hachul H, et al. Pre-eclampsia and nasal CPAP: part
    2. Hypertension during pregnancy, chronic snoring, and early nasal CPAP inter-
    vention. Sleep Med 2007;9:15–21.
43. Ding XX, Wu YL, Xu SJ, et al. A systematic review and quantitative assessment of
    sleep-disordered breathing during pregnancy and perinatal outcomes. Sleep
    Breath 2014;18:703–13.
44. Spence DL, Allen RC, Lutgendorf MA, et al. Association of obstructive sleep ap-
    nea with adverse pregnancy-related outcomes in military hospitals. Eur J Obstet
    Gynecol Reprod Biol 2017;210:166–72.
45. Pamidi S, Marc I, Simoneau G, et al. Maternal sleep-disordered breathing and the
    risk of delivering small for gestational age infants: a prospective cohort study.
    Thorax 2016;71:719–25.
46. Ge X, Tao F, Huang K, et al. Maternal snoring may predict adverse pregnancy
    outcomes: a cohort study in China. PLoS One 2016;11:e0148732.
47. Tauman R, Zuk L, Uliel-Sibony S, et al. The effect of maternal sleep-disordered breath-
    ing on the infant's neurodevelopment. Am J Obstet Gynecol 2015;212:656.e1–7.
48. Arnardottir ES, Mackiewicz M, Gislason T, et al. Molecular signatures of obstruc-
    tive sleep apnea in adults: a review and perspective. Sleep 2009;32:447–70.
49. Salihu HM, King L, Patel P, et al. Association between maternal symptoms of
    sleep disordered breathing and fetal telomere length. Sleep 2015;38:559–66.
50. Savolainen K, Eriksson JG, Kajantie E, et al. The history of sleep apnea is asso-
    ciated with shorter leukocyte telomere length: the Helsinki Birth Cohort Study.
    Sleep Med 2014;15:209–12.
51. Paz y Mar HL, Hazen SL, Tracy RP, et al. Effect of continuous positive airway pres-
    sure on cardiovascular biomarkers. Chest 2016;150:80–90.
52. Khan N, Lambert-Messerlian G, Monteiro JF, et al. Oxidative and carbonyl stress
    in pregnant women with obstructive sleep apnea. Sleep Breath 2017. [Epub
    ahead of print].
53. Dewan NA, Nieto FJ, Somers VK. Intermittent hypoxemia and OSA: implications
    for comorbidities. Chest 2015;147:266–74.
54. Chaiworapongsa T, Chaemsaithong P, Yeo L, et al. Pre-eclampsia part 1: current
    understanding of its pathophysiology. Nat Rev Nephrol 2014;10:466–80.
55. Bourjeily G, Curran P, Butterfield K, et al. Placenta-secreted circulating markers in
    pregnant women with obstructive sleep apnea. J Perinat Med 2015;43:81–7.
56. Izci-Balserak B, Pien GW. The relationship and potential mechanistic pathways
    between sleep disturbances and maternal hyperglycemia. Curr Diab Rep
    2014;14:459.
57. Ryan S. Adipose tissue inflammation by intermittent hypoxia: mechanistic link be-
    tween obstructive sleep apnoea and metabolic dysfunction. J Physiol 2017;595:
    2423–30.
58. Iturriaga R, Oyarce MP, Dias ACR. Role of carotid body in intermittent hypoxia-
    related hypertension. Curr Hypertens Rep 2017;19:38.
59. Ferguson KK, Meeker JD, McElrath TF, et al. Repeated measures of inflammation
    and oxidative stress biomarkers in preeclamptic and normotensive pregnancies.
    Am J Obstet Gynecol 2017;216:527.e1–9.

60. Schobel HP, Fischer T, Heuszer K, et al. Preeclampsia: a state of sympathetic overactivity. N Engl J Med 1996;335:1480–5.
61. Mohsenin V, Urbano F. Circulating antiangiogenic proteins in obstructive sleep apnea and hypertension. Respir Med 2011;105:801–7.
62. Jafari B, Mohsenin V. Endothelial dysfunction and hypertension in obstructive sleep apnea: is it due to intermittent hypoxia? J Cardiovasc Dis Res 2013;4: 87–91.
63. Maynard SE, Min JY, Merchan J, et al. Excess placental soluble fms-like tyrosine kinase 1 (sFlt1) may contribute to endothelial dysfunction, hypertension, and proteinuria in preeclampsia. J Clin Invest 2003;111:649–58.
64. Levine RJ, Maynard SE, Qian C, et al. Circulating angiogenic factors and the risk of preeclampsia. N Engl J Med 2004;350:672–83.
65. Palmer SK, Moore LG, Young D, et al. Altered blood pressure course during normal pregnancy and increased preeclampsia at high altitude (3100 meters) in Colorado. Am J Obstet Gynecol 1999;180:1161–8.
66. Keyes LE, Armaza JF, Niermeyer S, et al. Intrauterine growth restriction, preeclampsia, and intrauterine mortality at high altitude in Bolivia. Pediatr Res 2003;54:20–5.
67. Ilekis JV, Tsilou E, Fisher S, et al. Placental origins of adverse pregnancy outcomes: potential molecular targets: an Executive Workshop Summary of the Eunice Kennedy Shriver National Institute of Child Health and Human Development. Am J Obstet Gynecol 2016;215:S1–46.
68. Rosario GX, Konno T, Soares MJ. Maternal hypoxia activates endovascular trophoblast cell invasion. Dev Biol 2008;314:362–75.
69. Genbacev O, Joslin R, Damsky CH, et al. Hypoxia alters early gestation human cytotrophoblast differentiation/invasion in vitro and models the placental defects that occur in preeclampsia. J Clin Invest 1996;97:540–50.
70. Lai Z, Kalkunte S, Sharma S. A critical role of interleukin-10 in modulating hypoxia-induced preeclampsia-like disease in mice. Hypertension 2011;57: 505–14.
71. Adelman DM, Gertsenstein M, Nagy A, et al. Placental cell fates are regulated in vivo by HIF-mediated hypoxia responses. Genes Dev 2000;14:3191–203.
72. Gourvas V, Dalpa E, Konstantinidou A, et al. Angiogenic factors in placentas from pregnancies complicated by fetal growth restriction (review). Mol Med Rep 2012; 6:23–7.
73. Tal R. The role of hypoxia and hypoxia-inducible factor-1alpha in preeclampsia pathogenesis. Biol Reprod 2012;87:134.
74. Zamudio S, Wu Y, Ietta F, et al. Human placental hypoxia-inducible factor-1alpha expression correlates with clinical outcomes in chronic hypoxia in vivo. Am J Pathol 2007;170:2171–9.
75. Rajakumar A, Brandon HM, Daftary A, et al. Evidence for the functional activity of hypoxia-inducible transcription factors overexpressed in preeclamptic placentae. Placenta 2004;25:763–9.
76. Robb KP, Cotechini T, Allaire C, et al. Inflammation-induced fetal growth restriction in rats is associated with increased placental HIF-1alpha accumulation. PLoS One 2017;12:e0175805.
77. Nanduri J, Peng YJ, Yuan G, et al. Hypoxia-inducible factors and hypertension: lessons from sleep apnea syndrome. J Mol Med (Berl) 2015;93:473–80.
78. Nieto FJ, Young TB, Lind BK, et al. Association of sleep-disordered breathing, sleep apnea, and hypertension in a large community-based study. Sleep Heart Health Study. JAMA 2000;283:1829–36.

79. Marin JM, Carrizo SJ, Vicente E, et al. Long-term cardiovascular outcomes in men with obstructive sleep apnoea-hypopnoea with or without treatment with continuous positive airway pressure: an observational study. Lancet 2005;365:1046–53.

80. Aronsohn RS, Whitmore H, Van Cauter E, et al. Impact of untreated obstructive sleep apnea on glucose control in type 2 diabetes. Am J Respir Crit Care Med 2010;181:507–13.

81. Bokslag A, Teunissen PW, Franssen C, et al. Effect of early-onset preeclampsia on cardiovascular risk in the fifth decade of life. Am J Obstet Gynecol 2017; 216:523.e1–7.

82. Hermes W, Tamsma JT, Grootendorst DC, et al. Cardiovascular risk estimation in women with a history of hypertensive pregnancy disorders at term: a longitudinal follow-up study. BMC Pregnancy Childbirth 2013;13:126.

83. Tobias DK, Stuart JJ, Li S, et al. Association of history of gestational diabetes with long-term cardiovascular disease risk in a large prospective cohort of US women. JAMA Intern Med 2017;177(12):1735–42.

84. Kim C, Newton KM, Knopp RH. Gestational diabetes and the incidence of type 2 diabetes: a systematic review. Diabetes Care 2002;25:1862–8.

85. Dunietz GL, Chervin RD, O'Brien LM. Sleep-disordered breathing during pregnancy: future implications for cardiovascular health. Obstet Gynecol Surv 2014; 69:164–76.

86. Ahmed R, Dunford J, Mehran R, et al. Pre-eclampsia and future cardiovascular risk among women: a review. J Am Coll Cardiol 2014;63:1815–22.

87. Amaral LM, Cunningham MW Jr, Cornelius DC, et al. Preeclampsia: long-term consequences for vascular health. Vasc Health Risk Manag 2015;11:403–15.

88. O'Sullivan JB. Diabetes mellitus after GDM. Diabetes 1991;40(Suppl 2):131–5.

89. Louis J, Auckley D, Bolden N. Management of obstructive sleep apnea in pregnant women. Obstetrics Gynecol 2012;119:864–8.

90. Pien GW, Fife D, Pack AI, et al. Changes in symptoms of sleep-disordered breathing during pregnancy. Sleep 2005;28:1299–305.

91. American Society of Anesthesiologists Task Force on Perioperative Management of Patients with Obstructive Sleep Apnea. Practice guidelines for the perioperative management of patients with obstructive sleep apnea: an updated report by the American Society of Anesthesiologists Task Force on Perioperative Management of patients with obstructive sleep apnea. Anesthesiology 2014;120: 268–86.

92. Lamon AM, Habib AS. Managing anesthesia for cesarean section in obese patients: current perspectives. Local Reg Anesth 2016;9:45–57.

93. Chung F, Memtsoudis SG, Ramachandran SK, et al. Society of anesthesia and sleep medicine guidelines on preoperative screening and assessment of adult patients with obstructive sleep apnea. Anesth Analg 2016;123:452.

94. Mhyre JM, Riesner MN, Polley LS, et al. A series of anesthesia-related maternal deaths in Michigan, 1985-2003. Anesthesiology 2007;106:1096–104.

95. Zaremba S, Mueller N, Heisig AM, et al. Elevated upper body position improves pregnancy-related OSA without impairing sleep quality or sleep architecture early after delivery. Chest 2015;148:936–44.

96. Practice guidelines for the prevention, detection, and management of respiratory depression associated with neuraxial opioid administration: an updated report by the American Society of Anesthesiologists Task Force on Neuraxial Opioids and the American Society of Regional Anesthesia and Pain Medicine. Anesthesiology 2016;124:535–52.

97. Crowgey TR, Dominguez JE, Peterson-Layne C, et al. A retrospective assessment of the incidence of respiratory depression after neuraxial morphine administration for postcesarean delivery analgesia. Anesth Analg 2013;117:1368–70.
98. Lalmand M, Wilwerth M, Fils JF, et al. Continuous ropivacaine subfascial wound infusion compared with intrathecal morphine for postcesarean analgesia: a prospective, randomized controlled, double-blind study. Anesth Analg 2017; 125(3):907–12.

Maternal Genetic Disorders in Pregnancy

Sarah Harris, MS[a], Neeta L. Vora, MD[b],*

KEYWORDS

- Pregnancy • Management • Genetic disorders
- Hereditary hemorrhagic telangiectasia • Tuberous sclerosis • Myotonic dystrophy
- Ornithine transcarbamoylase deficiency

KEY POINTS

- Multidisciplinary management of pregnancy in women with genetic disorders is recommended.
- Discussions of maternal and fetal risks associated with pregnancy in women with genetic disorders, including options for genetic testing, are best completed before conception.
- Continued research of pregnancy outcomes in women with genetic disorders is needed.

INTRODUCTION

As the life expectancy and quality of life improves for individuals with genetic conditions, so does the need for information regarding the management of reproductive issues. A recent review article addressed pregnancy care in women with some of the more common genetic conditions, including phenylketonuria, Turner syndrome, cystic fibrosis, connective tissue disorders, and disorders of fatty oxidation.[1] The authors, therefore, focus their review on pregnancy management and outcomes in women with hereditary hemorrhagic telangiectasia (HHT), tuberous sclerosis complex (TSC), myotonic dystrophy, and ornithine transcarbamoylase (OTC) deficiency.

HEREDITARY HEMORRHAGIC TELANGIECTASIA

Hereditary Hemorrhagic Telangiectasia (HHT) is an autosomal dominant multisystem disease leading to the development of multiple arteriovenous malformations (AVMs). AVMs are abnormally formed vessels that lack capillaries, resulting in a direct connection of an artery with a vein. HHT is estimated to occur in approximately 1 in 5000 individuals.[2]

Disclosure Statement: The authors have no conflicts of interest.
[a] University of North Carolina at Chapel Hill School of Medicine, 3010 Old Clinic Building, CB 7516, Chapel Hill, NC 27516, USA; [b] Division of Maternal Fetal Medicine, Department of Obstetrics and Gynecology, University of North Carolina at Chapel Hill School of Medicine, 3010 Old Clinic Building, CB 7516, Chapel Hill, NC 27516, USA
* Corresponding author.
E-mail address: nvora@med.unc.edu

Obstet Gynecol Clin N Am 45 (2018) 249–265
https://doi.org/10.1016/j.ogc.2018.01.010
0889-8545/18/© 2018 Elsevier Inc. All rights reserved.

obgyn.theclinics.com

HHT is caused by mutations in genes that encode proteins for the transforming growth factor-beta (TGF-ß) signaling pathway, which is involved in angiogenesis.[3] It is estimated that 75% of patients who meet the clinical criteria for the diagnosis of HHT will have an identifiable mutation in one of 3 genes, *ACVRL1, ENG, SMAD4.*[4] Additional genes, including *GDF2*, are being investigated for their role in the pathogenesis of HHT.[5] Molecular genetic testing is available to establish a genetic diagnosis in clinically suspected cases.

The presentation of HHT is highly variable. Small AVMs, also called telangiectasia, can be found on the fingers, face, nasal mucosa, lips, tongue, and gastrointestinal mucosa.[3] Telangiectasias can range from small, blanchable, pink to red lesions to large, raised, purple lesions. Because of the abnormal formation of the vessels and the close proximity to the skin surface, telangiectasias can rupture and bleed.[3] The most common presenting symptom is recurrent episodes of epistaxis, occurring in more than 95% of patients. Large AVMs can also occur within the lungs, liver, or brain. The major concern with HHT is the risk of spontaneous rupture of a large AVM leading to a catastrophic bleed.[3]

HHT is typically a clinical diagnosis, for which diagnostic criteria have been developed[6] (**Table 1**). Current management guidelines recommend that individuals with HHT undergo screening for vascular malformations at the time of diagnosis, including MRI with and without contrast for the detection of cerebral AVMs, transthoracic contrast echocardiography for the detection of pulmonary AVM with follow-up for abnormalities with unenhanced thoracic computed tomography (CT), and liver ultrasound or abdominal CT for the detection of liver vascular malformations.[7]

Pregnancy in Women with Hereditary Hemorrhagic Telangiectasia

Fertility is not typically affected, and no increased risk of miscarriage has been reported in women with HHT.[8] Most pregnancies are uneventful. However, pregnancies in women with HHT should be considered high risk given the possibility of significant morbidity and mortality associated with the risk of bleeding from AVMs.

Table 1 The Curaçao criteria	
Diagnostic criteria for HHT *Definite diagnosis*: 3 criteria present *Possible or suspected diagnosis*: 2 criteria present *Unlikely*: <2 criteria present	
Criteria	
• Epistaxis	Spontaneous, recurrent nose bleeds
• Telangiectasias	Multiple, at characteristic sites • Lips • Oral cavity • Fingers • Nose
• Visceral lesions	Gastrointestinal telangiectasias Pulmonary AVM Hepatic AVM Cerebral AVM Spinal AVM
• Family history	First-degree relative with HHT

From Shovlin CL, Guttmacher AE, Buscarini E, et al. Diagnostic criteria for hereditary hemorrhagic telangiectasia (Rendu-Osler Weber syndrome). Am J Med Genet 2000;91(1):67; with permission.

An increase in development of new skin and mucosal telangiectasias has been reported in some women. The frequency of episodes of epistaxis may increase during pregnancy; however, these episodes are not typically associated with significant complications.[9]

A significant increase in pregnancy complications has been reported in women with pulmonary AVMs (PAVMs).[10] The abnormal, dilated vessels can create a right-to-left shunt between the pulmonary arterial and venous systems, which leads to arterial hypoxemia and an increased risk of ischemic and paradoxic embolic events.[11] PAVMs can also rupture leading to massive hemoptysis.

One retrospective series of 161 pregnancies in 47 women reported 6 cases of worsening right-to-left intrapulmonary shunting evident by increased hypoxemia and worsening dyspnea, 2 maternal deaths secondary to PAVM hemorrhage, and 3 strokes.[8] A second study including retrospective and prospective data of 484 pregnancies in 199 women reported life-threatening complications in 13 pregnancies, including 6 PAVM hemorrhages, 6 strokes, and 1 myocardial infarction. There were 5 maternal deaths. A statistically significant improvement in survival for women diagnosed with HHT or PAVM before pregnancy was noted.[12] In a separate study of 244 pregnancies in 87 women with HHT, 7 complications secondary to PAVMs were reported, including hemothorax, transient ischemic attack (TIA), myocardial infarction, and myocardial ischemia. Notably, all of the complications occurred in women who had not had screening or been treated for PAVMs. Most complications related to PAVMs have been reported in the second or third trimester, likely due to the increased maternal blood volume and cardiac output.[9]

Although cerebral AVMs (CAVMs)[13] and hepatic AVMs[14] are more prevalent in women with HHT, the risk of associated pregnancy complications seems to be low with only a few case reports in the literature.[8,12] Women who have had a previous CAMV rupture may be at increased risk for rebleeding during the second and third trimester of pregnancy. Spinal cord AVMs are rare in HHT[7]; however, some providers are hesitant to provide local anesthesia during labor given concern for potential spinal involvement.[9]

Pregnancy Management

Pregnancies in women with HHT should be managed by a multidisciplinary team, including obstetricians, pulmonologists, neurovascular specialists, anesthesiologists, and interventional radiologists. Consensus guidelines for the management of pregnant patients with HHT are not available. Clinical management guidelines based on expert opinion have been suggested.[12] Pregnancy-related risks and management recommendations for women with HHT are outlined in **Table 4**.

Severe epistaxis can lead to iron-deficient anemia. Conservative management for epistaxis includes the use of humidifiers and nasal lubricants. Refractory cases may require additional procedures.[7]

Recommendations for screening asymptomatic patients during pregnancy vary. Some experts stress that screening should be completed before conception to optimize outcomes and that asymptomatic patients should not undergo screening during pregnancy.[12] However, as some patients present for the first time during pregnancy, it may be necessary to offer additional screening. de Gussem and colleagues[9] suggest screening in the early second trimester with arterial blood gas analysis and transthoracic contrast echocardiography with follow-up chest CT for abnormal findings. If significant pulmonary AVMs are identified on CT, they recommend limited pulmonary angiography with embolization. Women with small AVMs are followed with arterial blood gas analysis in the second and third trimester to monitor for worsening hypoxemia, which would prompt a CT and treatment if indicated.

Screening for cerebral AVMs with MRI can be considered in the second or third trimester or delayed until after delivery. Delivery management for women identified to have a CAVM should be made in consultation with a neurosurgeon. Some experts argue that spinal AVM should be excluded by MRI.[12] However, others suggest MRI screening should be optional and that local anesthesia should be considered on a case-by-case basis given the low incidence of spinal AVMs in patients with HHT.[9]

Risk Assessment and Genetic Counseling

HHT is inherited in an autosomal dominant manner. Therefore, the offspring of an affected parent have a 1 in 2 (50%) chance of inheriting the condition. HHT is a highly variable condition, even within families, making it difficult to predict the phenotype prenatally.[7]

Prenatal and preimplantation genetic testing are technically feasible if a mutation has been identified in the family. However, the decision to undergo prenatal genetic testing is very personal and should be based on each individual patient's goals. Patients should be referred for formal genetic counseling to discuss the benefits and limitations of genetic testing.

TUBEROUS SCLEROSIS COMPLEX

Tuberous sclerosis complex (TSC) is an autosomal dominant, highly variable, multisystem disease involving the skin, brain, kidney, heart, and lungs. The condition is characterized by the growth of benign lesions that can disrupt normal functions leading to an increased risk of seizures, arrhythmias, renal failure, and lung disease. TSC occurs in approximately 1 in 6000 to 1 in 10,00 livebirths.[15]

Approximately 75% to 90% of patients with TSC will have a mutation in the *TSC1* or *TSC2* gene.[16] Hamartin and tuberin are the gene products of *TSC1* and *TSC2*, respectively. The two proteins form a heterodimer and control cell growth and proliferation through inhibition of the mammalian target of rapamycin (mTOR) pathway.[17] Mutations in the *TSC2* gene tend to be associated with a more severe phenotype, including younger age at presentation, seizures, and intellectual disability.[18]

Given the highly variable nature of this disease, diagnosis can be challenging. Diagnostic criteria have been developed based on genetic testing and the presence of major or minor criteria[6] (**Table 2**). TSC demonstrates age-dependent manifestations. In infancy and childhood, individuals are more likely to present with cardiac rhabdomyomas, brain hamartomas, and seizures. Characteristic skin lesions and TSC-associated neuropsychiatric disorders, including autism spectrum disorders, intellectual disabilities, psychiatric disorders, and neuropsychological deficits, may present throughout patients' lifetime. However, renal manifestations, such as angiomyolipomas, and the lung disease, lymphangioleiomyomatosis (LAM), are more likely to present in adulthood.[15]

mTOR inhibitors are a new oral medication that have been shown to reduce the growth of TSC-associated lesions. They are now considered the first-line therapy for asymptomatic angiomyolipomas measuring greater than 3 cm in diameter and can be used in patients with LAM who have moderate to severe lung disease.[19]

Pregnancy in Women with Tuberous Sclerosis Complex

Patients with TSC with a high disease burden, including those with significant TSC-associated neuropsychiatric disorders, may not reproduce. However, the phenotypic spectrum of TSC varies and can also present with milder features that are less life limiting. There are case reports of women diagnosed with TSC only after the birth of

Table 2	
Diagnostic criteria for tuberous sclerosis complex	
Genetic diagnostic criteria Identification of a pathogenic mutation in *TSC1* or *TSC2* is sufficient to make a definitive diagnosis of TSC Clinical diagnostic criteria Definite diagnosis: 2 major features or 1 major feature with >2 minor features Possible diagnosis: either 1 major feature or ≥2 minor features	
Major features	• Hypomelanotic macules (≥3, at least 5-mm diameter) • Angiofibromas (≥3) or fibrous cephalic plaque • Ungual fibromas (≥2) • Shagreen patch • Multiple retinal hamartomas • Cortical dysplasias • Subependymal nodules • Subependymal giant cell astrocytoma • Cardiac rhabdomyoma • Lymphangioleiomyomatosis • Angiomyolipomas (≥2)
Minor features	• Confetti skin lesions • Dental enamel pits (>3) • Intraoral fibromas (≥2) • Retinal achromic patch • Multiple renal cysts • Nonrenal hamartomas

Adapted from Northrup H, Krueger DA, International Tuberous Sclerosis Complex Consensus Group. Tuberous sclerosis complex diagnostic criteria update: recommendations of the 2012 international tuberous sclerosis complex consensus conference. Pediatr Neurol 2013;49(4):244; with permission.

affected children.[20] Current publications of pregnancy in women with TSC are limited to case reports and literature reviews.

King and Stamilio[20] completed a systematic review of TSC in pregnancy. They identified 23 pregnancies in 17 women with TSC. Complications were noted in 10 out of 23 (43%) pregnancies, including preeclampsia, oligohydramnios, polyhydramnios, intrauterine growth restriction, hemorrhage from ruptured angiomyolipomas, premature rupture of membranes, renal failure, placental abruption, and perinatal demise. Perinatal complications were found in all five of the women who had TSC-associated renal disease. No maternal deaths were reported. The authors concluded that pregnancies in women with TSC are at high risk for adverse outcomes.

Angiomyolipomas and LAM are 2 findings in TSC that can be associated with adverse outcomes in pregnancy. Angiomyolipomas are benign mesothelial tumors made up of mature adipose tissue, blood vessels, and smooth muscle cells that are observed in 80% of TSC patients.[16] They are typically asymptomatic, but can present with abdominal pain, hypotension, and shock secondary to rupture. It has been suggested that there is an increased risk of rupture during pregnancy.[21] LAM is a rare cystic lung disease that affects up to 80% of women with TSC.[22] It is characterized by smooth muscle cells infiltrating and destroying normal lung tissue. Patients typically present with dyspnea on exertion and multiple pneumothoraces.[16] It has been suggested that LAM may worsen during pregnancy secondary to the effects of estrogen.[23]

Fetuses affected with TSC are also at an increased risk for complications. Cardiac rhabdomyomas can be a presenting feature in TSC and may be diagnosed prenatally.

Although many rhabdomyomas will regress postnatally, they are associated with fetal dysrhythmias and the development of hydrops. In one case series of 37 cases of fetal cardiac rhabdomyomas associated with TSC, there were 6 cases of perinatal demise that were all preceded by in utero hydrops.[20]

Pregnancy Management

Consensus guidelines of the management of individuals with TSC do not provide guidance for pregnancy management.[19] Pregnancy management should include a multidisciplinary team given the multisystem nature of TSC and may include obstetrics, nephrology, neurology, pulmonology, intervention radiology, and anesthesiology. Pregnancy-related risks and management recommendations for women with TSC are outlined in **Table 4**.

In individuals with TSC, angiomyolipomas should be monitored every 1 to 3 years by MRI and renal function and blood pressure should be checked annually.[19] There are no specific recommendations for screening for angiomyolipomas during pregnancy. A ruptured angiomyolipoma should be high on the differential for pregnant women with TSC who present with acute-onset abdominal pain, hypotension, or shock. The first-line treatment of hemorrhaging angiomyolipoma is embolization followed by corticosteroids.[19] Referral to nephrology should be made if renal dysfunction is noted. Continued follow-up with nephrology postpartum is indicated, as patients with renal lesions associated with TSC are at risk of developing renal failure.

TSC management guidelines do not make recommendations on screening for LAM during pregnancy; however, it is recommended that asymptomatic patients have screening with high-resolution CT (HRCT) every 5 to 10 years.[19] Pregnant women who present with worsening dyspnea or recurrent pneumothoraces may need further evaluation, imaging, and referral to a pulmonologist.

Medications used to treat TSC may not be safe in pregnancy. mTOR inhibitors are a relatively new class of medication, so teratogenic effects are not well established. There are case reports of normal fetal outcomes, but the number of pregnancies limit the ability to generalize these results.[24] Certain antiepileptic medications are known to be associated with an increased risk for congenital anomalies, including open neural tube defects and cardiac anomalies.[25] Reviewing all medications before conception or early in pregnancy is recommended.

Targeted anatomic survey and fetal echocardiogram is warranted to evaluate for cardiac rhabdomyoma, which would be diagnostic of fetal TSC. Fetuses diagnosed with cardiac rhabdomyoma should have increased surveillance given the increased risk for the development of hydrops.[26] Weekly ultrasounds to screen for hydrops can be considered after a diagnosis of a fetal cardiac rhabdomyoma. The optimal gestational age to begin screening for hydrops depends on the family's wishes for intervention and resuscitation. Fetal MRI can be considered to further evaluate for brain lesions. Fetuses identified to have significant brain findings may be at an increased risk of seizures and intellectual disability. Prenatal consultation with a pediatric neurologist can be considered for a discussion of prognosis.

Risk Assessment and Genetic Counseling

Approximately 66% of cases of TSC result from a de novo mutation; of those that are inherited, TSC demonstrates an autosomal dominant pattern of inheritance.[15] Women with TSC have a 50% (1 in 2) chance of passing on the condition to their offspring.

Preimplantation genetic diagnosis and prenatal diagnosis with chorionic villus sampling (CVS) or amniocentesis is available if the mutation has been detected in the family. As discussed previously, imaging studies can also evaluate for features suggestive of TSC in the fetus. Fetal cardiac rhabdomyoma is diagnostic for fetal TSC in an at-risk pregnancy. Patients should be referred to genetic counseling to review the available testing options.

MYOTONIC DYSTROPHY

Myotonic dystrophy is an autosomal dominant multisystem neuromuscular disorder associated with slowly progressive muscle weakness and myotonia, or sustained muscle contractions. There are 2 types of myotonic dystrophy, myotonic dystrophy type 1 (DM1) and myotonic dystrophy type 2 (DM2). For this review, the authors focus on DM1, as it is the most common form of muscular dystrophy affecting pregnant women.[27] It is estimated that DM1 has a prevalence of between 3 and 10 per 100,000 live births.[28]

DM1 is a triplet repeat disorder caused by expansion of CTG repeats in the 3′ untranslated region of the *DMPK* gene. The diagnosis of DM1 is based on the finding of repeat length greater than 50 CTGs. Genotype-phenotype correlations have been established with larger repeat lengths associated with an earlier age of onset and a more severe clinical presentation (**Table 3**).[29] DM1 also demonstrates anticipation, with more significant clinical disease in successive generations due to expansion of CTG repeats. The most severe presentation, congenital myotonic dystrophy, is almost exclusively due to a maternally inherited repeat expansion.[30]

The clinical features of DM1 are variable and described along a continuum of 3 major types based on repeat length (see **Table 3**): mild, classic, and congenital.[29] Patients with mild DM1 typically have cataracts and mild myotonia with a normal life span. Patients with classic DM1 have cataracts, muscle weakness, myotonia, and cardiac conduction abnormalities. This type can be associated with physical limitations and a shortened life span. Congenital DM1, the most severe presentation, is characterized by severe generalized weakness, hypotonia, and respiratory insufficiency at birth. It is also associated with intellectual disability and early death.[31]

Table 3		
Genotype-phenotype correlations in myotonic dystrophy type 1		
Phenotype	**Clinical Features**[a]	**CTG Repeat Length**
Normal (unaffected)	None	5–34
Premutation	None	35–49
Mild	Cataracts Mild myotonia	50–150
Classic	Weakness Myotonia Cataracts Cardiac arrhythmia	100–1000
Congenital	Infantile hypotonia Respiratory difficulties Intellectual disability	>1000

[a] There is significant overlap of phenotypes and CTG repeats, making predictions of age of onset and severity for individual patients challenging.

Data from The International Myotonic Dystrophy Consortium (IDMC). New nomenclature and DNA testing guidelines for myotonic dystrophy type 1 (DM1). Neurology 2000;54(6):1218–1221.

Pregnancy in Women with Myotonic Dystrophy Type 1

Pregnancies in women with DM1 are considered to be high risk. Women with classic DM1 are more likely to have pregnancy complications than women with mild disease.[32] Available information regarding pregnancy outcomes is limited to small retrospective case series and literature reviews.

Two case series of women with DM1 reported that rates of miscarriage were not increased over the background population risk.[32,33] A registry-based study reported a higher rate of miscarriages (32.0% vs 16.9%) in women with DM1 as well as increased use of assistive reproductive technology, as compared with the general population.[34] Ectopic pregnancies were increased in one case series, which may represent impaired tube mobility.[32]

An increased rate of severe urinary tract infections during pregnancy has been noted, with rates between 9%[33] and 13%[32] of pregnancies. Some experts have hypothesized that this may be secondary to subtle pelvic floor muscle weakness in women with DM1.[35]

Polyhydramnios has been reported with a frequency of 10% to 20% but is exclusively seen in pregnancies affected by congenital myotonic dystrophy secondary to impaired fetal swallowing. Higher rates of stillbirth and neonatal deaths[32] are also attributed to fetuses affected with congenital myotonic dystrophy.

Uterine muscle abnormities have been suggested as a cause of pregnancy complications in women with DM1. An increased risk for placenta previa and abnormal vaginal bleeding has been noted, with a 10-fold increase more than the general population.[32,33] Prolonged labor due to uterine dysfunction and maternal weakness has been implicated as the reason for an increased rate of cesarean deliveries, instrumental deliveries, and nonvertex presentations. Increased rates of postpartum hemorrhage due to uterine atony or abnormal placentation have also been reported.[32,33]

Preterm birth, defined as delivery before 37 weeks' gestation, is more common in women with DM1 with rates reported at 34%,[32] 36.7%,[33] and 31%[34] compared with the baseline US population risk of 10%. Rudnik-Schöneborn and Zerres[32] reported that 15% to 20% of pregnancies delivered before 34 weeks' gestation, late preterm deliveries (34–37 weeks' gestation) occurred in about one-third of births, and only about half reached full term (after 37 weeks' gestation).

Johnson and colleagues[34] conducted a registry-based study to investigate the impact of pregnancy on women with myotonic dystrophy. Women with DM1 reported a significant increase in the impact of mobility limitations, activity limitations, pain, emotional issues, and myotonia from before pregnancy to after pregnancy. Although these results may suggest that pregnancy may lead to disease progression, this study relied on retrospective data and there was selection bias based on a low response rate of women with DM1 recruited through patient registries.

Pregnancy Management

The European Neuromuscular Center published recommendations for the management of pregnancy in women with neuromuscular disorders, including DM1.[36] They stress the importance of a multidisciplinary approach to the care of these women, which should include providers in obstetrics, neurology, anesthesiology, and genetics. Pregnancy-related risks and management recommendations for women with DM1 are outlined in **Table 4**.

Women with DM1 should plan to receive prenatal care and deliver at tertiary care centers given the increased risk for abnormal placentation, labor abnormalities, and

Table 4
Risks and management recommendations for specific genetic disorders

Genetic Condition	Pregnancy-Related Risks	Management Recommendations

HHT	• Increased episodes of epistaxis
	• Development of new skin and mucosa telangiectasias
	• Increased risk of hemorrhage from pulmonary AVMs
		Recommendations based on expert opinion[9,12]
		• PAVMs
		  ○ Preconception screening with chest CT and treatment if indicated
		  ○ Consider screening during pregnancy, if no previous screening completed
		  ○ Educate patients on concerning signs or symptoms, including hemoptysis and sudden, severe dyspnea
		• Cerebral AVM
		  ○ Cerebral MRI for women with family history of cerebral hemorrhage or symptoms
		  ○ No asymptomatic screening during pregnancy
		• Spinal AVM
		  ○ Consider spinal MRI to exclude spinal AMV
		• Delivery
		  ○ Provide prophylactic antibiotics
		  ○ Avoid prolonged second-stage labor when cerebral AVM has not been excluded
		• Genetic counseling

TSC	• Rupture and hemorrhage from renal angiomyolipomas • Dyspnea from lymphangioleiomyomatosis • Increased risk of preeclampsia • Teratogenic effects from commonly used medications • Fetal complications: preterm delivery, fetal growth restriction, preterm premature rupture of membranes	Recommendations based on expert opinion[20] • Referral to nephrologist if renal dysfunction noted • Referral to pulmonologist if worsening dyspnea or multiple pneumothoraces present • Review all medications for teratogenicity • Targeted ultrasound, fetal echocardiogram for evaluation of cardiac rhabdomyoma • Consider fetal MRI • Consider increased antenatal surveillance if concern for fetal TSC • Genetic counseling

Myotonic dystrophy	• Abnormal uterine muscle function leading to
	  ○ Increased risk of placenta previa, intrauterine and postpartum hemorrhage
	  ○ Increased rate of cesarean deliveries and instrumental deliveries
		Recommendations based on expert opinion[32,36]
		• Prenatal care and delivery at tertiary care center
		• Ultrasound to assess placental location
		• Consultation with anesthesiology

(continued on next page)

Table 4 (continued)		
Genetic Condition	**Pregnancy-Related Risks**	**Management Recommendations**
	• Increased rate of preterm delivery • Higher rate of complicated urinary tract infections • Anesthesia complications • Fetal complications: congenital DM, polyhydramnios, decreased fetal movement	• Regular maternal electrocardiogram screening, consider echocardiogram • Routine antenatal testing with increased surveillance if polyhydramnios is noted • Delivery ○ Cesarean delivery for routine obstetric indications • Genetic counseling
OTC deficiency	Increased risk for hyperammonemic episode in postpartum period	Recommendations based on expert opinion[46,52] • Baseline ammonia and plasmas amino acid levels • Referral to metabolic dietician to assure adequate oral intake • Maintenance fluids with 10% dextrose to avoid catabolism during labor and delivery • Monitor ammonia levels every 6 h during hospital course • Initiate therapy when ammonia levels are 1.5–2.0 times normal • Monitoring postpartum patients for 72 h with close follow-up as outpatient • Genetic counseling

complicated urinary tract infections. Additionally, some women with DM1 may have some associated cognitive delays that may limit their ability to understand risks, so close medical guidance is important.[32]

DM1 is associated with an increased risk for conduction disorders and arrhythmias, although the risk seems to be higher in men. A 2012 meta-analysis assessing the cardiac risks in patients with DM1 reported the risk for sudden cardiac death to be 0.56% per year.[37] Given this risk, echocardiogram and electrocardiogram screening may be warranted in pregnancy.[32]

Consultation with anesthesia is warranted for patients with significant muscle weakness to allow thoughtful planning for anesthetic needs during labor and delivery. Patients with DM1 may be at an increased risk for aspiration, excessive response to anesthetics, and increased myotonia with certain anesthetic agents.[38]

Risk Assessment and Genetic Counseling

DM1 is inherited in an autosomal dominant pattern. Offspring of affected individuals have a 50% (1 in 2) chance of inheriting the abnormal gene. An expanded DMPK gene has the potential to expand further during gametogenesis, resulting in children with earlier onset and more severe disease.[39] As noted previously, maternal transmission of the expansion of repeats may lead to congenital myotonic dystrophy. Cobo and colleagues[40] reported that the risk of congenital myotonic dystrophy increased with repeat length. Women with a CTG repeat less than 300 had a 10% risk of having a child with congenital myotonic dystrophy, whereas women with CTG repeat greater than 300 had a 59% risk for having an affected child.

Genetic testing for DM1 can be completed with prenatal genetic testing of the *DMPK* gene through CVS or amniocentesis. Preimplantation genetic testing is also an option for patients. Women with DM1 should be referred for genetic counseling to review the risks and testing options. Polyhydramnios and reduced fetal movement is suggestive of a diagnosis of congenital DM1 in an at-risk pregnancy.

ORNITHINE TRANSCARBAMOYLASE DEFICIENCY

Ornithine transcarbamylase deficiency (OTC) deficiency is an X-linked urea cycle disorder, a group of disorders caused by enzyme deficiencies that prevent the appropriate conversion of waste nitrogen to urea, leading to accumulation of toxic ammonia. In the most severe cases, urea cycle disorders present as encephalopathy and coma secondary to hyperammonemia.[41] OTC deficiency is the most common of the urea cycle disorders and is caused by a deficiency of the enzyme OTC (**Fig. 1**). Recent estimates suggest the overall birth prevalence for urea cycle disorders in the

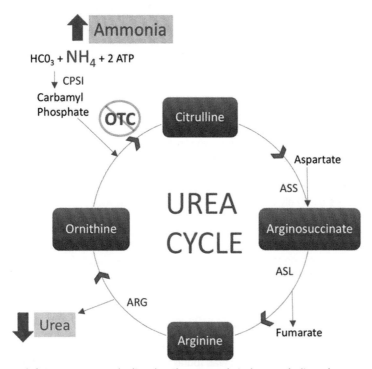

Fig. 1. OTC deficiency: a urea cycle disorder. The urea cycle is the metabolic pathway responsible for detoxification of excess and waste nitrogen. With each turn of the cycle, 2 nitrogen atoms are converted to urea, which can be safely excreted by the kidneys. Deficiency of the OTC enzyme, which catalyzes the production of citrulline from ornithine and carbamyl phosphate, prevents the formation of urea and leads to an accumulation of ammonium (NH_4). Systemic alkalosis converts NH_4 to the more toxic form, ammonia (NH_3). High levels of NH_3 are toxic to the brain and lead to the symptoms seen in OTC deficiency, including confusion, brain edema, and coma. ARG, arginase; ASL, argininosuccinate lyase; ASS, argininosuccinate synthase; CPSI, carbamoyl-phosphate synthase 1; HCO_3, bicarbonate.

United States is 1 in 35,000 and for OTC deficiencies the birth prevalence was estimated at 1 in 63,000 live births.[41]

OTC deficiency is caused by mutations in the *OTC* gene, which is located on the X-chromosome. Severe OTC deficiency typically affects boys who present within the first week of life with hyperammonemic coma. Milder symptoms or later age of presentation can also be seen in boys with partial enzyme activity.[42] Presenting symptoms can include nausea, vomiting, lethargy, confusion, ataxia, seizure, coma, and cerebral edema.

The phenotype of carrier females is highly variable, ranging from asymptomatic to neurologic compromise secondary to hyperammonemia. It has been hypothesized that the degree of symptoms is related to the level of skewed X-inactivation within the liver.[43] Catabolic states, which lead to an increase breakdown of protein and nitrogen release, cause elevated levels of ammonia. Various triggers have been implicated for hyperammonemic episodes in female carriers of OTC deficiency, including infection, surgery, trauma, decreased oral intake, and high protein intake. Symptomatic female carriers are typically treated with low-protein diets with amino acid supplementations in addition to sodium benzoate to assist with nitrogen excretion.

Pregnancy in Female Carriers of Ornithine Transcarbamoylase Deficiency

Most female carriers of OTC deficiency have uneventful pregnancies. However, they are at risk of hyperammonemic episodes during times of catabolic stress, including labor and delivery and the postpartum period. Data regarding pregnancies in women with OTC deficiency are limited to single case reports, small case series, and literature reviews.

Most studies suggest that the period associated with the highest risk for acute decompensation is between postpartum day 3 and 14.[44–46] Although the exact cause of postpartum hyperammonemia is not well understood, it is hypothesized that it may be secondary to increased protein catabolism that occurs with involution of the uterus.[46] Arn and colleagues[45] first reported adverse outcomes in women with OTC deficiency. Their case series included 2 known OTC carriers and one previously healthy woman who all developed hyperammonemic comas between postpartum days 3 and 8. Two of the women died secondary to cerebral edema. Many of the original case series are likely biased toward adverse outcomes.

Pregnancy is thought to be protective against the effects of hyperammonemic episodes secondary to the increased nitrogen needs of the placenta and fetus.[44] However, there have been case reports of hyperammonemic crisis in pregnancy. Schimanski and colleagues[47] reported the case of a previously healthy woman who presented with confusion and hyperemesis gravidarum at 14 weeks' gestation. Given concerns for malnutrition, she was treated with total parenteral nutrition (TPN) and 3 days later developed signs of encephalopathy and coma and subsequently died. The investigators conclude that the high protein load from TPN triggered the hyperammonemic episode. Lipskind and colleagues[48] reported the case of a known OTC carrier who was treated with corticosteroids for presumed preterm labor and subsequently became unresponsive and was found to be hyperammonemic. The investigators speculated that the corticosteroids in addition to low oral intake triggered an endogenous breakdown of protein, leading to hyperammonemia. The patient was treated with benzoate and a protein-restricted diet and her condition improved.

Maestri and colleagues[49] reported on a series of 175 women from 89 families with a family history of OTC deficiency. In their cohort, they identified 76 female carriers of OTC deficiency. Female carriers were more likely to report protein-restricted diets. Four women reported a personal history of coma, none of which occurred during the peripartum period. Among the 76 carriers, there were 260 pregnancies reported with no significant differences in fertility, number of miscarriages, or complications in pregnancies compared with the noncarrier women. However, limited data are presented about pregnancy outcomes. The investigators concluded that hyperammonemic encephalopathy is an uncommon finding in asymptomatic carriers of OTC deficiency but stressed the importance of educating women of this potential complication during times of physiologic stress.

Langendonk and colleagues[50] reported on a series of pregnancies in women with inborn errors of metabolism, including one full-term pregnancy in a woman with known OTC deficiency. The patient was treated with a protein-restricted diet with amino acid supplementation, sodium benzoate 6 g daily, citrulline 5 g daily, calcium 500 mg daily, folic acid 1 mg daily, and vitamin B6 100 mg daily and low-molecular-weight heparin. She reportedly had several episodes of elevated ammonia levels without significant clinical sequelae during pregnancy, triggered by a respiratory tract infection and nonadherence to her protein-restricted diet and amino acid supplementation. Her supplements were adjusted and her ammonia levels stabilized. She had mild hyperammonemia on postpartum day 1 and 3 and a sudden increase in ammonia at postpartum day 11, which was associated with agitation. She was treated with sodium benzoate and protein restriction and made a complete recovery. Additional case reports of women with known OTC deficiency carrier status have shown favorable outcomes when ammonia levels are monitored, allowing for early treatment and avoidance of a hyperammonemic coma.[44,46,51] These cases highlight the importance of a well-established management plan.

Pregnancy Management

Guidelines for the management of pregnancy in female carriers are based on expert opinion. Pregnancies in female carriers of OTC deficiency should be managed by a multidisciplinary team, including obstetricians, geneticists, metabolic dieticians, and anesthesiologists. Pregnancy-related risks and management recommendations for women with OTC deficiency are outlined in **Table 4**.

Patients should have serum ammonia levels and plasma amino acids drawn at the time of routine prenatal laboratory tests. Women should also be counseled on the importance of adequate nutrition to avoid increased catabolism.[46] Women who have significant nausea and vomiting or infections leading to decreased oral intake may require more regular monitoring of ammonia levels.

Women with OTC deficiency tend to be on protein-restricted diets, which can increase the risk of fetal growth restriction. Formal evaluation by a metabolic dietician is warranted for women who have a challenge meeting appropriate oral intake goals.[52] Increased antenatal surveillance is warranted if fetal growth restriction is identified.

The use of maintenance fluids, specifically 10% dextrose, has been recommended during labor and delivery given the increased energy demands.[52] Some experts recommend checking plasma ammonium levels every 6 hours during the hospital course, with increased frequency if levels are abnormal.[46]

Therapy should be initiated when ammonium levels are 1.5 to 2.0 times greater than normal and should be completed in consultation with an expert in urea cycle disorders. Mendez-Figueroa and colleagues[46] recommend oral sodium benzoate at 5 g/m^2/d divided in 3 doses. Intravenous (IV) sodium phenyl-acetate and sodium benzoate at 5.5 g/m^2/d with IV arginine at 3.5 g/m^2/d in 24 hours should be initiated if patients are not tolerating oral intake or if ammonia levels are rapidly increasing. Hemodialysis may be required if the ammonia levels do not decrease or rapidly increase to greater than 250 mg/dL.

Women should be monitored in the hospital for at least 72 hours after delivery, and close follow-up in an outpatient metabolic clinic should be recommended.

Risk Assessment for Offspring and Potential Prenatal Testing Options

OTC deficiency is inherited in an X-linked manner. A female carrier has a 50% (1 in 2) risk of passing the mutated gene to her offspring. Male children who inherit the mutation will be affected, whereas female children may develop symptoms or may remain asymptomatic. Affected male infants with severe OTC deficiency appear normal at birth but present within the first days of life with lethargy leading to a hyperammonemic coma. Surviving infants are at an increased risk for developmental delays and often require liver transplantation.[41] Individuals with partial OTC deficiency, which can include males and females, may present with hyperammonemic episodes from infancy to adulthood.[53]

Preimplantation genetic diagnosis or prenatal genetic testing through CVS or amniocentesis are available when the mutation has been identified in the family. Women should be referred for genetic counseling to review available testing options.

SUMMARY

Improvements in medical care for women with genetic disorders has led to an increased number of women reaching reproductive age. Preconception counseling regarding pregnancy-associated risks and genetic testing options should be made available to all women with genetic disorders.

Outcomes of pregnancies in rare genetic conditions are mainly limited to case reports, small case series, and literature reviews. Although these publications provide valuable information to obstetricians caring for women with genetic disorders, additional research is needed to better characterize pregnancy outcomes. Patient registries and continued publications of cases are needed to allow for the development of pregnancy management guidelines.

REFERENCES

1. Chetty S, Norton ME. Obstetric care in women with genetic disorders. Best Pract Res Clin Obstet Gynaecol 2017;42:86–99.
2. Guttmacher AE, Marchuk DA, White RI. Hereditary hemorrhagic telangiectasia. N Engl J Med 1995;333(14):918–24.
3. McDonald J, Bayrak-Toydemir P, Pyeritz RE. Hereditary hemorrhagic telangiectasia: an overview of diagnosis, management, and pathogenesis. Genet Med 2011; 13(7):607–16.
4. Richards-Yutz J, Grant K, Chao EC, et al. Update on molecular diagnosis of hereditary hemorrhagic telangiectasia. Hum Genet 2010;128(1):61–77.
5. Wooderchak-Donahue WL, McDonald J, O'Fallon B, et al. BMP9 mutations cause a vascular-anomaly syndrome with phenotypic overlap with hereditary hemorrhagic telangiectasia. Am J Hum Genet 2013;93(3):530–7.
6. Shovlin CL, Guttmacher AE, Buscarini E, et al. Diagnostic criteria for hereditary hemorrhagic telangiectasia (Rendu-Osler-Weber syndrome). Am J Med Genet 2000;91:66–7.
7. Faughnan ME, Palda VA, Garcia-Tsao G, et al. International guidelines for the diagnosis and management of hereditary haemorrhagic telangiectasia. J Med Genet 2011;48(2):73–87.
8. Shovlin CL, Winstock AR, Peters AM, et al. Medical complications of pregnancy in hereditary haemorrhagic telangiectasia. QJM 1995;88:879–87.
9. de Gussem EM, Lausman AY, Beder AJ, et al. Outcomes of pregnancy in women with hereditary hemorrhagic telangiectasia. Obstet Gynecol 2014;123(3):514–20.

10. Cottin V, Plauchu H, Bayle JY, et al. Pulmonary arteriovenous malformations in patients with hereditary hemorrhagic telangiectasia. Am J Respir Crit Care Med 2004;169(9):994–1000.

11. Shovlin CL, Jackson JE, Bamford KB, et al. Primary determinants of ischaemic stroke/brain abscess risks are independent of severity of pulmonary arteriovenous malformations in hereditary haemorrhagic telangiectasia. Thorax 2008; 63(3):259–66.

12. Shovlin CL, Sodhi V, McCarthy A, et al. Estimates of maternal risks of pregnancy for women with hereditary haemorrhagic telangiectasia (Osler-Weber-Rendu syndrome): suggested approach for obstetric services. BJOG 2008;115(9):1108–15.

13. Brinjikji W, Iyer VN, Wood CP, et al. Prevalence and characteristics of brain arteriovenous malformations in hereditary hemorrhagic telangiectasia: a systematic review and meta-analysis. J Neurosurg 2016;1–9. https://doi.org/10.3171/2016. 7.JNS16847.

14. Buscarini E, Plauchu H, Garcia Tsao G, et al. Liver involvement in hereditary hemorrhagic telangiectasia: consensus recommendations. Liver Int 2006;26(9): 1040–6.

15. Curatolo P, Bombardieri R, Jozwiak S. Tuberous sclerosis. Lancet 2008; 372(9639):657–68.

16. Northrup H, Krueger DA, International Tuberous Sclerosis Complex Consensus Group. Tuberous sclerosis complex diagnostic criteria update: recommendations of the 2012 international tuberous sclerosis complex consensus conference. Pediatr Neurol 2013;49(4):243–54.

17. van Slegtenhorst M, Nellist M, Nagelkerken B, et al. Interaction between hamartin and tuberin, the TSC1 and TSC2 gene products. Hum Mol Genet 1998;7(6): 1053–7.

18. Kothare SV, Singh K, Chalifoux JR, et al. Severity of manifestations in tuberous sclerosis complex in relation to genotype. Epilepsia 2014;55(7):1025–9.

19. Krueger DA, Northrup H, International Tuberous Sclerosis Complex Consensus Group. Tuberous sclerosis complex surveillance and management: recommendations of the 2012 International tuberous sclerosis complex consensus conference. Pediatr Neurol 2013;49(4):255–65.

20. King JA, Stamilio DM. Maternal and fetal tuberous sclerosis complicating pregnancy: a case report and overview of the literature. Am J Perinatol 2005;22(02): 103–8.

21. Zapardiel I, Delafuente-Valero J, Bajo-Arenas JM. Renal angiomyolipoma during pregnancy: review of the literature. Gynecol Obstet Invest 2011;72(4):217–9.

22. Cudzilo CJ, Szczesniak RD, Brody AS, et al. Lymphangioleiomyomatosis screening in women with tuberous sclerosis. Chest 2013;144(2):578–85.

23. McCartney R, Facey N, Chalmers G, et al. Multiple pneumothoraces during second and third trimesters as first presentation of lymphangioleiomyomatosis. Obstet Med 2009;2(2):84–6.

24. Yamamura M, Kojima T, Koyama M, et al. Everolimus in pregnancy: case report and literature review. J Obstet Gynaecol Res 2017;43(8):1350–2.

25. Bromley RL, Baker GA. Fetal antiepileptic drug exposure and cognitive outcomes. Seizure 2017;44:225–31.

26. Isaacs H. Perinatal (fetal and neonatal) tuberous sclerosis: a review. Am J Perinatol 2009;26(10):755–60.

27. Esplin MS, Hallam S, Farrington PF, et al. Myotonic dystrophy is a significant cause of idiopathic polyhydramnios. Am J Obstet Gynecol 1998;179(4):974–7.

28. Turner C, Hilton-Jones D. Myotonic dystrophy. Curr Opin Neurol 2014;27(5): 599–606.
29. The International Myotonic Dystropy Consortium (IDMC). New nomenclature and DNA testing guidelines for myotonic dystrophy type 1 (DM1). Neurology 2000;54: 1218–21.
30. Barbé L, Lanni S, López-Castel A, et al. CpG methylation, a parent-of-origin effect for maternal-biased transmission of congenital myotonic dystrophy. Am J Hum Genet 2017;100(3):488–505.
31. Udd B, Krahe R. The myotonic dystrophies: molecular, clinical, and therapeutic challenges. Lancet Neurol 2012;11(10):891–905.
32. Rudnik-Schöneborn S, Zerres K. Outcome in pregnancies complicated by myotonic dystrophy: a study of 31 patients and review of the literature. Eur J Obstet Gynecol Reprod Biol 2004;114(1):44–53.
33. Awater C, Zerres K, Rudnik-Schöneborn S. Pregnancy course and outcome in women with hereditary neuromuscular disorders: comparison of obstetric risks in 178 patients. Eur J Obstet Gynecol 2012;162(2):153–9.
34. Johnson NE, Hung M, Nasser E, et al. The impact of pregnancy on myotonic dystrophy: a registry-based study. J Neuromuscul Dis 2015;2(4):447–52.
35. Argov Z, de Visser M. What we do not know about pregnancy in hereditary neuromuscular disorders. Neuromuscul Disord 2009;19(10):675–9.
36. Norwood F, Rudnik-Schöneborn S. 179th ENMC international workshop: pregnancy in women with neuromuscular disorders: 5-7 November 2010, Naarden, The Netherlands. Neuromuscul Disord 2012;22(2):183–90.
37. Petri H, Vissing J, Witting N, et al. Cardiac manifestations of myotonic dystrophy type 1. Int J Cardiol 2012;160(2):82–8.
38. Hopkins AN, Alshaeri T, Akst SA, et al. Neurologic disease with pregnancy and considerations for the obstetric anesthesiologist. Semin Perinatol 2014;38(6): 359–69.
39. Harper PS, Harley HG, Reardon W, et al. Anticipation in myotonic dystrophy: new light on an old problem. Am J Hum Genet 1992;51:10–6.
40. Cobo AM, Poza JJ, Martorell L, et al. Contribution of molecular analyses to the estimation of the risk of congenital myotonic dystrophy. J Med Genet 2005;32: 105–8.
41. Batshaw ML, Tuchman M, Summar M, et al, Members of the Urea Cycle Disorders Consortium. A longitudinal study of urea cycle disorders. Mol Genet Metab 2014; 113(1–2):127–30.
42. Caldovic L, Abdikarim I, Narain S, et al. Genotype-phenotype correlations in ornithine transcarbamylase deficiency: a mutation update. J Genet Genomics 2015; 42(5):181–94.
43. Yorifuji T, Muroi J, Uematsu A, et al. X-inactivation pattern in the liver of a manifesting female with ornithine transcarbamylase. Clin Genet 1998;54:349–53.
44. Cordero DR, Baker J, Dorinzi D, et al. Ornithine transcarbamylase deficiency in pregnancy. J Inherit Metab Dis 2005;28:237–40.
45. Arn PH, Hauser ER, Thomas GH, et al. Hyperammonemia in women with a mutation at the ornithine carbamoyltransferase locus. A cause of postpartum coma. N Engl J Med 1990;322(23):1652–5.
46. Mendez-Figueroa H, Lamance K, Sutton V, et al. Management of ornithine transcarbamylase deficiency in pregnancy. Am J Perinatol 2010;27(10):775–84.
47. Schimanski U, Krieger D, Horn M, et al. A novel two-nucleotide deletion in the ornithine transcarbamylase gene causing fatal hyperammonia in early pregnancy. Hepatology 1998;24(6):1413–5.

48. Lipskind S, Loanzon S, Simi E, et al. Hyperammonemic coma in an ornithine trans-carbamylase mutation carrier following antepartum corticosteroids. J Perinatol 2011;31(10):682–4.

49. Maestri NE, Lord C, Glynn M, et al. The phenotype of ostensibly healthy women who are carriers for ornithine transcarbamylase deficiency. Medicine 1998;77: 387–97.

50. Langendonk JG, Roos JC, Angus L, et al. A series of pregnancies in women with inherited metabolic disease. J Inherit Metab Dis 2011;35(3):419–24.

51. Lamb S, Aye CYL, Murphy E, et al. Multidisciplinary management of ornithine transcarbamylase (OTC) deficiency in pregnancy: essential to prevent hyperammonemic complications. BMJ Case Rep 2013. https://doi.org/10.1136/bcr-2012-007416.

52. Murphy E. Pregnancy in women with inherited metabolic disease. Obstet Med 2015;8(2):61–7.

53. McCullough BA, Yudkoff M, Batshaw ML, et al. Genotype spectrum of ornithine transcarbamylase deficiency: correlation with the clinical and biochemical phenotype. Am J Med Genet 2000;93:313–9.

Maternal Congenital Heart Disease in Pregnancy

Megan E. Foeller, MD[a],*, Timothy M. Foeller, MD[b], Maurice Druzin, MD[a]

KEYWORDS

- Congenital heart disease • Pregnancy • Tetralogy of Fallot
- Transposition of great arteries • Pulmonary hypertension

KEY POINTS

- Most maternal heart diseases in pregnancy result from congenital heart disease.
- Pregnancy is contraindicated in certain cardiac conditions, such as dilated aortopathy, severe aortic stenosis, primary pulmonary hypertension, and severe mitral stenosis.
- Pregnancy can be safely accomplished in most individuals with careful risk assessment before conception and multidisciplinary care throughout pregnancy and the postpartum period.

INTRODUCTION

Maternal cardiac disease is present in 1% of the pregnant population,[1] most of which originates from congenital heart disease.[2] Global advances in recognizing and surgically correcting congenital heart disease has resulted in more women living to childbearing ages and the option to pursue future fertility. Despite these advances, pregnancy is often complicated in this population because of the profound physiologic hemodynamic changes associated with pregnancy. Cardiovascular disease has recently been identified as a leading cause of maternal mortality in the United States, although this increase is not primarily related to congenital cardiac disease.[3] Pregnancies complicated by cardiac conditions of any cause require coordinated, multidisciplinary care to achieve optimal outcomes. This approach should begin in the preconception period.

MATERNAL PHYSIOLOGIC CHANGES IN PREGNANCY

Normal physiologic alterations in pregnancy often result in significant hemodynamic changes to the cardiovascular system. By 24 weeks of pregnancy, maternal blood

Disclosure Statement: The authors have no disclosures.
[a] Obstetrics and Gynecology, Stanford University, Stanford Hospital, 300 Pasteur Drive, Room G302, 5317, Stanford, CA 94305-5317, USA; [b] Internal Medicine, Stanford Health Care–ValleyCare, 5555 West Positas Boulevard, 1 West Hospitalist Room 1, Pleasanton, CA 94588, USA
* Corresponding author.
E-mail address: mfoeller@stanford.edu

Obstet Gynecol Clin N Am 45 (2018) 267–280
https://doi.org/10.1016/j.ogc.2018.01.011
0889-8545/18/© 2018 Elsevier Inc. All rights reserved.

volume often increases by 40% and is accompanied by marked maternal systemic vasodilation.[2] In response to these profound changes, heart size expands by 30%, heart rate increases, and cardiac output increases by nearly 50%.[2]

Delivery poses a particularly challenging situation, as systolic and diastolic blood pressure increases; cardiac output may increase by 25% during active labor and 50% during the second stage with pushing.[2] Immediately post partum, an auto-transfusion of about 500 mL from the uterus into the systemic circulation occurs, resulting in an incremental increase in cardiac output following delivery of the placenta.[1,2]

These physiologic stressors are typically well tolerated by most women; however, they can pose a serious challenge for women with cardiac disorders and limited ability to adapt to significant hemodynamic changes.

GENERAL CONSIDERATIONS
Maternal Risk and Risk Stratification

Although most women with structural heart disease will tolerate pregnancy without major complications, this population remains at high risk for maternal, fetal, and neonatal adverse outcomes.[4] Complications tend to be lower for women with congenital heart disease when compared with acquired heart disease,[5] and as many as 25% of patients require hospitalization during pregnancy.[6] The most common cardiac events during pregnancy include atrial arrhythmia, heart failure, and ventricular arrhythmia.[2] The International Registry of Heart Disease in Pregnancy (ROPAC), with data on structural and ischemic heart disease, found a high rate of maternal heart failure, most often occurring around 31 weeks' gestation.[7] Cardiac-related medications were used in 32% of women in this registry, most commonly beta-blockers.[8] Patients with prior cardiac surgery, New York Heart Association (NYHA) classes I and II, and those on no medication tended to experience more favorable outcomes.[9]

Multiple classification and risk prediction models have been applied to maternal cardiac disease to aid clinicians in counseling and clinical management. The Cardiac Disease in Pregnancy (CARPREG) study prospectively enrolled 562 pregnant women with congenital or acquired cardiac disease and created a maternal cardiac risk index based on the history of arrhythmia, prior cardiac event, baseline NYHA functional class, cyanosis, and systemic heart obstruction.[10] The NYHA and World Health Organization (WHO) created 2 commonly used scoring systems in pregnancy. The NYHA risk classification system is based on functional status (**Table 1**), and the WHO risk classification integrates maternal cardiac risk factors with underlying cardiac disease (**Table 2**). Advancing WHO class has been clearly associated with increased maternal and fetal adverse outcomes.[9] In an analysis of the ROPAC database,

Table 1		
New York Heart Association classification system		
NYHA Class	**Functional Status**	**Pregnancy Risk Factor**
I	Asymptomatic	Expect favorable outcome
II	Symptoms with greater than normal activity	Expect favorable outcome
III	Symptoms with normal activity	Pregnancy not advised
IV	Symptoms at rest	Pregnancy not advised

Data from Simpson LL. Maternal cardiac disease: update for the clinician. Obstet Gynecol 2012;119(2 Pt 1):346.

Table 2
World Health Organization pregnancy risk

Risk Class	Maternal Congenital Cardiac Condition	Risk of Maternal Morbidity	Risk of Maternal Mortality
I	• Mild/uncomplicated pulmonary stenosis, PDA, mitral valve prolapse • Repaired ASD, VSD, PDA, anomalous pulmonary venous drainage • Isolated ectopic beats	None to small morbidity	None
II	• Repaired TOF • Most arrhythmias • Unrepaired ASD/VSD	Moderate morbidity	Small increase
II/III	• Mild left ventricular impairment • Hypertrophic cardiomyopathy • Marfan syndrome without aortic dilation • Aorta <45 mm (bicuspid aortic valve) • Repaired coarctation	—	—
III	• Mechanical valve • Systemic right ventricle • Fontan circulation • Unrepaired cyanotic heart disease • Aortic dilation 40–45 mm (Marfan) • Aortic dilation 45–50 mm (bicuspid aortic valve)	Severe morbidity	Significant increase
IV	• Pulmonary arterial hypertension • LVEF<30%, NYHA III–IV • History of PPCM with residual impairment • Severe mitral stenosis or aortic stenosis • Aortic dilation >45 mm (Marfan) • Aortic dilation >50 mm (bicuspid aortic valve) • Native severe coarctation	Severe morbidity, pregnancy contraindicated	Extreme increase, pregnancy contraindicated

Abbreviations: ASD, atrial septal defect; LVEF, left ventricular ejection fraction; PDA, patent ductus arteriosus; PPCM, peripartum cardiomyopathy; TOF, tetralogy of Fallot; VSD, ventricular septal defect.

Adapted from Thorne S, MacGregor A, Nelson-Piercy C. Risks of contraception and pregnancy in heart disease. Heart 2006;92(10):1521; with permission.

Pijuan-Domènech and colleagues[5] found that the modified version of the WHO classification was the best predictor of cardiac complications in pregnancies compared with other risk prediction models. Independent risk factors for adverse outcomes included ejection fraction of less than 40%[11] and an abnormal exercise stress test.[12] Certain structural heart conditions are associated with an unacceptably high risk of maternal mortality; therefore, pregnancy is contraindicated. These conditions include the following:

• Pulmonary arterial hypertension
• Marfan syndrome with aortic root measuring greater than 45 mm
• Bicuspid valve with aortic root measuring greater than 50 mm
• Severe mitral stenosis
• Severe symptomatic aortic stenosis

- Severe systemic ventricular dysfunction (left ventricular ejection fraction <30%, NYHA III–IV)[13]

Fetal and Neonatal Risk

Fetal and neonatal outcomes are closely correlated with the severity of the maternal congenital cardiac disease. Studies have demonstrated increased early pregnancy loss rates and intrauterine growth restriction during pregnancy.[6,14,15] Predictors of adverse neonatal outcomes include NYHA class greater than II, maternal cyanosis and left heart obstruction, and anticoagulant use.[11] Neonatal complication rates are estimated to be twice the general population, and as many as 25% of women will deliver small-for-gestational age neonates.[16]

Women with heart disease experience higher rates of preterm delivery, often as a result of medical indications.[16] Individualization of care and choice of route of delivery should be followed for each patient.[2]

Preconception Counseling and Management

Specific management recommendations often depend on the maternal cardiac structural anomaly and related complications, but general principles of management may guide care and optimize pregnancy outcomes.[17,18] Ideally, preconception consultation and coordinated multidisciplinary care to evaluate maternal status should be undertaken in all women for risk stratification and pregnancy planning. Unfortunately, this is often not possible, as 45% of all pregnancies in women with congenital cardiac disease are unplanned.[19]

Genetic counseling is of particular importance, as maternal congenital cardiac increases the risk of congenital heart disease in the offspring by 4% (if no chromosomal abnormality identified) to 50% based on the lesion and inheritance pattern.[20,21] The highest rates of transmission occur in autosomal dominant conditions, such as Marfan syndrome, Loeys-Dietz, and vascular Ehlers-Danlos.[22]

A thorough evaluation of maternal hemodynamic status should be performed for risk stratification. Most often, this evaluation includes echocardiogram, electrocardiogram, and exercise stress testing, with consideration for MRI and cardiac catheterization. Corrective surgery, if performed before conception, can often dramatically improve outcomes during pregnancy and may be recommended in certain clinical scenarios.

Antepartum Care

A coordinated multidisciplinary team consisting of cardiology, maternal fetal medicine, anesthesia, and neonatology is recommended in the management of maternal cardiac disease during pregnancy. Frequency of visits and monitoring of maternal cardiac status should be individualized, but close follow-up is recommended.[17,18]

The risk of thrombotic events in women with structural heart disease is 2%, compared with a 0.1% baseline risk.[4] Anticoagulation may be considered in certain individuals, especially those with mechanical heart valves, certain arrhythmias, and pulmonary hypertension.[1] A collaborative effort involving cardiology and hematology is helpful in guiding management decisions related to anticoagulation initiation, therapeutic approaches, and intrapartum and postpartum management.

Given the increased risk of adverse fetal and neonatal risks in this population,[6,14–16] antepartum evaluation and serial growth ultrasounds are recommended. Because structural heart disease is often associated with genetic conditions and carries an increased risk of inheritance to offspring,[11] genetic counseling, targeted fetal anatomy scans, and fetal echocardiograms should be performed.

Intrapartum Care

The intrapartum and immediate postpartum time period poses the highest risk for women with cardiac disease secondary to profound hemodynamic changes and fluid shifts. Intrapartum care needs to be individualized but may range from standard obstetric care to invasive hemodynamic monitoring, telemetry, anticoagulation, endocarditis prophylaxis, and intensive care unit admission. These decisions should be made in close collaboration with cardiology, maternal-fetal medicine, anesthesia, and any other relevant specialty. General principles for many patients include an early epidural and a shortened second stage. Cesarean delivery should be reserved for obstetric indications, with some exceptions.[17,18] Important exceptions in which primary cesarean delivery is preferred include pulmonary hypertension,[23] Marfan syndrome with aortic diameter greater than 45 mm, and bicuspid aortic valve with aortic diameter greater than 50 mm.[22]

There are few indications for endocarditis prophylaxis for congenital heart disease during labor that are recommended by the American Heart Association[24] and the American College of Obstetrics and Gynecology.[25] These indications include prosthetic cardiac valves, prosthetic material used for cardiac valve repair, and cyanotic congenital heart disease. Typically, treatment includes ampicillin, cefazolin, ceftriaxone, or clindamycin administered 30 to 60 minutes before delivery.[25]

SPECIFIC CARDIAC CONDITIONS
Thoracic Aortic Disease

There are multiple thoracic aortic diseases that can be impacted by pregnancy, including Marfan syndrome, Ehlers-Danlos, Loeys-Dietz, Turner syndrome, bicuspid aortic valve, and coarctation of the aorta. Studies have shown that, even in healthy individuals, pregnancy may predispose women to aortic weakening and dissection.[26,27] Increased susceptibility to aortic dissection during pregnancy in certain individuals may stem from physiologic structural changes to the aortic wall structure,[26] physiologic increases in aortic diameter,[27] and increased vascular stress. Importantly, pregnancy increases the rate of aortic dissection by 100-fold from 6 per 100,000 (general population) to 0.6%.[28]

In general, pregnancy is contraindicated in women with Marfan syndrome and an aortic root diameter greater than 45 mm, prior aortic dissection, and Ehlers-Danlos affecting the vascular system.[22] Optimal management of gravid women with thoracic aortic disease includes prepregnancy MRI of the aorta, consideration of aortic repair if dilatation is present, initiation of beta-blocker therapy, and discontinuation of angiotensin-receptor blocker therapy.[22]

Most thoracic aortic conditions during pregnancy warrant serial ultrasound surveillance of the ascending aorta and consideration of full aorta imaging if dilatation is present. In the rare event of a type A aortic dissection (dissection into ascending aorta), immediate cardiac surgery is needed with consideration of cesarean delivery based on gestational age. In contrast, type B dissections (dissection not into ascending aorta) are treated medically with close imaging surveillance. Cesarean delivery is recommended in patients with Marfan syndrome with an aortic diameter greater than 45 mm and bicuspid aortic diameter greater than 50 mm.[22] Early epidural anesthesia, consideration of assisted second stage, and left lateral decubitus positioning in between contractions is usually recommended for attempted vaginal delivery.[22]

Marfan Syndrome

Marfan syndrome is an autosomal dominant connective tissue disorder found in approximately 1 in 3000 individuals. The most significant risk during pregnancy is aortic dissection, which seems to be related to the diameter of the aorta. In women with aortic dilatation measuring 45 to 49 mm, the rate of dissection was 0.3% and 1.3% in 50 to 54 mm.[22] Risk of aortic dissection, aortic rupture, or other serious cardiac complications increased with aortic root dilation (greater than 40–45 mm in diameter), increasing aortic size,[29] and valvular disease. It is difficult to quantify the exact risk of cardiac complications with aortic root dilation or increasing aortic size, and cesarean delivery should be considered in the highest-risk individuals.[2] The American Heart Association recommends that women with aortic roots measuring greater than 40 mm in diameter should consider replacement of the aortic root before pregnancy, but the residual aorta remains at risk for dissection.[2] Mortality rates following aortic dissection are as high as 30% for mothers and up to 50% for the fetus.[22]

Aortic Coarctation

Aortic coarctation is found in approximately 4% to 6% of congenital cardiac anomalies and can be associated with aortic dilatation, bicuspid aortic valve, and aortic stenosis.[30] Typically, coarctation repair is recommended early in life or at the time of diagnosis in order to prevent systemic hypertension[31]; thus, most pregnant women will have a repaired coarctation. Signs of significant aortic coarctation include hypertension isolated to the upper body or decreased femoral pulses.[30]

In women with repaired coarctation, pregnancy is generally well tolerated and considered WHO risk class II.[2] However, chronic hypertension and hypertensive diseases of pregnancy are increased, especially in women with hemodynamically significant coarctation.[32] In women with unrepaired coarctation, there is an increased risk for aortic aneurysm and aortic rupture.[32] Intervention to alleviate the obstruction during pregnancy may be recommended in those with unrepaired lesions and poorly controlled blood pressure, but this decision should be individualized. In a retrospective study of 126 pregnancies complicated by maternal coarctation, 5 individuals experienced a 15 mm Hg or greater gradient increase during pregnancy and one required postpartum surgical intervention.[33]

Recurrence risk for offspring with maternal aortic coarctation has been estimated to be as high as 10%.[34]

Tetralogy of Fallot

Tetralogy of Fallot (TOF) is the most common cyanotic heart condition and is responsible for an estimated 5% of congenital heart disease.[35] TOF refers to a tetrad of features, including the following:

- Right ventricular outflow obstruction
- Ventricular septal defect
- Overriding aorta
- Right ventricular hypertrophy

Although unrepaired TOF was historically associated with a 44% mortality risk within the first year of life,[36] modern medicine now allows for increasing rates of recognition during the fetal period and typically surgical repair within 6 months of life.[35]

Pregnancy is generally well tolerated in women with repaired TOF and is considered WHO risk class II to III, depending on the individual.[2,6] In a large series of women with corrected TOF, complications from arrhythmias occurred in 19% of patients, with a subsequent risk for right heart failure.[37] Studies demonstrate that this risk may be related to residual disease, including valvular regurgitation and right ventricular outflow tract obstruction.[35] Because right-sided heart failure may be increased with severe pulmonary regurgitation,[37] preconception valve revision should be considered.[35]

Management during pregnancy should be tailored to the individual. In most patients with repaired TOF, cardiology visits every trimester is sufficient. However, some organizations recommend monthly maternal echocardiograms in cases of residual disease, such as severe pulmonary regurgitation.[2] For most patients, vaginal delivery is recommended.[37]

Although TOF is most commonly sporadic in nature, the recurrence risk for congenital heart disease is estimated to be 2%[37] compared with a baseline risk of 0.08%. It is recommended that women with TOF and other conotruncal lesions be screened for 22q11[6] mutations, as microdeletions of 22q11 underlie 15% to 20% of congenital cardiac anomalies involving the aortic arch and ventricular outflow tracts.[38]

Transposition of the Great Arteries

Transposition of the great arteries (TGA) involves a cardiac configuration in which the aorta inserts into the right ventricle and the pulmonary artery inserts into the left ventricle. The more common configuration of TGA is the dextra type (d-TGA), which can result in cyanosis.[17] In patients with d-TGA, a connection between the two separate circuits in the form of a ventricular septal defect (VSD) or patent ductus arteriosus (PDA) needs to be present to be compatible with life.[1] The more rare form of TGA, levo type is congenitally corrected and, therefore, not associated with cyanosis.[17]

Most adults will have undergone corrective surgery early in life, most commonly via an arterial switch operation. This procedure restores normal physiologic connections for the aorta and pulmonary artery, and is associated with low rates of stenosis at surgical sites, pulmonary or aortic regurgitation, and aortic root dilation.[17] Tobler and colleagues[39] found that after an atrial switch operation, the adult complication rate was up to 11% and reduced exercise capacity occurred in 82% of individuals. Patients who underwent corrective surgery via an atrial baffle procedure (typically before 1980) had a long-term risk of systemic right ventricle failure and tricuspid regurgitation.[17] Those treated with a Rastelli operation often required surgical revisions into adulthood and were at risk for obstruction of the outflow tracts from the heart, arrhythmias, aortic dilation, and aortic regurgitation.[17]

Most women with repaired TGA tolerate pregnancy fairly well if they have undergone corrective surgery and lack complications or residual disease.[17] This condition is considered WHO class III.[2] However, increasing evidence suggests an increased risk for long-term dysfunction after pregnancy.[2] Unlike other congenital cardiac conditions, TGA is not associated with genetic abnormalities and seems sporadic in nature.[20]

Fontan Circulation

The Fontan procedure is a common palliative procedure for individuals with single ventricle hearts.[17] Additionally, the Fontan procedure can be performed for tricuspid and pulmonary atresia, unbalanced atrioventricular canal defects, and double inlet left ventricle. The procedure is complex in nature and uses central venous pressure and intrathoracic pressure to allow systemic venous blood to directly enter the pulmonary artery.[1,17] Therefore, complications are common (including arrhythmia and increased risk of thrombosis); one study demonstrated a 76% survival at 25 years after the procedure.[40] Hypoplastic left heart was one of the major risk factors for heart failure.[40]

Pregnancies in mothers with a Fontan circuit in place are typically considered high risk with a WHO risk class of III to IV.[2] Indications to avoid pregnancy include moderate to severe aortic valve regurgitation, decreased oxygen saturation levels, impaired ventricular function, and moderate to severe valvular regurgitation.[2]

Gouton and colleagues[41] studied maternal and fetal outcomes in 37 patients and 59 pregnancies complicated by Fontan circulation. In this study, 10% of patients experienced cardiac events of which atrial arrhythmia was most common. In a review of the literature, Drenthen and colleagues[4] noted a 16% risk of cardiac arrhythmia and 4% risk of heart failure associated with maternal Fontal circulation. Because of an increased rate of thromboembolic complications in adults with Fontan circulation,[42] consideration of anticoagulation during pregnancy and post partum should be made.[2]

Obstetric complications are markedly increased in this population, with a prematurity rate up to 69%.[41] In most cases, vaginal delivery is the preferred mode of delivery in the absence of significant ventricular dysfunction.[2] Although data are limited, there is an estimated 5% risk of recurrent cardiac anomalies in offspring.[41]

Atrial Septal Defects

Atrial septal defect (ASD) accounts for 10% of congenital heart defects and has a female preponderonce.[17,43] The hemodynamic changes from an ASD is due to the left atrial to right atrial shunt created by the defect. This shunt initially increases right atrial pressures due to increased blood volume shunting to the right atrium; however, it can eventually cause right atrial dilation and pulmonary hypertension.[17] Rarely, the pulmonary hypertension (PH) leads to increased right atrial pressures that can cause a reversal of this shunt called Eisenmenger syndrome, with a high maternal mortality rate.[44]

Most patients will initially have few to no symptoms until later in life. When symptoms initially occur, they can include exercise intolerance, shortness of breath, and fatigue. Occasionally, right atrial dilation can cause atrial fibrillation or flutter. Rarely, a transient ischemic event or paradoxic embolus can occur through the ASD.[43] Echocardiogram with bubble study can diagnose ASDs and provide information on the size and direction of the shunt.[45]

In nonpregnant individuals, treatment is offered when there are any symptoms or signs of right atrial dilation or other hemodynamic pathology on echocardiogram.[17] Although medical therapy is sometimes used, surgical management is significantly superior and is composed of open or endovascular closure.[46] Contraindications to closure of ASD include a lack of hemodynamic significance (no symptoms or signs of right atrial dysfunction), severe pulmonary hypertension, and severe left ventricular dysfunction. If none of the aforementioned contraindications to closure exist, closure of the ASD before pregnancy is recommended.[43]

In the event of an unplanned pregnancy or discovery of the ASD during pregnancy, which often occurs because of the accentuated pulmonary flow murmur, management is more variable. If PH or ventricular dysfunction exist, patients should be counseled on the significant risks to the mother and fetus, including maternal mortality, and early termination of the pregnancy should be recommended.[17,43] If the mother chooses to continue the pregnancy, referral to a tertiary care setting is recommended. Closure of the ASD can be performed, if necessary, via echocardiographic-guided percutaneous endovascular catheter-directed closure.[43] This procedure, however, is only recommended in the setting of worsening symptoms and worsening hemodynamics on echocardiogram.[2]

Pregnancy is generally well tolerated in women with an ASD in the absence of PH or ventricular dysfunction.[47] The most common significant complication is thromboembolic disease, specifically paradoxic emboli, which has been noted in up to 5% of pregnancies complicated by ASD.[4] The recommended management is aimed to prevent embolic phenomena and consists of heparin prophylaxis when immobilized, early ambulation following delivery, and the use of compression stockings.[2]

Pregnancy-related complications typically occur in women with unrepaired ASDs and include increased risk for preeclampsia and small-for-gestational age neonates.[47] Yap and colleagues[47] did not find an increased risk of preeclampsia, growth restriction, or fetal mortality in women with repaired ASD. For most patients, spontaneous vaginal delivery is appropriate care and cesarean delivery should be reserved for obstetric indications.

The risk of inheritance with maternal ASD to offspring is as high as 10%[17] in sporadic cases; but because of commonly associated genetic conditions associated with ASD, genetic counseling and a thorough investigation into family history should be performed.[17]

Atrioventricular Septal Defect (Endocardial Cushion Defect)

An atrioventricular septal defect (AVSD) is a congenital defect in the endocardial cushion with direct communication between all 4 chambers of the heart.[17] This defect occurs in 1 in 2130 births and is substantially increased in individuals with Down syndrome.[48] Although it is almost invariably identified in infancy or early childhood and surgically repaired, residual complications often include ASD, atrioventricular valvular insufficiency including stenosis and regurgitation, arrhythmias, and congestive heart failure.[4] The most significant comorbidity associated with this defect is persistent regurgitation through the atrioventricular valves. In a retrospective study of 116 individuals, 68% of patients had at least mild mitral valve regurgitation, 3% developed moderate to severe mitral stenosis, and 8% required additional operations within 2 years for mitral valve regurgitation or stenosis.[49]

In pregnancy, the maternal risk is generally low in those who have undergone surgical correction and lack persistent severe mitral valve regurgitation, mitral stenosis, or residual ASD.[17] AVSD is commonly seen in individuals with Down syndrome and may have up to a 50% risk of transmission to offspring.[17]

Ventricular Septal Defect

VSD is the most common cardiac malformation in neonates.[17] Although many will close spontaneously by adulthood, it remains one of the most frequent forms of congenital heart defects encountered in pregnancy. Most women with a history of isolated VSD with successful closure have pregnancies that are well tolerated.[17,47] However, VSDs with hemodynamically significant left to right shunts that are accompanied by pulmonary hypertension[17] are associated with unacceptably high maternal risks during pregnancy, and termination of pregnancy should be recommended.[13] All individuals with repaired or unrepaired VSDs should undergo prepregnancy evaluation and, in select cases, consider VSD closure before pregnancy.[2]

In a study of 202 pregnancies of mothers with VSDs, preeclampsia was significantly increased in women with VSDs, especially unrepaired VSDs.[50] Recurrence of congenital heart disease in offspring was present in 2% of the indviduals.[50]

Patent Ductus Arteriosus

PDA is a common congenital heart defect with an incidence of 1 in 2000 births, comprising 5% to 10% of all congenital heart disease.[51] The ductus arteriosus, which connects the aorta to the main pulmonary artery, can cause a physiologic left to right shunt when patent and unrepaired.[17] The significance of the shunt varies from patient to patient. Large and uncorrected PDAs can lead to Eisenmenger syndrome over time.[17] Treatment of PDA in nonpregnant individuals can include medical therapy targeted at afterload reduction, diuresis, and digoxin therapy. However, definitive treatment of a hemodynamically significant or symptomatic PDA is surgical or endovascular closure.[17,51]

There is very little maternal or neonatal risk in pregnancy with closed PDAs and in individuals with mild asymptomatic shunts. However, clinical decisions on whether or not to close moderate to severe shunts need to be made in conjunction with cardiology.[6]

Pulmonary Stenosis and Regurgitation

The incidence of congenital pulmonic stenosis is 729 per 1 million births and accounts for 10% to 12% of congenital heart defects.[30] The condition is defined as a pulmonary valvular gradient greater than 25 mm Hg.[52] Pulmonic valve stenosis is generally treated with balloon valvotomy if it is associated with exertional dyspnea, angina, syncope, presyncope, or a right ventricle to pulmonary artery pressure greater than 30 mm Hg catheterization in symptomatic individuals.[53]

Pregnancy-related complications are more frequent in women with pulmonary stenosis and regurgitation. In a review of 81 cases of maternal congenital pulmonic stenosis, Drenthen and colleagues[4] identified 14.6% with hypertension-related disorders, 3.7% with thromboembolic events, and 16.0% with preterm birth. Cardiac complications included temporary worsening of congestive heart failure in 2 of 81 studied pregnancies.[4]

In pregnancy, referral to a cardiologist for evaluation is recommended. If treatment is indicated (generally for NYHA classification of III–IV or other symptomatic valvular disease) percutaneous balloon valvotomy/valvuloplasty can be performed.[53] Vaginal delivery is generally preferred in individuals without severe pulmonic stenosis. If pulmonic stenosis or regurgitation is associated with significant heart failure (NYHA class III–IV), a cesarean delivery may be indicated.[2]

Pulmonary Hypertension

PH is a condition in which pulmonary vascular resistance increases and is defined as a mean pulmonary artery pressure greater than 30 mm Hg with exertion or 25 mm Hg or greater at rest.[17] PH is categorized into different WHO classes based on the underlying cause, which range from idiopathic PH to congenital heart disease and thromboembolic disease.[17] In nonpregnant individuals, Lowe and colleagues[54] found a 5.8% prevalence of PH in adults with congenital heart disease.

Numerous cardiac structural defects have been identified as risk factors for PH, including complex cardiac anatomy (such as TGA and single ventricle systems), pulmonary vein stenosis, and unrepaired large left to right shunts (such as ASD and VSD).[17] A systematic review by Bédard and colleagues[55] identified isolated ASD and VSD as the most common lesions associated with congenital heart disease–associated PH (CHD-PH) in pregnancy through a pathologic mechanism termed Eisenmenger physiology.

Eisenmenger physiology occurs when individuals with preexisting left to right shunts (such as unrepaired truncus arteriosus, VSD, ASD, and PDA) experience shunt reversal due to increased pulmonary vascular resistance. This physiology can lead to life-threatening complications, including chronic hypoxemia, erythrocytosis, cardiac ischemia, and pulmonary ventricular failure.[17]

PH remains associated with a prohibitively high risk of maternal mortality despite recent therapeutic advances. In a systematic review of women with PH from congenital heart disease, advanced therapy has contributed to decreasing the maternal mortality rate to 28%[55] from historical rates of 50%.[56] Although decreasing, PH continues to pose an unacceptably high risk of maternal death. It is considered WHO class IV and pregnancy is contraindicated.[2] Bédard and colleagues[55] identified severe heart failure as the inciting cause of death among most women who died, and most deaths occurred within 4 weeks of delivery. Other common complications in this cohort included bleeding/transfusion (38%), pulmonary hypertensive crisis (7%), and pulmonary thromboembolism (14%).[55]

Comprehensive multidisciplinary counseling is of utmost importance for pregnant women with PH. Pregnancy termination should be recommended, given the maternal, fetal, and neonatal risk. For individuals who continue their pregnancies, close multidisciplinary care should be undertaken with PH specialists, cardiologists, maternal-fetal medicine specialists, and anesthesiologists.

Advanced therapies should be considered in women with CHD-PH who present during pregnancy, as this may improve outcomes in certain individuals. In a study by Bédard and colleagues,[55] more than 50% of women were treated with advanced therapy during the pregnancy, most commonly nitric oxide, prostacyclin analogues, sildenafil, and calcium channel blockers. Management considerations for pregnancy should include anticoagulation, discontinuation of endothelin receptor antagonists (teratogenic to humans), and treatment with phosphodiesterase type 5 inhibitors and prostacyclins.[57]

Some experts recommend scheduled cesarean delivery with neuraxial anesthesia at 34 weeks' gestation,[23,57] although the optimal delivery mode and timing remains controversial. General anesthesia should be avoided if possible, as one study indicated that it was associated with a 4-fold increase in maternal death in patients with CHD-PH.[58]

Obstetric complications are common in pregnancies complicated by maternal CHD-PH. In a study of 28 mothers with CHD-PH, Ladouceur and colleagues[58] noted an increased risk of postpartum hemorrhage (often related to anticoagulation) and small-for-gestational age neonates. In this study, more than 75% of deliveries were premature (often indicated), with a mean gestational age of 33 weeks.

SUMMARY

Clinicians are caring for an ever-increasing number of mothers with structural heart disease because of advances in the recognition and surgical management of congenital malformations. Pregnancy outcomes are generally favorable in mothers with mild disease; however, preconception consultation and risk assessment is of utmost importance, as pregnancy may pose an unacceptably high risk of maternal mortality and related complications in certain individuals. Further, preconception consultation allows providers the opportunity to recognize and surgically correct maternal cardiac disease in some individuals, thereby drastically improving pregnancy outcomes. Overall, thoughtful multidisciplinary management and close follow-up can optimize outcomes for the mother and child and lead to successful and healthy pregnancies in most individuals.

REFERENCES

1. Simpson LL, Cauldwell M, Gatzoulis M, et al. Maternal cardiac disease update for the clinician. Obstet Gynecol 2012;119(2):345–59.
2. Regitz-Zagrosek V, Blomstrom Lundqvist C, Borghi C, et al. ESC guidelines on the management of cardiovascular diseases during pregnancy. Eur Heart J 2011;32(24):3147–97.
3. Creanga AA, Syverson C, Callaghan WM, et al. Pregnancy-related mortality in the United States. Obstet Gynecol 2017;130(2):2011–3.

4. Drenthen W, Pieper PG, Roos-Hesselink JW, et al. Outcome of pregnancy in women with congenital heart disease. A literature review. J Am Coll Cardiol 2007;49(24):2303–11.

5. Pijuan-Domènech A, Galian L, Goya M, et al. Cardiac complications during pregnancy are better predicted with the modified WHO risk score. Int J Cardiol 2015; 195:149–54.

6. Rao S, Ginns JN. Adult congenital heart disease and pregnancy. Semin Perinatol 2014;38(5):260–72.

7. Ruys TP, Roos-Hesselink JW, Hall R, et al. Heart failure in pregnant women with cardiac disease: data from the ROPAC. Heart 2014;100:231–8.

8. Ruys TPE, Maggioni A, Johnson MR, et al. Cardiac medication during pregnancy, data from the ROPAC. Int J Cardiol 2014;177(1):124–8.

9. Roos-Hesselink JW, Ruys TPE, Stein JI, et al. Outcome of pregnancy in patients with structural or ischaemic heart disease: results of a registry of the European Society of Cardiology. Eur Heart J 2013;34(9):657–65.

10. Siu SC, Sermer M, Colman JM, et al. Prospective multicenter study of pregnancy outcomes in women with heart disease. Circulation 2001;104(5):515–21.

11. Lindley K, Conner S, Cahill A. Adult congenital heart disease in pregnancy. Obstet Gynecol Surv 2015;70(6):397–407.

12. Lui GK, Silversides CK, Khairy P, et al. Heart rate response during exercise and pregnancy outcome in women with congenital heart disease. Circulation 2011; 123(3):242–8.

13. Thorne S. Risks of contraception and pregnancy in heart disease. Heart 2006; 92(10):1520–5.

14. Siu SC, Colman JM, Sorensen S, et al. Adverse neonatal and cardiac outcomes are more common in pregnant women with cardiac disease. Circulation 2002; 105(18):2179–84.

15. Khairy P, Ouyang DW, Fernandes SM, et al. Pregnancy outcomes in women with congenital heart disease. Circulation 2006;113(4):517–24.

16. Gelson E, Curry R, Gatzoulis MA, et al. Effect of maternal heart disease on fetal growth. Obstet Gynecol 2011;117(4):886–91.

17. Warnes CA, Williams RG, Bashore TM, et al. ACC/AHA 2008 guidelines for the management of adults with congenital heart disease. J Am Coll Cardiol 2008; 52(23):1890–947.

18. Cauldwell M, Gatzoulis M, Steer P. Congenital heart disease and pregnancy: a contemporary approach to counselling, pre-pregnancy investigations and the impact of pregnancy on heart function. Obstet Med 2017;10(2):53–7.

19. Lindley K, Tessa M, Cahill A, et al. Contraceptive use and unintended pregnancy in women with congenital heart disease. Obstet Gynecol 2015;126(2): 363–9.

20. Burn J, Brennan P, Little J, et al. Recurrence risks in offspring of adults with major heart defects: results from first cohort of British collaborative study. Lancet 1998; 351(9099):311–6.

21. Bowater SE, Thorne SA. Management of pregnancy in women with acquired and congenital heart disease. Postgrad Med J 2010;86(1012):100–5.

22. Wanga S, Silversides C, Dore A, et al. Pregnancy and thoracic aortic disease: managing the risks. Can J Cardiol 2016;32(1):78–85.

23. Rex S, Devroe S. Anesthesia for pregnant women with pulmonary hypertension. Curr Opin Anaesthesiol 2016;29:273–81.

24. Wilson W, Taubert KA, Gewitz M, et al. Prevention of infective endocarditis: guidelines from the American Heart Association. Circulation 2007;116(15):1736–54.

25. American College of Obstetricians and Gynecologists. ACOG Practice Bulletin No. 120: Use of Prophylactic Antibiotics in Labor and Delivery. Obstet Gynecol 2011;117(6):1472–83. Reaffirmed 2016.
26. Manalo-Estrella P, Barker A. Histopathologic findings in human aortic media associated with pregnancy. Arch Pathol 1967;83:336–41.
27. Easterling TR, Benedetti TJ, Schmucker BC, et al. Maternal hemodynamics and aortic diameter in normal and hypertensive pregnancies. Obstet Gynecol 1991; 78(6):1073–7.
28. Nienaber CA, Fattori R, Mehta RH, et al. Gender-related differences in acute aortic dissection. Circulation 2004;109(24):3014–21.
29. Kuperstein R, Cahan T, Yoeli-Ullman R, et al. Risk of aortic dissection in pregnant patients with the Marfan syndrome. Am J Cardiol 2017;119(1):132–7.
30. Hoffman JIE, Kaplan S. The incidence of congenital heart disease. J Am Coll Cardiol 2002;39(12):1890–900.
31. Seirafi PA, Warner KG, Geggel RL, et al. Repair of coarctation of the aorta during infancy minimizes the risk of late hypertension. Ann Thorac Surg 1998;66(4):1378–82.
32. Beauchesne LM, Connolly HM, Ammash NM, et al. Coarctation of the aorta: outcome of pregnancy. J Am Coll Cardiol 2001;38(6):1728–33.
33. Vriend JWJ, Drenthen W, Pieper PG, et al. Outcome of pregnancy in patients after repair of aortic coarctation. Eur Heart J 2005;26(20):2173–8.
34. Whittemore R, Wells JA, Castellsague X. A second-generation study of 427 probands with congenital heart defects and their 837 children. J Am Coll Cardiol 1994;23(6):1459–67.
35. Apitz C, Webb GD, Redington AN. Tetralogy of Fallot. Lancet 2009;374(9699): 1462–71.
36. Bertranou EG, Blackstone EH, Hazelrig JB, et al. Life expectancy without surgery in tetralogy of Fallot. Am J Cardiol 1978;42(3):458–66.
37. Meijer JM, Pieper PG, Drenthen W, et al. Pregnancy, fertility, and recurrence risk in corrected tetralogy of Fallot. Heart 2005;91(6):801–5.
38. Webber SA, Hatchwell E, Barber JC, et al. Importance of microdeletions of chromosomal region 22q11 as a cause of selected malformations of the ventricular outflow tracts and aortic arch: a three-year prospective study. J Pediatr 1996; 129(1):26–32.
39. Tobler D, Williams WG, Jegatheeswaran A, et al. Cardiac outcomes in young adult survivors of the arterial switch operation for transposition of the great arteries. J Am Coll Cardiol 2010;56(1):58–64.
40. d'Udekem Y, Iyengar AJ, Galati JC, et al. Redefining expectations of long-term survival after the Fontan procedure: twenty-five years of follow-up from the entire population of Australia and New Zealand. Circulation 2014;130(11 Suppl 1):32–9.
41. Gouton M, Nizard J, Patel M, et al. Maternal and fetal outcomes of pregnancy with Fontan circulation: a multicentric observational study. Int J Cardiol 2015;187(1): 84–9.
42. van den Bosch AE, Roos-Hesselink JW, Van Domburg R, et al. Long-term outcome and quality of life in adult patients after the Fontan operation. Am J Cardiol 2004;93(9):1141–5.
43. Webb G, Gatzoulis MA. Atrial septal defects in the adult: recent progress and overview. Circulation 2006;114(15):1645–53.
44. Beghetti M, Galiè N. Eisenmenger syndrome. A clinical perspective in a new therapeutic era of pulmonary arterial hypertension. J Am Coll Cardiol 2009;53(9):733–40.
45. Krasuski RA. When and how to fix a "hole in the heart": approach to ASD and PFO. Cleve Clin J Med 2007;74(2):137–47.

46. Konstantinides S, Geibel A, Olschewski M, et al. A comparison of surgical and medical therapy for atrial septal defect in adults. N Engl J Med 1995;333(8): 469–73.

47. Yap SC, Drenthen W, Meijboom FJ, et al. Comparison of pregnancy outcomes in women with repaired versus unrepaired atrial septal defect. BJOG 2009;116(12): 1593–601.

48. Parker SE, Mai CT, Canfield MA, et al. Updated national birth prevalence estimates for selected birth defects in the United States, 2004-2006. Birth Defects Res A Clin Mol Teratol 2010;88(12):1008–16.

49. Suzuki T, Bove EL, Devaney EJ, et al. Results of definitive repair of complete atrioventricular septal defect in neonates and infants. Ann Thorac Surg 2008;86(2): 596–602.

50. Yap SC, Drenthen W, Pieper PG, et al. Pregnancy outcome in women with repaired versus unrepaired isolated ventricular septal defect. BJOG 2010;117(6):683–9.

51. Schneider DJ, Moore JW. Patent ductus arteriosus. Circulation 2006;114(17): 1873–82.

52. Bound JP, Logan WF. Incidence of congenital heart disease in Blackpool 1957-1971. Br Heart J 1977;39(4):445–50.

53. Bonow RO, Carabello BA, Chatterjee K, et al. 2008 focused update incorporated into the ACC/AHA 2006 guidelines for the management of patients with valvular heart disease. J Am Coll Cardiol 2008;52(13):e1–142.

54. Lowe BS, Therrien J, Ionescu-Ittu R, et al. Diagnosis of pulmonary hypertension in the congenital heart disease adult population: impact on outcomes. J Am Coll Cardiol 2011;58(5):538–46.

55. Bédard E, Dimopoulos K, Gatzoulis MA. Has there been any progress made on pregnancy outcomes among women with pulmonary arterial hypertension? Eur Heart J 2009;30(3):256–65.

56. Kahn ML. Eisenmenger's syndrome in pregnancy. N Engl J Med 1993;329(12):887.

57. McLaughlin VV, Shah SJ, Souza R, et al. Management of pulmonary arterial hypertension. J Am Coll Cardiol 2015;65(18):1976–97.

58. Ladouceur M, Benoit L, Radojevic J, et al. Pregnancy outcomes in patients with pulmonary arterial hypertension associated with congenital heart disease. Heart 2017;103:287–92.

New Insights in Peripartum Cardiomyopathy

Meredith O. Cruz, MD, MPH, MBA[a],*, Joan Briller, MD[b,c], Judith U. Hibbard, MD[a]

KEYWORDS

- Peripartum cardiomyopathy • Pregnancy • Cardiac disease
- Congestive heart failure

KEY POINTS

- Specific diagnostic criteria should be used to diagnose peripartum cardiomyopathy (PPCM), but this is a diagnosis of exclusion.
- Although rare, PPCM is a leading cause of maternal mortality.
- Significant advances have been made in understanding PPCM pathophysiology, especially hormonal and genetic mechanisms.
- Long-term and recurrent pregnancy prognosis depends on recovery of cardiac function.

INTRODUCTION

Peripartum cardiomyopathy (PPCM), or heart failure (HF) associated with pregnancy, was first described in 1937.[1] The syndrome was poorly defined until 1971 when specifically noted as occurring in the peripartum period.[2] Hibbard and colleagues[3] included echocardiographic (ECHO) criteria for PPCM in 1999, stressing reduced ejection fraction (EF <45%) toward the end of pregnancy or in the months postpartum in women without structural heart disease,[4] although some women may present earlier.[5] Incidence, 1:1000 to 1:4000 live births in the United States,[6] varies by geographic location[7,8] and has been increasing in the United States.[9–12] PPCM is a leading cause of maternal mortality.[13–17] Long-term consequences include chronic HF and transplantation. Recent advances based on animal models, registries, and genetic/biomarker testing have shed light on pathways promising more specific diagnosis, improved risk stratification, and targets for specific therapy.

No financial disclosures.
[a] Division of Maternal Fetal Medicine, Department of Obstetrics and Gynecology, Medical College of Wisconsin, 9200 West Wisconsin Avenue, Milwaukee, WI 53226-3522, USA; [b] Division of Cardiology, University of Illinois at Chicago, 840 South Wood Street, M/C 715, Chicago, IL 60612, USA; [c] Department of Obstetrics and Gynecology, University of Illinois at Chicago, 1740 W. Taylor Street, Chicago, IL 60612, USA
* Corresponding author.
E-mail address: mocruz@mcw.edu

PROPOSED PATHOGENIC MECHANISMS

Investigation of the pathophysiology of PPCM is limited by its rare incidence and lack of specific diagnostic markers. Postulated mechanisms include hemodynamic stress of pregnancy, viral myocarditis, fetal microchimerism, and malnutrition.[18]

The theory that PPCM results from idiopathic dilated cardiomyopathy (DCM) precipitated by the hemodynamic stress of pregnancy is limited by the fact that hemodynamic changes reach near maximum by the end of the second or early third trimester before peak PPCM incidence.[19] Similarly, although myocarditis was proposed as an important mediator, the prevalence of abnormal endomyocardial biopsy specimens has varied widely and is not clearly different from controls.[20,21]

An autoimmune hypothesis developed from evidence that hematopoietic cells introduced into maternal circulation due to pregnancy-related immunosuppression are attracted to cardiac tissue, later recognized as non-self, leading to a pathologic response.[22] However, migration of multipotential fetal stem cells may mitigate injury.[23] Malnutrition (eg, selenium deficiency) could magnify PPCM development in some populations but has not been described widely.[24] Other associations include prolonged tocolysis, although β-mimetic tocolysis has diminished.[25] Novel proposed associations include anemia, asthma, and substance abuse,[26] but these may provoke HF through different mechanisms.

Hormonal/Vascular Derangements

Current research focuses on hormonal shifts occurring peripartum coinciding with the peak incidence of PPCM.[6] Both prolactin and soluble FMs-like tyrosine kinase-1 (sFlt1) have been implicated in PPCM pathogenesis.[27,28] An imbalance in angiogenic factors appears to promote PPCM.

Antiangiogenic fragments of prolactin derived from pituitary gland can result in cardiac apoptosis, vascular dropout, and systolic dysfunction.[28] Hilfiker-Kleiner and colleagues[27] noted that female mice with cardiomyocyte-specific deletion of the STAT3 gene developed PPCM. The role of STAT3 is cardioprotective, upregulating antioxidant enzymes such as manganese superoxide dismutase (MnSOD). In the absence of STAT3, cathepsin D cleaves prolactin into a 16-kDa fragment, which promotes apoptosis with subsequent left ventricular (LV) dysfunction. The 16-kDa fragments induce endothelial cells to package microRNAs into lipid-encapsulated particles, which suppress the neuregulin/ErbB pathway, required for cardiomyocyte function and viability.[29] Treatment with bromocriptine, inhibiting prolactin production, rescued the mice, thus preventing PPCM.[27] Biopsy tissue from PPCM patients undergoing transplant showed lower levels of STAT3 activity, and 16-kDa fragments were detected in serum of patients with PPCM.[27]

In a second model, mice lacking proliferator-activated receptor-gamma coactivator-1α (PGC1-α) developed PPCM.[28] PGC1-α, a transcriptional coactivator that drives mitochondrial biogenesis, is highly expressed in the heart, upregulates MnSOD, and regulates angiogenic factors, including vascular endothelial growth factor (VEGF).[30] Absence of PGC1-α leads to reduced antioxidant activity and increased reactive oxygen species with cleavage of prolactin into the 16-kDa fragment.[28] Treatment with VEGF in this model improves outcomes, but treatment with both VEGF and bromocriptine is required for complete rescue. In this model, 2 pathways lead to PPCM.[28]

Late pregnancy is associated with an antiangiogenic environment due to placental secretion of factors such as sFlt1.[28] The heart secretes local VEGF, but this is insufficient to prevent development of PPCM. In this model, administration of sFlt1 is sufficient to cause cardiomyopathy outside of pregnancy.[28] Placental secretion of sFlt1 is markedly increased in preeclampsia[31] and twin gestation,[32] which may explain correlation with these conditions and PPCM presentation times. SFlt1 levels are elevated in PPCM[33] and in the Investigations of Pregnancy-Associated Cardiomyopathy (IPAC) registry correlated with adverse outcomes.[34]

The vasculohormonal model is shown in **Fig. 1**.[6] Continued understanding of the pathogenic pathways should spur development of treatment-specific modalities.

Genetics

Several studies have found familial clustering of PPCM.[35–37] The TTN gene encodes the largest human protein, titin, and is involved in structural, developmental, mechanical, and regulatory functions of cardiac muscle.[38] TTN mutations are found in patients with DCM.[38] Ware and colleagues[39] recently sequenced DNA from 43 genes in 172 women with PPCM, including 83 from the IPAC cohort. Fifteen percent had truncating variants, many in the TTN gene, significantly higher than a reference cohort but similar to a DCM cohort. Moreover, the presence of a TTN gene truncation correlated with lower EF at 1-year follow-up.[39]

Other genetic changes may contribute to development of PPCM. A genome-wide association study in 41 women with PPCM discovered a single nucleotide polymorphism near a parathyroid hormone–related gene locus linked to calcium transfer in the placenta and uterus.[40] The guanine nucleotide–binding protein β3 C825T is

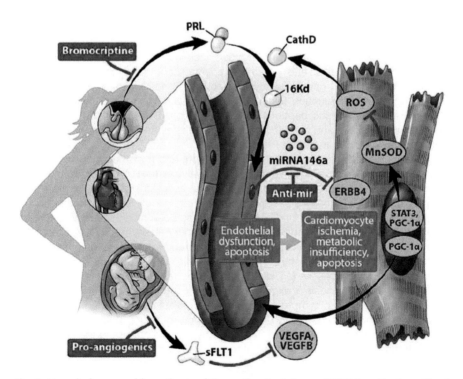

Fig. 1. Vasculo-hormonal hypothesis of the pathophysiology of PPCM. anti-mir, antibody to miRNA146a; CathD, cathepsinD; ERBB4, avian erythroblastic leukemia viral oncogene homolog 4; miRNA, microRNA; PRL, prolactin; ROS, reactive oxygen species; STAT3, signal transducer and activator of transcription 3. (*From* Arany Z, Elkayam U. Peripartum cardiomyopathy. Circulation 2016;133(14):1404; with permission.)

associated with cardiac remodeling and documented to have an increased prevalence in African Americans (AAs) in the IPAC cohort, and moreover, associated with reduced recovery at long-term follow-up.[41] Such findings support genetic foundations to PPCM in addition to a vasculotoxic milieu.

Risk Factors

Several risk factors are implicated in development of PPCM, including older age, the majority $\geq$30 years old.[9,10,42] PPCM is significantly more prevalent in women of African descent, almost 50% in the United States in AAs.[9,12] Multiple gestations have an increased likelihood of PPCM, with 9% prevalence of twins in one meta-analysis.[43] PPCM also occurs more often in women with higher gravidity and parity.[5,44] Hypertensive disorders of pregnancy are strongly associated, and a recent meta-analysis of 979 cases of PPCM found preeclampsia prevalence to be 22% and gestational hypertension to be 37%.[43]

Diagnosis

HF is a syndrome resulting from impaired ventricular ejection and filling. Symptoms include dyspnea and fatigue, fluid retention, edema, and impaired exercise tolerance. Thorough history and physical examination are required to address contributing disorders and potential causes. History of underlying hypertension, diabetes, dyslipidemia, coronary, rheumatic, or valvular heart disease, prior chemotherapy or mediastinal radiation, sleep disorders, alcohol or drug use, collagen vascular disease, sexually transmitted diseases, thyroid disease, arrhythmias, and family history of cardiomyopathy or sudden death should be obtained, and functional status should be assessed. Physical examination often reveals tachycardia, elevated jugular venous pressure, pulmonary rales, and peripheral edema. Laboratory assessment should include complete blood count, urinalysis, electrolytes, fasting glucose, hemoglobin A1c, lipid profile, liver function tests, thyroid-stimulating hormone, and HIV status. Measurement of natriuretic peptides (BNP and NT pro-BNP), seen with LV volume and pressure overload, and cardiac troponins can be helpful assessing volume status and risk stratification, but are not PPCM specific.[45,46]

Twelve-lead electrocardiogram, chest radiograph, and transthoracic with Doppler should be performed to assess ventricular and valvular function. Cardiac magnetic resonance (CMR) imaging can provide additional assessment of morphology and help predict adverse outcomes based on extent of late gadolinium enhancement.[45,46] Prevalence of abnormal CMR findings in PPCM has been highly variable; a PPCM-specific pattern has not been described.[47,48] Coronary arteriography or noninvasive imaging for myocardial ischemia should be considered for women at risk of coronary disease.[45] Endomyocardial biopsy is not performed routinely, although may be used to confirm some other causes (eg, giant cell myocarditis).[45,46]

PPCM remains a diagnosis of exclusion (**Box 1**). Recognition is challenging because HF symptoms can mimic symptoms of pregnancy,[49] but paroxysmal nocturnal dyspnea, chest pain, nocturnal cough, new regurgitant murmurs, pulmonary crackles, elevated jugular venous pressure, or hepatomegaly should prompt further evaluation. Demonstrating LV dysfunction is integral to the diagnosis.[3]

Management of Heart Failure in Pregnancy

Therapy is directed at improving symptoms, slowing progression of LV dysfunction, and improving survival (**Box 2**). Generally, HF guideline-directed medical therapy (GDMT) recommendations should be followed with modifications based on pregnancy and/or breastfeeding status. Interventions should be selected with known benefit.[45,46]

Box 1
Clinical criteria for the diagnosis of peripartum cardiomyopathy

- Cardiac failure in the last month of pregnancy or within a few months postpartum
- Absence of another identifiable cause
- Absence of underlying structural heart disease
- LV systolic dysfunction by echocardiographic data:
  1. EF less than 45%
  2. M-mode fractional shortening less than 30% or both
  3. LV end-diastolic dimension greater than 2.7 cm/m^2

Data from Refs.[4–6,95]

Goals include fluid management, afterload reduction, β-blockade, treatment of hypertension, and consideration of aldosterone antagonists, anticoagulation, and sudden death prevention. Cardiac rehabilitation is recommended once stable.[45] Advanced HF interventions should be addressed in the absence of improvement.[45] Novel therapeutic modalities have been used in some circumstances.[46] Medical management of PPCM should occur in conjunction with a cardiologist versant in the use of cardiac drugs during pregnancy. Indications and cautions for agents are shown in **Table 1**.

Fluid management is achieved by restricting fluid and dietary salt intake in combination with diuretics. Diuretics are indicated for volume overload because they improve pulmonary and peripheral edema.[45] However, caution needs to be exercised to avoid overdiuresis during pregnancy with reduced fetal blood flow.[50] The authors

---

Box 2
Recommended therapy for peripartum cardiomyopathy

- Goals
  - Treat hypertension
  - Fluid restriction
  - Dietary salt restriction
  - Routine exercise postpartum if stable

- Drugs for routine use
  - Diuretics
  - β-Blockers
  - Vasodilators

- Therapies in selected patients
  - Aldosterone antagonists
  - Digoxin
  - Anticoagulation
  - Implantable defibrillators
  - Biventricular pacing
  - Inotropes
  - LVAD/cardiac transplantation

Data from Yancy CW, Jessup M, Bozkurt B, et al. 2013 ACCF/AHA guideline for the management of heart failure: executive summary: a report of the American College of Cardiology Foundation/American Heart Association Task Force on Practice Guidelines. Circulation 2013;128(16):1810–52; and Bozkurt B, Colvin M, Cook J, et al. Current diagnostic and treatment strategies for specific dilated cardiomyopathies: a scientific statement from the American Heart Association. Circulation 2016;134(23):e579–646.

Table 1
Common medications in the treatment of peripartum cardiomyopathy

Medication	Indication	Drug Effect	Precautions		
			Maternal	Fetal	
Diuretics Furosemide[L3] (1st line) Thiazides[L2] (2nd line)	Volume overload or fluid retention	↓ Preload Decreased lung congestion and edema Improved symptoms and exercise tolerance	Electrolyte abnormalities Fluid depletion Hypotension Azotemia	Decreased placental perfusion Neonatal hyponatremia or hyperuricemia Compatible with normal development if electrolytes balanced	
ACEIs[a] Lisinopril[L3] Enalapril[L2] Captopril[L2]	Nonpregnant state LV dysfunction All classes HF	↓ Preload & afterload Mortality benefit Morbidity benefit Reduced hospitalization	Electrolyte abnormalities Hypotension Cough Angioedema Worsening renal function	Skull hypoplasia, anuria, renal failure, limb contractures, craniofacial deformation, hypoplastic lungs, death	
ARBS[a] Valsartan[L3] Losartan[L3] Sacubitril[b,58]/valsartan	Intolerance to ACEIs LV dysfunction All classes HF	↓ Preload & afterload Mortality benefit Morbidity benefit Reduced hospitalization	Similar to ACEIs	Similar to ACEIs	
β-Blockers Metoprolol[L2] Carvedilol[L3] Bisoprolol[L3]	LV dysfunction unless contraindicated	Improves myocardial contractility by ↓ sympathetic tone Reduces mortality	Avoid initiation or increased dose in decompensated HF		
Peripheral vasodilators Hydralazine[L2] Nitrates[L4]	First-line vasodilator in pregnancy or when ACE and ARBS are contraindicated; additional intervention postpartum in selected patients	↓ Preload & afterload Mortality benefit Morbidity benefit especially in AAs	Hypotension Tolerance w/long-term nitrate therapy Headache with nitrates Lupuslike reaction with hydralazine	Bradycardia, hypoglycemia, growth restriction	

Drug	Indication	Benefit	Adverse effects	Pregnancy/lactation comments
Aldosterone antagonists Spironolactone[L2] Eplerenone[L3]	LV dysfunction NYHA class II–IV on β-blocker/ACE Creatinine Clearance >30 mL/min and K+ <5 mEq/dL	Mortality benefit Mortality benefit Morbidity benefit	Little data in pregnancy Hyperkalemia Worsening renal function	Little data in humans Feminizaton of male rat fetuses
Selective sinus node inhibitor Ivabradine[b,58]	Symptomatic chronic HF with reduced EF <35% Sinus rhythm and HR >70 bpm on maximal β-blocker	Reduced composite hospitalization and death	Bradycardia Visual side effects Hypotension Atrial fibrillation Should not be used in decompensated HF	Embryofetal toxicity and cardiac teratogenic effects in animal studies. Should not be used in pregnancy
Calcium channel blocker Amlodipine[L3] Felodipine[L3]	Blood pressure control	Peripheral vasodilation	Peripheral edema Hypotension	
Inotropes Digoxin[L2]	Persistent symptoms despite therapy Experience during pregnancy Palliation with refractory HF	↑ Myocontractility	Arrhythmias Gastrointestinal symptoms Narrow therapeutic index	
Dopamine[c,L2] Dobutamine[c,L2] Milrinone[c,L4]			Arrhythmias Hypotension with dobutamine and milrinone	

Dr Hale's Lactation Risk Category: L1-Compatible: Drug that has been taken by a large number of breastfeeding mothers without any observed increase in adverse effects in the infant. Controlled studies in breastfeeding women fail to demonstrate a risk to the infant and the possibility of harm to the breastfeeding infant is remote, or the product is not orally bioavailable in an infant. L2-Probably Compatible: Drug that has been studied in a limited number of breastfeeding women without an increase in adverse effects in the infant, and/or the evidence of a demonstrated risk that is likely to follow use of this medication in a breastfeeding woman is remote. L3-Probably Compatible: There are no controlled studies in breastfeeding women; however, the risk of untoward effects to a breastfed infant is possible, or controlled studies show only minimal nonthreatening adverse effects. Drugs should be given only if the potential benefit justifies the potential risk to the infant. L4-Possibly Hazardous: There is positive evidence of risk to a breastfed infant or to breast-milk production, but the benefits of use in breastfeeding mothers may be acceptable despite the risk to the infant (eg, if the drug is needed in a life-threatening situation or for a serious disease for which safer drugs cannot be used or are ineffective). L5-Hazardous: Studies in breastfeeding mothers have demonstrated that there is significant and documented risk to the infant based on human experience, or it is a medication that has a high risk of causing significant damage to an infant. The risk of using the drug in breastfeeding women clearly outweighs any possible benefit from breastfeeding. The drug is contraindicated in women who are breastfeeding an infant.[96]

a Not safe in pregnancy based on limited evidence.
b No pregnancy or lactation data.
c Reserved for refractory HF and palliation.

typically use furosemide in gravidas with volume overload and after delivery when intravascular volume increases because of relief of aortocaval compression, auto-transfusion of uteroplacental blood, and mobilization of extravascular fluid.[51] Thiazide diuretics may be added for additional therapy. Aldosterone antagonists improve survival in selected HF patients and should be added postpartum for women who are New York Heart Association (NYHA) functional class II or worse,[45] but the authors have not used them during pregnancy.

ACE inhibitors (ACEIs) improve survival for patients with all classes of HF but are avoided during pregnancy because of teratogenicity.[52] When patients are started on ACEIs postpartum, the authors counsel patients about teratogenicity should subsequent pregnancy occur, and they stress the need for appropriate birth control. The authors start with low-dose ACEI uptitrating at intervals to maximal tolerated dose. Angiotensin receptor antagonists (ARBs) are used when ACEIs are not tolerated; teratogenic risks are similar. A combination of sacubritril, a neprilysin inhibitor, and valsartan, an ARB, enhances the heart's neurohormonal axis while suppressing the renin-angiotensin-aldosterone axis, resulting in reduced mortality in comparison with enalapril alone.[53] The combination is indicated in the United States for NYHA class II to IV HF with systolic dysfunction.[54] Risk/benefit ratio of infant exposure to medications compared with improvement in LV function should be weighed for use in lactating mothers, although the authors have often prescribed ACEIs in this setting.

Rationale for combined use of hydralazine, an arterial vasodilator, and nitrates, predominantly venodilators, is reduced afterload and preload, leading to improved symptoms and mortality benefit in some racial groups.[45] Nitrates also enhance nitric oxide bioavailability, enhancing hydralazine's activity.[55] A large clinical experience with hydralazine in pregnancy suggests that it is safe and compatible with breastfeeding. This combination is the vasodilator therapy of choice during pregnancy or if medications acting on the renin-angiotensin system are contraindicated. However, ACEIs remain first-line agents outside of pregnancy.

Three β-blockers (sustained release metoprolol succinate, carvedilol, and bisoprolol) reduce morbidity and mortality with HF with reduced EF.[45] β-Blocker therapy is recommended for all stable patients unless contraindicated.[45] The authors recommend monitoring exposed neonates for bradycardia, hypoglycemia, or growth restriction.[50,56] Transient worsening of HF symptoms has been reported; therefore, patients should have minimal fluid retention and not be on inotropic agents.[45] Therapy is started at low dose and uptitrated until maximal dose used in trials is achieved or the patient has symptoms.[45]

Treatment of hypertension is an important component of GDMT.[45] Calcium channel blocking agents are not recommended routinely for patients with reduced EF.[45] However, second-generation dihydropyridine channel blockers, such as amlodipine, can be added for additional control.[45] Blood pressure goals should follow current established guidelines, but the authors do not decrease doses of vasodilators or β-blockers for asymptomatic hypotension.[45]

Digoxin improves symptoms, quality of life, and exercise tolerance by attenuation of the neurohormonal system and inhibition of sodium potassium adenosine triphosphatase, increasing myocontractility.[45] Benefit occurs regardless of underlying rhythm, cause of HF, or concomitant therapy but does not clearly reduce mortality.[45] Digoxin has a narrow therapeutic dosing window; therefore, attention is required to avoid toxicity.[45] Digoxin has been used safely in pregnancy; the authors typically add digoxin during pregnancy when ACEIs and ARBs are contraindicated.

Ivabradine, a sinus node inhibitor, improves outcomes in patients with reduced EF and elevated heart rates.[54] It is recommended for stable chronic class II to III

HF, EF $\leq$35%, and sinus rhythm with heart rate greater than 70 bpm on maximum tolerated β-blocker.[54] In a small retrospective analysis of 20 women in the German PPCM registry, the medication was well tolerated, and EFs improved in the majority.[57] There are no adequate studies in pregnant women; embryotoxicity was seen in animal models.[58]

LV dysfunction is associated with thromboembolic risk, estimated at approximately 1% to 3% per year.[45] Thromboembolic complications correlate with severity of LV dysfunction, atrial fibrillation, and thrombus is noted on transthoracic.[45] However, thromboembolic risk in PPCM is higher: 6.6% and 6.8%, respectively, in the Nationwide Inpatient Sample and in more than 400 women in the EURObservational Research Programme (EURObRP).[12,42] A recent Nigerian study documented 21.4% incidence of LV thrombi. The authors have used full anticoagulation in the setting of the above complications or EF $\leq$30% until the thrombophilia of pregnancy resolves. Optimal anticoagulation strategy after that time is less clear.[45] The authors use low-molecular-weight heparin or continuous unfractionated heparin during pregnancy depending on whether antepartum or intrapartum, along with warfarin postpartum. All agents are compatible with breastfeeding.[52] There are limited data on direct oral anticoagulants (direct thrombin inhibitors and antifactor Xa inhibitors) during pregnancy and lactation; current recommendations advise against use.[59]

Drugs known to adversely affect clinical status in HF should be avoided. These drugs include nonsteroidal anti-inflammatory agents, thiazolidinediones, and non-dihydropyridene calcium channel blockers other than amlodipine.[45] Statins are not beneficial in HF in the absence of another indication.[45] Prolonged intravenous inotropic therapy may shorten survival, but may be used as palliation or bridge to advanced interventions.[45] Exercise can be an adjunct to improving status in stable postpartum patients.[45]

For patients with persistent LV dysfunction (EF $\leq$35%), class II or III symptoms, and with an expected survival of >1 year, implantable cardioverter defibrillators may be warranted for primary prevention of sudden cardiac death.[60] Relatively high rate of recovery in PPCM should be considered before a defibrillator is placed. Moreover, delayed recovery after 6 months is reported in a significant minority of patients, which may modify the decision for placement.[61] Women should have received a minimum of 3 months of GDMT with β-blockers and ACEIs before deciding.[60] Wearable cardiac defibrillators have been used successfully for primary prevention in anticipation of ventricular function recovery, especially with high-risk features.[62] Cardiac resynchronization therapy is recommended for some patients.[60] LV assist devices (LVADs) and transplantation are therapeutic options in the most critical patients, with the former associated with subsequent improvement of ventricular function in a few patients.[45,63]

Impact of breastfeeding on outcomes has been controversial, especially given the proposed role of prolactin in disease development.[50,64,65] Fear of adverse effects of medication transmission to the child via breast milk or increased hemodynamic demands of lactation in sick women sometimes lead to recommendations to discontinue lactation. Fifteen percent of women in the IPAC registry breastfed.[64] No effect was seen on myocardial recovery at 12 months. In a retrospective review of PPCM women recruited via the Internet, 67.3% of women breastfed, and this was associated with increased recovery.[65] However, it is unknown if women had better initial EFs or other reasons for improved survival.

Other Novel Therapies

In mouse models, proapoptotic fragments of prolactin lead to myocardial injury.[27,28] Bromocriptine stimulates hypothalamic dopaminergic receptors inhibiting prolactin secretion, suggesting theoretic treatment benefit.[66] A randomized controlled trial with bromocriptine as adjunctive therapy in 20 South African women showed improved ventricular recovery as proof of concept, although adverse outcomes in the control group were high.[67] A nonrandomized German registry found bromocriptine use twice as common in women with improved LV function, although the percentage of women receiving advanced HF interventions in both groups was similar.[68] A recent multicenter trial of 63 PPCM patients with EFs less than 35% randomized women to 1 week or 8 weeks of bromocriptine therapy.[69] No patient required advanced HF interventions or died. There was a nonsignificant trend toward greater recovery in the 8-week therapy group, but both groups showed improvement. Therapy was well tolerated. A major limitation to the study was lack of a placebo control group. An accompanying editorial suggested that bromocriptine could be added to usual GDMT.[70] Small numbers of patients, validity of comparing outcomes to a historical control groups with large numbers of AAs who have worse outcomes, concerns about potential hypertensive or thrombotic complications with bromocriptine treatment, and loss of ability to lactate in treated women, especially in developing countries, are among the reasons dampening enthusiasm for widespread use in the United States in the absence of a placebo-controlled trial.[6] When bromocriptine is used, patients should receive concomitant anticoagulant therapy.[69] Although approved for other indications, bromocriptine is not currently approved for treatment of PPCM in the United States.

Evidence regarding treatment with intravenous immune globulin has been inconsistent.[71,72] A South African study demonstrated improved outcomes in PPCM women treated with pentoxyfylline. Tumor necrosis factor-α levels decreased in patients and controls, but there was greater survival, EF improvement, and NYHA class in the pentoxyfilline group.[73] A randomized trial of Levosimendan, a calcium sensitizer, in 24 women with PPCM showed no difference in clinical or outcomes.[74]

GDMT should continue with persistent LV dysfunction. There are no well-controlled studies to advise duration of therapy when LV function improves, but most experts recommend continuing for 6 months after recovery.[6,75] Ivabradine could be discontinued first, followed by aldosterone antagonists before downtitration of ACEIs or β-blockers, observing for recurrence.[75]

Management of Delivery

Most women present postpartum, but for women who present during pregnancy, it is not known if early delivery will diminish progression of LV dysfunction.[6] Timing and mode of delivery decisions are best made by a team approach, including the maternal fetal medicine, cardiology, obstetric-anesthesia, and neonatology providers caring for the patient. Labor is not contraindicated for stable patients. Administration of steroids to promote fetal lung maturity can increase fluid retention.[45] In the authors' practice, labor induction can be conducted with minimal risk; cervical ripening with prostaglandins and oxytocin can be administered safely. Early epidural will minimize sympathetic output however, but caution must be exercised with fluid boluses to avoid overload.[51] Shortening the second stage of labor and the use of low-forceps or vacuum device will also decrease cardiac work.[76] Given the surgical risks encountered with cesarean delivery, such as infection, blood loss, fluid shifts, and postoperative complications, the authors believe cardiovascular benefits from vaginal delivery most often outweigh that of surgical delivery. The authors reserve cesarean delivery for obstetric indications; however, need for prompt delivery may influence the decision. Placement of a pulmonary artery catheter for hemodynamic monitoring is rarely recommended,[50] but strict monitoring of fluid status is critical. The authors often administer diuretics after delivery in the absence of bleeding to prevent volume overload.

It is important to continue monitoring volume status postpartum because fluid is mobilized. Additional diuretic therapy may be required. Therapy with medications contraindicated during pregnancy, such as ACEIs or ARBs, can now be started. Thromboprophylaxis needs to be addressed. Women need early evaluation after discharge to ensure they are not decompensating. It is also crucial to consider contraceptive options. In a recent survey of 177 PPCM patients, almost 30% of sexually active PPCM patients reported contraceptive nonuse and 27% nonusers reported no contraceptive discussion with health care providers.[77] Lack of social support is also associated with increased hospitalization and mortality risk.[78]

Neonates of mothers with PPCM had worse outcomes than neonates of mothers without: they were born earlier, born smaller, and had more smaller-for-gestational age infants, and APGAR scores were lower.[11] In the EURObRP, neonatal death rate was 3.1%.[42]

Maternal Prognosis

Maternal prognosis is variable but better than other causes of cardiomyopathy.[79] Improvement occurs in most patients.[64] Most women improve in the first 2 to 6 months, with complete recovery for many.[6,64] Delayed recovery has also been reported.[80] In EURObRP, enrollment at 411 with PPCM, 2.4% mortality was seen at 1 month with most deaths due to HF, followed by sudden cardiac death and stroke; device placement (automatic implantable cardioverter-defibrillator or resynchronization therapy) occurred in 2.1% and an LVAD was placed in 2%.[42] Almost 87% of women were still classified as having HF.[42] The IPAC registry had 13% major events or persistent cardiomyopathy at 1 year. Mortality at 1 year was 4%; LVADs were placed in 4%, and 1 patient (1.1%) underwent heart transplantation.[64] Of 27 women with an initial EF <30%, more than one-third (37%) still had severe LV dysfunction at study end.[64]

AA race is associated with worse outcomes.[10,64,81–83] Harper and colleagues[81] found a 4-fold increased prevalence and fatality in non-Hispanic AAs when compared with Caucasians. Irizarry and colleagues[83] found AAs were younger, diagnosed later, had worse EF, and were less likely to recover, and EF was more likely to worsen after diagnosis despite adequate therapy. Worse outcomes in AAs relative to non-AAs may reflect socioeconomic factors, genetic and epigenetic factors, or access to medical care.

Baseline LV function is a strong predictor of eventual recovery. Goland and colleagues[84] found an inverse correlation between presenting EF and outcome. Seventy-nine percent of women with an EF greater than 30% achieved full recovery in comparison with only 37% who presented with an EF less than 20%. Larger LV size at presentation is also a marker for poor recovery, along with reduced right ventricular function.[64,68,84–86] The combination of LVEF with increased LV size resulted in more accurate assessment of recovery.[64]

The presence of hypertensive disorders is associated with increased likelihood of recovery in some studies, but not all.[43,64,68,87] The ongoing worldwide registry of PPCM (EURObRP) may shed further light on this.[42] Elevation of cardiac troponins is associated with myocardial injury and reduced EF (<35% at 6-month follow-up).[88]

The recent focus on the vascular-hormonal causes has led to an interest in whether vascular biomarkers provide prognostic information. Higher Relaxin 2 levels, which have anti-inflammatory, angiogenic, and antifibrotic effects, were associated with improved 2-month recovery.[34] In contrast, higher sFLT1 levels were associated with worse NYHA functional class and death.[34] There was no relationship between prolactin level or VEGF levels and LV recovery or adverse clinical events.[34] Routine use of these biomarkers, or others such as cathepsin D, 16-kDa Prolactin fragment, microRNA-146, in evaluating prognosis is an area for additional investigation. Similarly, genetic variants assessed in the IPAC cohort correlated with 1-year EF, suggesting genetic analysis may play a future clinical prognostic role.[41]

Prognosis with Subsequent Pregnancies

Many women with PPCM desire a subsequent pregnancy. Recurrence risk is based on retrospective reviews. Elkayam and colleagues[89] reviewed the risk of recurrent cardiomyopathy dividing women into those with recovered compared with depressed LV function. Mean EF decreased in both groups, but HF symptoms were seen in 21% of gravidas with normal function and 44% of those with persistent LV dysfunction. Other studies have shown similar findings.[90] Elkayam[91] recently performed a meta-analysis of published case series. In the normalized group, 27% of women developed deterioration of function and 32% of women had symptomatic HF. Outcomes in women with persistent dysfunction were significantly worse. Almost half had deterioration of LV function and symptomatic HF; LV dysfunction was persistent in 39%, and 16% died.[91] In women with more than one subsequent pregnancy, outcome of the first subsequent pregnancy did not predict outcome of further pregnancies.[91] Exercise stress ECHO or dobutamine stress ECHO may help define risk in women with recovered function.[90] Some patients with improved LV function based on EF have decreased contractile reserve only evident with stress testing.[92] Elkayam[91] also found that fetal complications were more common in women with persistent LV dysfunction. Fifty percent of births were premature, and 25% of women had therapeutic abortions in the persistent LV dysfunction group. In contrast, 13% of women had premature deliveries, and only 4% of women had a therapeutic abortion in those with normalized LV function.[91]

Currently, no biomarkers define the group of women who will develop recurrent HF. Proangiogenic and antiangiogenic factors, such as sFLT1, sFLT1:PlGF ratio, relaxin-2, and genetic markers seen in PPCM, such as TTN truncating gene variants and GNB3TT genotype, are avenues for future investigation. Similarly, it is unknown if prophylactic β-blockade has a role in preventing recurrence in recovered function.

All women with subsequent pregnancies should be considered high risk, necessitating close communication between the treating physicians. The authors perform frequent evaluations, including physical examination, transthoracic, and BNP levels at baseline, second and third trimesters, 1-month and 6-months postpartum, or if concerns about relapse. The authors typically perform a sonogram at 20 weeks' gestation to assess fetal anatomy and then serially assess for fetal intrauterine growth restriction. In their practice, the authors routinely perform antenatal testing in the third trimester, regardless of the EF (eg, nonstress test and amniotic fluid index or biophysical profile starting at 32 weeks and then weekly thereafter), although benefit is not proven.

Fett[93,94] developed a simple periodic self-assessment tool validated on women with PPCM recruited from support groups, which the authors have found helpful in identifying women with potential relapse (**Table 2**). Elevated scores prompt additional evaluation. In Fett's study, all PPCM patients had scores greater than 5 and control women had scores less than 4 (mean score 8.93 with PPCM; 1.5 in controls).[94] The authors have typically continued β-blockade in women with continued LV dysfunction and substituted the combination of hydralazine/nitrates for ACEIs or ARBs during pregnancy.

Table 2
Self-assessment tool in identifying women at risk for potential relapse

Symptom/Sign	0 Points	1 Point	2 Points
Orthopnea	None	Need to elevate head only	Need to elevate body >45°
Dyspnea	None	When climbing ≥8 stairs	Walking level
Unexplained cough	None	Night time	Day and night
Pitting edema	None	Below knee	Above and below knee
Weight gain (9th mo)	≤907 g/wk	907–1814 g/wk	>1814 lbs/wk
Palpitations	None	When lying down	Any position day and night

Scoring and action: 0 to 2 low risk, observe. 3 to 4 mild risk, consider BNP/Hs-CRP → ECHO if abnormal. ≥5 high risk, BNP, Hs-CRP, ECHO.

From Fett JD. Personal commentary: monitoring subsequent pregnancy in recovered peripartum cardiomyopathy mothers. Crit Pathw Cardiol 2009;8(4):174; with permission.

SUMMARY

Significant progress in understanding the pathophysiology of PPCM, especially the underlying contribution of hormonal and genetic mechanism, has been made recently. Although diagnostic criteria should be used to diagnose PPCM, it remains a diagnosis of exclusion. Both long-term and recurrent pregnancy prognosis depend on recovery of cardiac function. Risk stratification from large registries such as IPAC and EURObRP together with randomized controlled trials of evidence-based therapeutics from translational studies holds promise of improved clinical outcomes in the future.

REFERENCES

1. Gouley BA, McMillan TM, Bellet S. Idiopathic myocardial degeneration associated with pregnancy and especially the puerperium. Am J Med Sci 1937;19:185–99.
2. Demakis JG, Rahimtoola SH. Peripartum cardiomyopathy. Circulation 1971;44(5): 964–8.
3. Hibbard JU, Lindheimer M, Lang RM. A modified definition for peripartum cardiomyopathy and prognosis based on echocardiography. Obstetrics Gynecol 1999; 94(2):311–6.
4. Sliwa K, Hilfiker-Kleiner D, Petrie MC, et al. Current state of knowledge on aetiology, diagnosis, management, and therapy of peripartum cardiomyopathy: a position statement from the Heart Failure Association of the European Society of Cardiology Working Group on peripartum cardiomyopathy. Eur J Heart Fail 2010;12(8):767–78.
5. Elkayam U, Akhter MW, Singh H, et al. Pregnancy-associated cardiomyopathy: clinical characteristics and a comparison between early and late presentation. Circulation 2005;111(16):2050–5.
6. Arany Z, Elkayam U. Peripartum cardiomyopathy. Circulation 2016;133(14): 1397–409.
7. Kuklina EV, Callaghan WM. Cardiomyopathy and other myocardial disorders among hospitalizations for pregnancy in the United States: 2004-2006. Obstetrics Gynecol 2010;115(1):93–100.
8. Whitehead SJ, Berg CJ, Chang J. Pregnancy-related mortality due to cardiomyopathy: United States, 1991-1997. Obstetrics Gynecol 2003;102(6):1326–31.
9. Mielniczuk LM, Williams K, Davis DR, et al. Frequency of peripartum cardiomyopathy. Am J Cardiol 2006;97(12):1765–8.

10. Brar SS, Khan SS, Sandhu GK, et al. Incidence, mortality, and racial differences in peripartum cardiomyopathy. Am J Cardiol 2007;100(2):302–4.

11. Gunderson EP, Croen LA, Chiang V, et al. Epidemiology of peripartum cardiomyopathy: incidence, predictors, and outcomes. Obstetrics Gynecol 2011;118(3): 583–91.

12. Kolte D, Khera S, Aronow WS, et al. Temporal trends in incidence and outcomes of peripartum cardiomyopathy in the United States: a nationwide population-based study. J Am Heart Assoc 2014;3(3):e001056.

13. CDC. Severe maternal morbidity in the United States 2017. Available at: www. cdc.gov/reproductivehealth/maternalinfanthealth/pmss.html. Accessed July 25, 2017.

14. Briller J, Koch AR, Geller SE. Maternal cardiovascular mortality in Illinois, 2002-2011. Obstetrics Gynecol 2017;129(5):819–26.

15. Main EK, McCain CL, Morton CH, et al. Pregnancy-related mortality in California: causes, characteristics, and improvement opportunities. Obstetrics Gynecol 2015;125(4):938–47.

16. Hameed AB, Lawton ES, McCain CL, et al. Pregnancy-related cardiovascular deaths in California: beyond peripartum cardiomyopathy. Am J Obstet Gynecol 2015;213(3):379.e1-10.

17. Cantwell R, Clutton-Brock T, Cooper G, et al. Saving mothers' lives: reviewing maternal deaths to make motherhood safer: 2006-2008. The Eighth Report of the Confidential Enquiries into Maternal Deaths in the United Kingdom. BJOG 2011;118(Suppl 1):1–203.

18. Ntusi NB, Mayosi BM. Aetiology and risk factors of peripartum cardiomyopathy: a systematic review. Int J Cardiol 2009;131(2):168–79.

19. Robson SC, Hunter S, Boys RJ, et al. Serial study of factors influencing changes in cardiac output during human pregnancy. Am J Physiol 1989;256(4 Pt 2): H1060–5.

20. Rizeq MN, Rickenbacher PR, Fowler MB, et al. Incidence of myocarditis in peripartum cardiomyopathy. Am J Cardiol 1994;74(5):474–7.

21. Felker GM, Jaeger CJ, Klodas E, et al. Myocarditis and long-term survival in peripartum cardiomyopathy. Am Heart J 2000;140(5):785–91.

22. Ansari AA, Fett JD, Carraway RE, et al. Autoimmune mechanisms as the basis for human peripartum cardiomyopathy. Clin Rev Allergy Immunol 2002;23(3): 301–24.

23. Kara RJ, Bolli P, Karakikes I, et al. Fetal cells traffic to injured maternal myocardium and undergo cardiac differentiation. Circ Res 2012;110(1):82–93.

24. Karaye KM, Yahaya IA, Lindmark K, et al. Serum selenium and ceruloplasmin in nigerians with peripartum cardiomyopathy. Int J Mol Sci 2015;16(4):7644–54.

25. Lampert MB, Hibbard J, Weinert L, et al. Peripartum heart failure associated with prolonged tocolytic therapy. Am J Obstet Gynecol 1993;168(2):493–5.

26. Kao DP, Hsich E, Lindenfeld J. Characteristics, adverse events, and racial differences among delivering mothers with peripartum cardiomyopathy. JACC Heart Fail 2013;1(5):409–16.

27. Hilfiker-Kleiner D, Kaminski K, Podewski E, et al. A cathepsin D-cleaved 16 kDa form of prolactin mediates postpartum cardiomyopathy. Cell 2007;128(3): 589–600.

28. Patten IS, Rana S, Shahul S, et al. Cardiac angiogenic imbalance leads to peripartum cardiomyopathy. Nature 2012;485(7398):333–8.

29. Halkein J, Tabruyn SP, Ricke-Hoch M, et al. MicroRNA-146a is a therapeutic target and biomarker for peripartum cardiomyopathy. J Clin Invest 2013;123(5): 2143–54.
30. Arany Z, Foo SY, Ma Y, et al. HIF-independent regulation of VEGF and angiogenesis by the transcriptional coactivator PGC-1alpha. Nature 2008;451(7181): 1008–12.
31. Powe CE, Levine RJ, Karumanchi SA. Preeclampsia, a disease of the maternal endothelium: the role of antiangiogenic factors and implications for later cardiovascular disease. Circulation 2011;123(24):2856–69.
32. Bdolah Y, Lam C, Rajakumar A, et al. Twin pregnancy and the risk of preeclampsia: bigger placenta or relative ischemia? Am J Obstet Gynecol 2008;198(4): 428.e1-6.
33. Goland S, Weinstein JM, Zalik A, et al. Angiogenic imbalance and residual myocardial injury in recovered peripartum cardiomyopathy patients. Circ Heart Fail 2016;9(11) [pii:e003349].
34. Damp J, Givertz MM, Semigran M, et al. Relaxin-2 and soluble Flt1 levels in peripartum cardiomyopathy: results of the multicenter IPAC study. JACC Heart Fail 2016;4(5):380–8.
35. Fett JD, Sundstrom BJ, Etta King M, et al. Mother-daughter peripartum cardiomyopathy. Int J Cardiol 2002;86(2–3):331–2.
36. van Spaendonck-Zwarts KY, van Tintelen JP, van Veldhuisen DJ, et al. Peripartum cardiomyopathy as a part of familial dilated cardiomyopathy. Circulation 2010; 121(20):2169–75.
37. Morales A, Painter T, Li R, et al. Rare variant mutations in pregnancy-associated or peripartum cardiomyopathy. Circulation 2010;121(20):2176–82.
38. Herman DS, Lam L, Taylor MR, et al. Truncations of titin causing dilated cardiomyopathy. N Engl J Med 2012;366(7):619–28.
39. Ware JS, Li J, Mazaika E, et al. Shared genetic predisposition in peripartum and dilated cardiomyopathies. N Engl J Med 2016;374(26):2601–2.
40. Horne BD, Rasmusson KD, Alharethi R, et al. Genome-wide significance and replication of the chromosome 12p11.22 locus near the PTHLH gene for peripartum cardiomyopathy. Circ Cardiovasc Genet 2011;4(4):359–66.
41. Sheppard R, Hsich E, Damp J, et al. GNB3 C825T polymorphism and myocardial recovery in peripartum cardiomyopathy: results of the multicenter investigations of pregnancy-associated cardiomyopathy study. Circ Heart Fail 2016;9(3): e002683.
42. Sliwa K, Mebazaa A, Hilfiker-Kleiner D, et al. Clinical characteristics of patients from the worldwide registry on peripartum cardiomyopathy (PPCM): EURObservational Research Programme in conjunction with the Heart Failure Association of the European Society of Cardiology Study Group on PPCM. Eur J Heart Fail 2017; 19(9):1131–41.
43. Bello N, Rendon IS, Arany Z. The relationship between pre-eclampsia and peripartum cardiomyopathy: a systematic review and meta-analysis. J Am Coll Cardiol 2013;62(18):1715–23.
44. Fett JD, Christie LG, Carraway RD, et al. Five-year prospective study of the incidence and prognosis of peripartum cardiomyopathy at a single institution. Mayo Clinic Proc 2005;80(12):1602–6.
45. Yancy CW, Jessup M, Bozkurt B, et al. 2013 ACCF/AHA guideline for the management of heart failure: executive summary: a report of the American College of Cardiology Foundation/American Heart Association Task Force on Practice Guidelines. Circulation 2013;128(16):1810–52.

46. Bozkurt B, Colvin M, Cook J, et al. Current diagnostic and treatment strategies for specific dilated cardiomyopathies: a scientific statement from the American Heart Association. Circulation 2016;134(23):e579–646.

47. Mouquet F, Lions C, de Groote P, et al. Characterisation of peripartum cardiomyopathy by cardiac magnetic resonance imaging. Eur Radiol 2008;18(12):2765–9.

48. Schelbert EB, Elkayam U, Cooper LT, et al. Myocardial damage detected by late gadolinium enhancement cardiac magnetic resonance is uncommon in peripartum cardiomyopathy. J Am Heart Assoc 2017;6(4) [pii:e005472].

49. Sliwa K, Fett J, Elkayam U. Peripartum cardiomyopathy. Lancet 2006;368(9536): 687–93.

50. Regitz-Zagrosek V, Blomstrom Lundqvist C, Borghi C, et al. ESC guidelines on the management of cardiovascular diseases during pregnancy: the task force on the management of cardiovascular diseases during pregnancy of the European Society of Cardiology (ESC). Eur Heart J 2011;32(24):3147–97.

51. Ueland K. Maternal cardiovascular dynamics. VII. Intrapartum blood volume changes. Am J Obstet Gynecol 1976;126(6):671–7.

52. Briggs GG, Freeman RK. Drugs in pregnancy and lactation: a reference guide to fetal and neonatal risk. 11th edition. Philadelphia: Lippincott Williams & Wilkins; 2017.

53. McMurray JJ, Packer M, Desai AS, et al. Angiotensin-neprilysin inhibition versus enalapril in heart failure. N Engl J Med 2014;371(11):993–1004.

54. Yancy CW, Jessup M, Bozkurt B, et al. 2017 ACC/AHA/HFSA focused update of the 2013 ACCF/AHA guideline for the management of heart failure: a report of the American College of Cardiology/American Heart Association Task Force on Clinical Practice Guidelines and the Heart Failure Society of America. J Am Coll Cardiol 2017;70(6):776–803.

55. Cole RT, Kalogeropoulos AP, Georgiopoulou VV, et al. Hydralazine and isosorbide dinitrate in heart failure: historical perspective, mechanisms, and future directions. Circulation 2011;123(21):2414–22.

56. Ersboll AS, Hedegaard M, Sondergaard L, et al. Treatment with oral betablockers during pregnancy complicated by maternal heart disease increases the risk of fetal growth restriction. BJOG 2014;121(5):618–26.

57. Haghikia A, Tongers J, Berliner D, et al. Early ivabradine treatment in patients with acute peripartum cardiomyopathy: subanalysis of the German PPCM registry. Int J Cardiol 2016;216:165–7.

58. Amgen C. What is Corlanor? 2016. Available at: https://www.corlanor.com/what-is-corlanor-chronichf-treatment/. Accessed September 30, 2017.

59. Cohen H, Arachchillage DR, Middeldorp S, et al. Management of direct oral anticoagulants in women of childbearing potential: guidance from the SSC of the ISTH. J Thromb Haemost 2016;14(8):1673–6.

60. Russo AM, Stainback RF, Bailey SR, et al. ACCF/HRS/AHA/ASE/HFSA/SCAI/SCCT/SCMR 2013 appropriate use criteria for implantable cardioverter-defibrillators and cardiac resynchronization therapy: a report of the American College of Cardiology Foundation appropriate use criteria task force, Heart Rhythm Society, American Heart Association, American Society of Echocardiography, Heart Failure Society of America, Society for Cardiovascular Angiography and Interventions, Society of Cardiovascular Computed Tomography, and Society for Cardiovascular Magnetic Resonance. Heart Rhythm 2013;10(4):e11–58.

61. Pillarisetti J, Kondur A, Alani A, et al. Peripartum cardiomyopathy: predictors of recovery and current state of implantable cardioverter-defibrillator use. J Am Coll Cardiol 2014;63(25 Pt A):2831–9.

62. Duncker D, Haghikia A, Konig T, et al. Risk for ventricular fibrillation in peripartum cardiomyopathy with severely reduced left ventricular function-value of the wearable cardioverter/defibrillator. Eur J Heart Fail 2014;16(12):1331–6.

63. Cook JL, Colvin M, Francis GS, et al. Recommendations for the use of mechanical circulatory support: ambulatory and community patient care: a scientific statement from the American Heart Association. Circulation 2017;135(25):e1145–58.

64. McNamara DM, Elkayam U, Alharethi R, et al. Clinical outcomes for peripartum cardiomyopathy in North America: results of the IPAC study (Investigations of Pregnancy-Associated Cardiomyopathy). J Am Coll Cardiol 2015;66(8):905–14.

65. Safirstein JG, Ro AS, Grandhi S, et al. Predictors of left ventricular recovery in a cohort of peripartum cardiomyopathy patients recruited via the internet. Int J Cardiol 2012;154(1):27–31.

66. Spark RF, Pallotta J, Naftolin F, et al. Galactorrhea-amenorrhea syndromes: etiology and treatment. Ann Intern Med 1976;84(5):532–7.

67. Sliwa K, Blauwet L, Tibazarwa K, et al. Evaluation of bromocriptine in the treatment of acute severe peripartum cardiomyopathy: a proof-of-concept pilot study. Circulation 2010;121(13):1465–73.

68. Haghikia A, Podewski E, Libhaber E, et al. Phenotyping and outcome on contemporary management in a German cohort of patients with peripartum cardiomyopathy. Basic Res Cardiol 2013;108(4):366.

69. Hilfiker-Kleiner D, Haghikia A, Berliner D, et al. Bromocriptine for the treatment of peripartum cardiomyopathy: a multicentre randomized study. Eur Heart J 2017; 38(35):2671–9.

70. Arrigo M, Blet A, Mebazaa A. Bromocriptine for the treatment of peripartum cardiomyopathy: welcome on BOARD. Eur Heart J 2017;38(35):2680–2.

71. Bozkurt B, Villaneuva FS, Holubkov R, et al. Intravenous immune globulin in the therapy of peripartum cardiomyopathy. J Am Coll Cardiol 1999;34(1):177–80.

72. McNamara DM, Holubkov R, Starling RC, et al. Controlled trial of intravenous immune globulin in recent-onset dilated cardiomyopathy. Circulation 2001;103(18): 2254–9.

73. Sliwa K, Skudicky D, Candy G, et al. The addition of pentoxifylline to conventional therapy improves outcome in patients with peripartum cardiomyopathy. Eur J Heart Fail 2002;4(3):305–9.

74. Biteker M, Duran NE, Kaya H, et al. Effect of levosimendan and predictors of recovery in patients with peripartum cardiomyopathy, a randomized clinical trial. Clin Res Cardiol 2011;100(7):571–7.

75. Hilfiker-Kleiner D, Haghikia A, Nonhoff J, et al. Peripartum cardiomyopathy: current management and future perspectives. Eur Heart J 2015;36(18):1090–7.

76. Cruz MO, Briller J, Hibbard JU. Update on peripartum cardiomyopathy. Obstet Gynecol Clin North Am 2010;37(2):283–303.

77. Rosman L, Salmoirago-Blotcher E, Wuensch KL, et al. Contraception and reproductive counseling in women with peripartum cardiomyopathy. Contraception 2017;96(1):36–40.

78. Luttik ML, Jaarsma T, Moser D, et al. The importance and impact of social support on outcomes in patients with heart failure: an overview of the literature. J Cardiovasc Nurs 2005;20(3):162–9.

79. Lu CH, Lee WC, Wu M, et al. Comparison of clinical outcomes in peripartum cardiomyopathy and age-matched dilated cardiomyopathy: a 15-year nationwide population-based study in Asia. Medicine (Baltimore) 2017;96(19):e6898.

80. Biteker M, Ilhan E, Biteker G, et al. Delayed recovery in peripartum cardiomyopathy: an indication for long-term follow-up and sustained therapy. Eur J Heart Fail 2012;14(8):895–901.

81. Harper MA, Meyer RE, Berg CJ. Peripartum cardiomyopathy: population-based birth prevalence and 7-year mortality. Obstetrics Gynecol 2012;120(5):1013–9.

82. Goland S, Modi K, Hatamizadeh P, et al. Differences in clinical profile of African-American women with peripartum cardiomyopathy in the United States. J Card Fail 2013;19(4):214–8.

83. Irizarry OC, Levine LD, Lewey J, et al. Comparison of clinical characteristics and outcomes of peripartum cardiomyopathy between African American and non-African American women. JAMA Cardiol 2017;2(11):1256–60.

84. Goland S, Modi K, Bitar F, et al. Clinical profile and predictors of complications in peripartum cardiomyopathy. J Card Fail 2009;15(8):645–50.

85. Blauwet LA, Libhaber E, Forster O, et al. Predictors of outcome in 176 South African patients with peripartum cardiomyopathy. Heart 2013;99(5):308–13.

86. Blauwet LA, Delgado-Montero A, Ryo K, et al. Right ventricular function in peripartum cardiomyopathy at presentation is associated with subsequent left ventricular recovery and clinical outcomes. Circ Heart Fail 2016;9(5) [pii:e002756].

87. Kamiya CA, Kitakaze M, Ishibashi-Ueda H, et al. Different characteristics of peripartum cardiomyopathy between patients complicated with and without hypertensive disorders. Results from the Japanese nationwide survey of peripartum cardiomyopathy. Circ J 2011;75(8):1975–81.

88. Hu CL, Li YB, Zou YG, et al. Troponin T measurement can predict persistent left ventricular dysfunction in peripartum cardiomyopathy. Heart 2007;93(4):488–90.

89. Elkayam U, Tummala PP, Rao K, et al. Maternal and fetal outcomes of subsequent pregnancies in women with peripartum cardiomyopathy. N Engl J Med 2001; 344(21):1567–71.

90. Fett JD, Fristoe KL, Welsh SN. Risk of heart failure relapse in subsequent pregnancy among peripartum cardiomyopathy mothers. Int J Gynaecol Obstet 2010;109(1):34–6.

91. Elkayam U. Risk of subsequent pregnancy in women with a history of peripartum cardiomyopathy. J Am Coll Cardiol 2014;64(15):1629–36.

92. Lampert MB, Weinert L, Hibbard J, et al. Contractile reserve in patients with peripartum cardiomyopathy and recovered left ventricular function. Am J Obstet Gynecol 1997;176(1 Pt 1):189–95.

93. Fett JD. Personal commentary: monitoring subsequent pregnancy in recovered peripartum cardiomyopathy mothers. Crit Pathw Cardiol 2009;8(4):172–4.

94. Fett JD. Validation of a self-test for early diagnosis of heart failure in peripartum cardiomyopathy. Crit pathways Cardiol 2011;10(1):44–5.

95. Pearson GD, Veille JC, Rahimtoola S, et al. Peripartum cardiomyopathy: National Heart, Lung, and Blood Institute and Office of Rare Diseases (National Institutes of Health) workshop recommendations and review. JAMA 2000;283(9):1183–8.

96. Hale TW. Medications and mother's milk. 17th edition. New York: Springer Publishing; 2017.

Gestational Diabetes

Underpinning Principles, Surveillance, and Management

Jeffrey M. Denney, MD, MS*, Kristen H. Quinn, MD, MS

KEYWORDS

- Gestational diabetes • Glycemic intolerance • Fetal programming • Macrosomia
- Neonatal hypoglycemia • Maternal glucose control • Antenatal testing • Pregnancy

KEY POINTS

- Gestational diabetes mellitus (GDM) is defined as glycemic intolerance diagnosed at or beyond the achievement of 20 completed weeks of gestation.
- In women who ultimately develop GDM, pancreatic beta-cell compensation fails to meet the metabolic demands, creating a hyperglycemic state.
- Observational data demonstrate risks with poorly controlled GDM, including abnormal fetal growth, hypertensive disorders of pregnancy, difficult labor and vaginal delivery, increased risk of cesarean section, and the neonatal metabolic complications, including hypoglycemia, hyperbilirubinemia, and the potential for delayed pulmonary maturity.
- Poorly controlled GDM places the fetus at risk for adult-onset metabolic diseases (obesity, diabetes, hypertension, cardiovascular disease).
- Seventy percent of women with GDM will develop DM at some point in their life, and 40% to 50% of those women will develop DM within 10 years.

INTRODUCTION

The objective of this review is to provide the clinician with a working framework to evaluate and manage gestational diabetes mellitus (GDM). The American Congress of Obstetricians and Gynecologists (ACOG) defines gestational diabetes as onset of carbohydrate intolerance in pregnancy.[1] Groups such as the American Diabetes Association (ADA), World Health Organization (WHO), and International Federation of Gynecology and Obstetrics have attempted to distinguish women with likely preexisting diabetes that are first recognized in pregnancy from women whose carbohydrate intolerance is a transient condition due to pregnancy-related

Disclosure Statement: The authors have no conflicts of interest to report.
Department of Obstetrics and Gynecology, Section on Maternal-Fetal Medicine, Wake Forest University School of Medicine, Medical Center Boulevard, Winston-Salem, NC 27157, USA
* Corresponding author.
E-mail address: jdenney@wakehealth.edu

Obstet Gynecol Clin N Am 45 (2018) 299–314
https://doi.org/10.1016/j.ogc.2018.01.003
0889-8545/18/© 2018 Elsevier Inc. All rights reserved.

obgyn.theclinics.com

insulin resistance.[2,3] Thus, these organizations define GDM as glycemic intolerance diagnosed at or beyond the achievement of 20 completed weeks of gestation.[1-3]

Depending on the population sampled, GDM affects 3% to 25% of pregnancies.[1-4] There is an increased prevalence of GDM among African American, Pacific Islander, Hispanic, and Native American women.[2] The global prevalence of GDM has been increasing likely because of the increase of maternal obesity, delayed child bearing, and sedative lifestyles.[1-3]

Observational data demonstrate risks with poorly controlled GDM, including abnormal fetal growth, hypertensive disorders of pregnancy, difficult labor and vaginal delivery, increased risk of cesarean section, and the neonatal metabolic complications, including hypoglycemia, hyperbilirubinemia, and the potential for delayed pulmonary maturity.[1] Risks for the fetus are not limited to the gestation and subsequent neonatal period. Because of imprinting and environmental effect on gene activation, these babies are at risk for adult onset of metabolic disorders, diabetes, hypertension, obesity, cardiovascular disease, and shorter lifespan[1-4] (Table 1). These risks highlight the need for accurate diagnosis and proper management of GDM.[4] In the course of this review, the authors additionally discuss the emphasis on diet and activity/exercise as means of controlling blood sugars, the usual schedule of glucose monitoring, indications for medical treatment, fetal surveillance, timing of delivery, neonatal care, and postpartum care.

Physiology

In normal pregnancy, a myriad of physiologic alterations occur to promote the growth and development of the conceptus. A euglycemic state is maintained despite the fetus' energy demands via a compensatory and proliferative response within the maternal pancreas, namely the beta islet cells.[5] Conversely, in women who ultimately develop GDM, the beta-cell compensation fails to meet the metabolic demands, creating a hyperglycemic state. Data obtained from observational studies in humans and animal models have generated insights into the molecular biology leading to glycemic intolerance. Such studies demonstrate a down-regulation of insulin receptors on maternal cell surfaces in GDM.[5,6] Accordingly, these same women are biologically predisposed toward development of diabetes mellitus, type 2 later in life.[5-7] The underlying processes all lead to the assortment of metabolic derangements affecting both mother and baby that are called GDM.

Table 1	
Risks associated with gestational diabetes	
Maternal	**Fetal**
Labor dystocia	Macrosomia
Cesarean section	Hypoglycemia
Vaginal laceration	Shoulder dystocia/brachial plexus injury
Preeclampsia/gestational hypertension	Preterm delivery
Increased gestational weight gain	Delayed pulmonary maturity
DM	Metabolic syndrome in adulthood (obesity, hypertension, DM)
Cardiovascular disease	Polyhydramnios
Postpartum weight retention	Polycythemia
	Hyperbilirubinemia

Fetal Programming

Alterations of the maternal physiologic milieu inherently alter the environment for fetal development. Although lifestyle choices (smoking, diet high in fat/sugar, and sedentary lifestyle) have been widely accepted as causative in cardiovascular disease as one ages, evidence for the maternal environment having such effects on the fetus well into adulthood continues to mount.[8–11] It is now known that changes in the fetal environment alter telomere and subtelomere acetylation and methylation.[10] The flux of histone acetylation and DNA methylation impacts whether chromatin is in an open configuration and as such available for interaction with telomerase to facilitate gene transcription and/or recombination.[11] Such changes in gene activation affect predisposition toward developing chronic disease (eg, hypertension, diabetes, obesity) as the child ages.[11] In addition, there is a clear association with adulthood glucose intolerance and insulin resistance, and adaptive changes in the fetal pancreas.[12] Hence, it is imperative that clinicians provide guidance to their patients that strike the perfect balance for fetal well-being for delivery, the immediate neonatal period, and beyond.[12,13]

Last, telomere length of fetal DNA is likewise impacted by environmental insults in the maternal unit. Maternal stress and endocrine dysfunction impact fetal telomere length.[13,14] Such stressors induce telomere attrition, in turn, impacting length of the fetus' ultimate lifespan.[14] Epidemiologic data show that maternal stress leads to higher incidence of adulthood obesity, diabetes, and cardiovascular disease for their babies. As adults, these same individuals show lower cortisol, higher ACTH levels, and less prefrontal cortex and memory function when measured in stressful conditions.[14] Hence, the fetal programming phenomenon impacts the subsequent ex utero aging process and lifespan of the child well after delivery.[9]

Diagnosis

Given the lack of clear inflection point with respect to degree of gestational hyperglycemia and onset of or risk for adverse outcome, commonly cited professional organizations (eg, ACOG, ADA, WHO) vary in algorithms for diagnostic methods and interpretation of screening tests.[1–4,15] Several studies have highlighted the lack of ability to declare a clear demarcation along the continuum of hyperglycemia and outcomes.[16,17] Occult or previously undiagnosed diabetes affecting pregnancy is an issue of increasing incidence given the general trend of obesity and diabetes in the general population.[18–20] Accordingly, women identified with glycemic intolerance in the first half or before the completion of 20 weeks' gestation are diagnosed with pregestational diabetes (see Ronan Sugrue and Chloe Zera's article, "Pregestational Diabetes in Pregnancy," in this issue).[21] Women identified as having onset of glycemic intolerance in the last half of pregnancy—any time after completing 20 weeks' gestation—are classified as having GDM.[21]

Given that 90% of pregnant women in the United States present with at least one risk factor for GDM (**Fig. 1**) and 20% of those with no risk factors (**Fig. 2**) develop GDM (**Box 1**),[1,15,16,21] universal screening appears most appropriate.[1,15,16,21] Two approaches to identifying GDM exist. The most commonly used is the 2-step approach using an initial 1-hour screening 50-g glucose challenge test.[1,4,16] If negative, no further testing is required. However, screen positive individuals must undergo a formal diagnostic evaluation with a 100-g 3-hour oral glucose tolerance test (GTT). The other approach uses a singular 75-g, 2-hour GTT.[16]

Either approach is reasonable, and the choice may be made by the provider, depending on their ability to consistently implement an approach for their patient

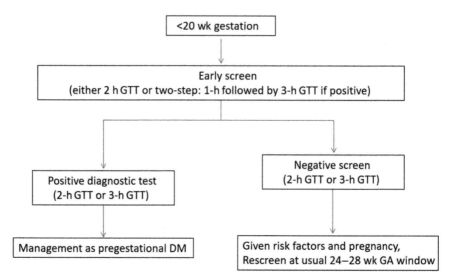

Fig. 1. Glycemic intolerance screening for patients at increased risk for insulin resistance. GA, gestational age.

population with available resources. The US Preventative Services Task Force (USPSTF) performed a systematic review on screening and deemed sufficient evidence to support universal screening but only after the achievement of 24 completed weeks' gestation.[2] Accordingly, conventional timing for screening per ACOG guidelines remains between 24 and 28 weeks, provided there is no reason to suspect underlying pregestational DM (see **Fig. 2**).[1] For those suspected to be at increased risk for underlying DM, screening should not be delayed and may be performed as early as the first prenatal visit (see **Fig. 1**).[1–4]

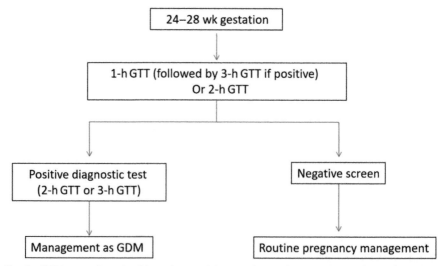

Fig. 2. GDM screening. At-risk patients with negative early screening or low-risk patients with no prior screening.

Box 1
Risk factors for gestational diabetes mellitus

- Glucosuria
- Multiple gestation
- Maternal age greater than 25 years old
- Prior pregnancy affected by GDM
- History of impaired glucose tolerance
- Prior unexplained perinatal loss or child with congenital anomaly
- Hypertension
- Obesity
- Use of glucocorticoids
- Polycystic ovarian syndrome
- Family history of diabetes
- Excessive gestational weight gain
- Significant weight gain in early adulthood
- Intergestational weight retention

Glucose Challenge Tests

The 50-g oral glucose challenge can be taken regardless of fasting or postprandial state with assessment of plasma glucose 1 hour after consumption. The 3 commonly used thresholds for "positive screens" are $\geq$130 mg/dL (7.2 mmol/L), $\geq$135 mg/dL (7.5 mmol/L), and $\geq$140 mg/dL (7.8 mmol/L).[1,2] The USPSTF published a systematic review citing sensitivities and specificities at the low end and the high end for proposed thresholds[2]: 130 mg/dL yielded 88% to 99% sensitivity and 66% to 77% specificity, whereas 140 mg/dL demonstrated 70% to 88% sensitivity and 69% to 89% specificity.[16] In the authors' academic obstetric group, they have adopted a threshold of 135 mg/dL. Upon positive screening, several criteria are used depending on the provider's preference and interpretation of the data's generalizability for implementation in their own population.[16–21] For the 2-step screen ending in a 100-g glucose challenge, Carpenter and Coustan[21] recommend the following cut points (mg/dL): fasting, 95; 1 hour, 180; 2 hours, 155; 3 hours, 140. For the same 100-g challenge, National Diabetes Data Group (NDDG) recommends using the following cut points (mg/dL): fasting, 105; 1 hour, 190; 2 hours, 165; 3 hours, 145.[22] There are others used as well (**Table 2**).

In women with markedly elevated oral glucose challenge screens, a high probability of abnormal diagnostic GTT exists.[23] That being said, the positive predictive value (PPV) depends on both the population's prevalence of GDM and the criteria for diagnosis, for example, NDDG or Carpenter-Coustan.[21–24] Carpenter and Coustan[21] report greater than 95% probability of GDM with 1 hour plasma glucose of greater than 182 mg/dL (10.1 mmol/L) following the 50-g challenge.[21] Other studies report PPV of 200 mg/dL to range from 69% to 80%.[23–25] The authors use 200 mg/dL as a threshold for GDM diagnosis and not requiring exposure to the 100-g GTT. Granted, a patient who prefers the 3-hour GTT in lieu of committing to the diagnosis may do so, as long as the provider is not concerned with risk for clinically significant diabetic ketosis in the patient. Expert opinion has defined

Table 2
Criteria for GDM diagnosis

Plasma Glucose	Carpenter-Coustan (100 gm; Two-Step)	NDDG (100 gm; Two-Step)	CDA (75 gm; Two-Step)	WHO (75 gm; One Step)	IADPSG (75 gm; One Step)
Fasting (mg/dL)	95	105	95	92–125	92–125
One-hour (mg/dL)	180	190	191	180	180
Two-hour (mg/dL)	155	165	160	153–199	153
Three-hour (mg/dL)	140	145	—	—	—

Abbreviations: CDA, Canadian Diabetes Association; IADPSG, International Association of Diabetes and Pregnancy Study Groups; NDDG, National Diabetes Data Group; WHO, World Health Organization.

GDM as diagnosed on GTT by a list of criteria either by the 1-step or by the 2-step approaches (see **Table 2**).[25] The authors' group uses a 2-step approach with the Carpenter-Coustan cut points.[21]

The Eunice Kennedy Shriver National Institute of Child Health and Human Development Consensus Development Conference on Diagnosing Gestational Diabetes recommended the continued use of the 2-step approach to screen for and diagnose GDM.[26] This recommendation was based on the lack of evidence for improved clinical maternal or neonatal outcomes with the 1-step approach (75-g 2-hour GTT) and the increase in health care costs that would result. Based on this recommendation and a *Cochrane Review* that reported no specific screening strategy has shown to be optimal, ACOG supports the 2-step approach.[1,4]

Management (Glucose Monitoring)

Several studies have evaluated the utility of glucose monitoring and treatment of GDM. The 2005 Australian Carbohydrate Intolerance Study in Pregnant Women trial randomized women with GDM to receive treatment or routine care.[27] The study found that treatment was associated with a reduction in serious newborn complications, preeclampsia, and frequency of large for gestational age (LGA) infants. A subsequent randomized controlled trial done in the United States showed a decrease in frequency of LGA infants, reduced neonatal fat mass, and decreased rates of cesarean delivery, shoulder dystocia, and hypertensive disorders of pregnancy with treatment of GDM.[28] Given these observed benefits with treatment, it is recommended that patients monitor their glucose levels, and treatment should be initiated upon diagnosis as appropriate.

Home serum glucose monitoring is the crux of outpatient maternal surveillance with GDM. Patients are routinely instructed on glucometer use and the importance of steadfast maintenance of a glucose log as derived from fasting and either 1-hour or 2-hour postprandial glucose levels.[1] Such monitoring facilitates ease of review by the patient's obstetric provider and in the identification of deviations from target glycemic measures. In patients with poor control, providers may additionally ask patients to monitor preprandial glucose levels, whenever sensing high or low glucose, and at 2 to 3 AM in the morning to better characterize the overall control of the patient's glucose throughout the day. Current standard of care for target blood glucose values are fasting blood glucose concentration ≤95 mg/dL (5.3 mmol/L), 1-hour postprandial blood glucose concentration ≤140 mg/dL (7.8 mmol/L), and 2-hour postprandial glucose concentration ≤120 mg/dL (6.7 mmol/L) (**Fig. 3**).[1,28]

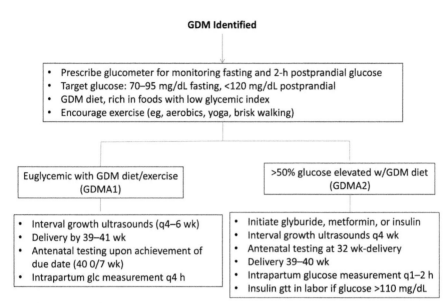

GDM Identified

- Prescribe glucometer for monitoring fasting and 2-h postprandial glucose
- Target glucose: 70–95 mg/dL fasting, <120 mg/dL postprandial
- GDM diet, rich in foods with low glycemic index
- Encourage exercise (eg, aerobics, yoga, brisk walking)

Euglycemic with GDM diet/exercise
(GDMA1)

>50% glucose elevated w/GDM diet
(GDMA2)

- Interval growth ultrasounds (q4–6 wk)
- Delivery by 39–41 wk
- Antenatal testing upon achievement of due date (40 0/7 wk)
- Intrapartum glc measurement q4 h

- Initiate glyburide, metformin, or insulin
- Interval growth ultrasounds q4 wk
- Antenatal testing at 32 wk-delivery
- Delivery 39–40 wk
- Intrapartum glucose measurement q1–2 h
- Insulin gtt in labor if glucose >110 mg/dL

Fig. 3. GDM identified. Rx, prescription; u/s, ultrasound.

Management (Diet Control)

Dietary changes are the mainstay of initial attempts in glycemic control following the diagnosis of GDM. Data demonstrate a clear association of postprandial hyperglycemia and diet high (>55%) in carbohydrate content.[28,29] Because carbohydrates are the sole macronutrient to significantly raise postprandial blood glucose, dietary modification predominantly consists of carbohydrate restriction and distribution evenly throughout the 3 main meals of the day.[30,31] Glycemic control is improved by avoiding processed/red meat, high-fat dairy, refined grains while favoring vegetables, fruit, whole grains, and fish[31–36] (**Box 2**). For patients achieving target measures for glucose control with GDM diet, the diagnosis remains diet-controlled GDM or GDMA1 per the widely used White Classification that stratifies diabetes by pregestational diabetes mellitus (DM) with or without organ involvement and GDM, either controlled by diet alone or requiring medication.[37] Some patients will consistently demonstrate fasting blood glucose greater than 100 mg/dL along with a persistent pattern of postprandial glucose measures greater than 120 mg/dL despite the GDM diet; these patients

---

Box 2
Gestational diabetes mellitus diet

- Review IOM guidelines for weight gain as based on patient's BMI
- Limit carbohydrates to 40% to 45% of calories
- Avoid processed sugar (eg, soda, candy)
- Avoid fruit and juice at breakfast
- Encourage increased fiber intake and foods with low glycemic index
- Move fruit and milk servings to snack time
- Keep starchy carbohydrates at meal
- Encourage exercise plan

require medical therapy and have GDMA2.[30,37] Some of these patients may have occult diabetes simply diagnosed during pregnancy and may also fail to achieve euglycemia with institution of the GDM diet.

Recently, investigators have evaluated the impact of a diet with low glycemic index (GI) for improvement of outcomes in GDM.[29] The GI is a systematic and physiologically based measurement of the dietary carbohydrate load and its inherent glycemic burden.[30] GI is the number associated with the carbohydrates in a particular type of food, indicating the individual's response (assessed by blood sugar level) relative to the reference food—pure glucose.[30–34] High GI diets result in more gestational weight gain, whereas low GI foods are associated with lower birth weight, improved insulin sensitivity, and potentially lowered risk for development of GDM, better adherence to Institute of Medicine (IOM) weight gain guidelines in pregnancy, and lower onset of obesity later in life.[29–36] Low GI diet effectively reduces postprandial blood glucose spikes, appears to be safe in pregnancy, and shows promise for improving the outcomes with GDM.[34–36]

Gestational Weight Gain and Gestational Diabetes Mellitus

Because obesity and insulin resistance parallel one another in terms of comorbidity, the 2 conditions are somewhat inseparable in terms of clinical considerations. Both, if not well controlled, lead to increased risk of indicated preterm delivery, gestational hypertension, preeclampsia, delivery by cesarean, and fetal growth abnormalities.[1,2,26–28] Excessive gestational weight gain correlates well with onset of GDM.[38] Accordingly, 2009 IOM Guidelines for weight gain in pregnancy provide direction for target weight gain as based on intake body mass index (BMI).[39] Online calculators based on IOM guidelines to individualize the approach are available.[40] Regardless of BMI, a typical goal for a patient's calorie intake would be 30 to 35 calories per kilogram ideal body weight. Five hundred of those daily calories should be protein (125 g).[41] The remainder of the calories may then be equally halved between fat and carbohydrate while avoiding processed carbohydrates. A good recommendation for calorie distribution by meal would be 24% at breakfast, 30% at lunch, 33% at dinner, and the remaining 13% from between-meal snacks.[41] Keeping gestational weight gain to within the IOM guidelines can reduce the risk of developing GDM and improve glycemic control in women with GDM.[29–35,38,41]

Management (Pharmacologic Control: Oral Hypoglycemic Agents and Insulin)

When diet fails to achieve euglycemia, defined as no more than 50% of glycemic measures above the target ranges, medication is required and the patient is classified as GDMA2.[1,36] Both oral hypoglycemic agents and insulin therapy are acceptable and used. Insulin therapy has been the most well-studied and used treatment of both GDMA2 and DM and continues to be endorsed by the ADA and ACOG as an accepted therapy.[1] Insulin does not cross the placenta and is the only regimen approved by the US Food and Drug Adminstration for treatment of GDM.[1] Insulin regimens typically consist of a long-acting and a short-acting insulin; however, insulin dosing and regimens must be individualized. Given that insulin resistance increases with increasing placental mass, total insulin requirements increase with increasing gestational age. A commonly used protocol uses maternal weight and gestational age to calculate starting daily insulin requirements (**Table 3**).[1] The total daily insulin requirement is then divided into two-thirds long-acting and one-third short-acting insulin. The short-acting insulin (one-third of total dose) is further subdivided into 3 doses taken with meals.[1] Commonly used long- and short-acting insulins are listed in **Table 4**.

In addition, close surveillance of glucose values is also indicated in patients with GDM who are receiving a course of antenatal corticosteroids for fetal lung maturity.

Table 3	
Weight-based guidelines for starting/adjusting total daily insulin therapy by gestational age	
Weeks Gestational Age	**Insulin (Units/kg/d)**
0–13 6/7	0.7
14–27 6/7	0.8
28–35 6/7	0.9
36–delivery	1.0

Corticosteroids are known to increase the risk of transient hyperglycemia, thus more frequent assessments of maternal glucose in this setting (eg, every 4 hours depending on initial starting glucose level) are appropriate.[42] In the setting of post–corticosteroid hyperglycemia, patients often require insulin coverage even if they were previously well controlled with diet.[43]

Oral Hypoglycemic Agents

Commonly used oral hypoglycemic agents include both glyburide and metformin. Glyburide is a second-generation sulfonylurea that was investigated using single-cotyledon placental models to assess placental transfer. Initial studies demonstrated no significant transfer of glyburide in both therapeutic and supratherapeutic dosing concentrations.[44,45] The subsequent landmark randomized controlled trial compared the insulin therapy to glyburide in the management of GDM. Not only was there no detectable glyburide in cord blood but also maternal and neonatal outcomes were similar with respect to glycemic control and adverse events.[46] Notably, subsequent data conflict the initial Langer randomized controlled trial reporting glyburide being actively transported from the fetus to the mother.[47] Although the range of fetal exposure varied widely, 9% to 70% maternal glyburide concentration, these data create pause for consideration of possible fetal risks. A 2015 meta-analysis showed therapeutic glyburide use resulted in a 2-fold increase in neonatal hypoglycemia, a 2-fold increase in macrosomia, and a 100-g increase in mean birth weight compared with traditional insulin therapy.[47] In addition, 4% to 16% of women who took glyburide as initial therapy eventually required the addition of insulin.[1,47]

Metformin is a biguanide used to improve both fertility and glycemic control by way of increasing insulin sensitivity.[48] Insulin sensitivity is heightened by metformin via an inhibitory effect on hepatic glucose production and intestinal glucose absorption.[48] Pharmacologic studies demonstrate that metformin freely crosses the placenta, rendering a circulating fetal concentration roughly 50% that found in maternal circulation.[48] Accordingly, a landmark trial published by Rowan and colleagues[49] called the Metformin in Gestational Diabetes (MIG) trial compared the outcomes of 751 women and fetuses allocated to either traditional insulin therapy or metformin for the treatment of GDM. Although there were no differences in congenital malformations, serious

Table 4	
Long- and short-acting insulins used for gestational diabetes mellitus treatment	
Long Acting	**Short Acting**
Glargine (Lantus)	Aspart
Protamine Hagedorn (NPH, Novolin)	Lispro
Detemir	Regular

maternal events, or serious neonatal events, significant variance in outcome was shown with use of metformin. Namely, metformin use resulted in significantly less neonatal hypoglycemia (3.3% vs 8.1%; P<.008) and an unexpected higher rate of preterm delivery (12.1% vs 7.6%; P = .04). A 2-year follow-up report on the MIG trial babies showed those in the metformin arm had more subcutaneous fat in upper arm and shoulder compared with those in the insulin arm.[50] In addition, 26% to 46% of patients who took metformin alone eventually required insulin.[50]

Although insulin therapy remains the standard therapy recommended by most, oral antihyperglycemic agents are a reasonable alternative in patients who refuse to take or are unable to comply with insulin therapy. Providers should have a thorough discussion of the published outcome data and unknown long-term effects of transplacental passage of oral agents.[1]

Fetal Surveillance

Given the effect of hyperglycemia on fetal growth and well-being, women diagnosed with GDM are typically followed with serial biometry and amniotic fluid volume assessment. Frequency of such assessments is typically performed every 4 to 6 weeks from time of diagnosis of GDM to delivery. Indications for antepartum fetal testing include insulin or oral hypoglycemic requirement, polyhydramnios, onset of gestational hypertension, or, less commonly in the setting of GDM, growth restriction. Although a consequence of poorly controlled GDM, testing is not indicated for macrosomia. Either weekly biophysical profile or twice weekly nonstress tests with weekly amniotic fluid indices after 32 weeks are acceptable and equivalent for ensuring fetal well-being when indicated (see **Fig. 3**).[1] There is currently no consensus regarding antepartum fetal testing for women with GDMA1 because studies have not demonstrated an increased risk of stillbirth in these patients before 40 weeks.[1,49,51]

Intrapartum Management and Delivery Timing

Provided glucose measures demonstrate good control with diet alone and serial ultrasound demonstrates normal growth and amniotic fluid volume, the patient essentially has uncomplicated GDMA1 and does not require timed delivery before 41 weeks 0 days. Notably, ACOG does allow for the role of elective delivery in term patients with good dating following the achievement of 39 weeks' gestational age.[51,52] Hence, timing for delivery in those who are term albeit less than 41 weeks can be individualized with patient and the obstetric provider. Upon surpassing the due date, a good practice would be to initiate antenatal testing and weekly amniotic fluid volume measurements. On the contrary, patients with GDMA2 are likely best served by delivery at 39 0/7 to 39 6/7 weeks of gestation given increased risk of stillbirth in patients who require insulin or oral hypoglycemic medication for glucose control.[50,51] Moreover, recent data indicate inducing labor actually does not increase risk for cesarean delivery and that induction at 39 weeks yields lower failure rate (as defined by cesarean) than induction at 40 or 41 weeks.[53,54] In women with poor glycemic control despite medical intervention, delivery before 39 weeks may be warranted. Recommendations for delivery timing should incorporate consideration for risks of prematurity and ongoing risk of stillbirth (see **Fig. 3**).[1,55]

Delivery Mode

Simply stated, GDM is not an indication for cesarean delivery. That being said, GDM places a fetus at greater risk for macrosomia as defined by an estimated fetal weight (EFW) in excess of 4500 g for pregnancies affected by GDM/DM per the most recent ACOG Practice Bulletin.[1] In addition, fetuses often show an accelerated growth pattern with abnormally low head circumference/abdominal circumference ratio even in the absence of macrosomia. These growth patterns are important risk factors for complications, such as shoulder dystocia, Erb palsy, and third/fourth degree lacerations.[56–58] Scheduled cesarean section is typically offered to women with GDM whose fetuses are estimated to be ≥4500 g.[1] Risks of birth trauma, shoulder dystocia, errors in estimating fetal weight, and risks of cesarean section both immediate and for future pregnancies should be included in the counseling. In women undergoing a trial of labor, caution should be exercised in the second stage especially in the scenario of an operative vaginal delivery because even appropriately grown fetuses of mothers with GDM are at increased risk of shoulder dystocia.[1,56–58]

Insulin Glucose Tolerance Test Protocol and Glycemic Monitoring Protocol Intrapartum

Given that labor increases glucose utilization, hyperglycemia in women not requiring medical control of GDM is rare. Hence, practitioners may periodically monitor glucose every 4 hours intrapartum for GDMA1.[1,58] On the contrary, gestational diabetics requiring either oral hypoglycemic medications or insulin (GDMA2) respond similarly to DM in labor and are best served by every 1- to 2-hour glucose assessments in the intrapartum period. Although ketoacidosis is rare in GDMA2, intrapartum maternal hyperglycemia may cause an acute increase in fetal insulin, placing the fetus at heightened risk for neonatal hypoglycemia.[58] The authors' group initiates an insulin drip upon maternal blood glucose at or greater than 120 mg/dL, with the addition of D5 (dextrose 5%) ½ NS (normal saline) at 125 cc/h provided glucose levels are less than 200 mg/dL. Similarly, in a survey of academic medical centers, 60% aimed to maintain maternal glucose less than 110 mg/dL, whereas 30% targeted a value between 110 and 150 mg/dL.[1,42]

Postpartum Screening

Many women with GDM are pregestational diabetics that were first detected in pregnancy, and women with true GDM are at risk for the development of DM later in life.[59,60] Seventy percent of women with GDM will develop DM at some point in their life, and 40% to 50% of those women will develop DM within 10 years.[61] Hence, all women should receive screening for DM with a 75-g GTT at 6 to 12 weeks postpartum. If negative, they should continue to be rescreened every 3 years with their primary care provider.[61] Women with a positive 2-hour GTT are diagnosed with DM and should be managed or referred for long-term management accordingly.[61]

Encouraging breastfeeding, regular physical activity, and formal nutrition programs focusing on decreased gestational weight retention are recommended by the ADA.[59–61] However, given that 44.9% of US births are covered by Medicaid and many of these women experience coverage lapses due to Medicaid coverage ending at 60 days' postpartum, cost becomes an issue. Research shows that obstetricians have much room for improvement in their rates of nutrition referrals and postpartum screening for patients who had GDM.[59–61] Unfortunately, women seeing a primary care physician after delivery often fail to disclose the fact their recent pregnancy was complicated by GDM.

Martinez and colleagues[61] recently recommended Situation Background Assessment Recommendation strategy to help bridge the gap between GDM and postpartum care. This model reinforces recommendations through reminders to both patient and provider to facilitate communication, screening, and care (**Box 3**).

> **Box 3**
> **Postpartum management and situation background assessment recommendation**
>
> - Discontinue insulin or oral hypoglycemic
> - Encourage breast-feeding
> - Encourage enrollment in formal exercise program or encourage exercise as patients progress through convalescence and recovery in the puerperium
> - Encourage referral to formal nutrition program
> - Routine contraceptive recommendations (no change based on GDM)
> - 75-g GTT at 6 to 12 weeks' postpartum
> - "Warm handoff" to primary care provider replete with notification of pregnancy complication by GDM
> - Repeat 75-g GTT every 3 years until positive (then manage as DM)

SUMMARY

GDM is a common complication in pregnancy. Risks associated with occult or unmanaged GDM are detrimental to both maternal and fetal well-being. Sufficient evidence exists to warrant screening and management strategies once diagnosed. Although many variations in both screening and management may be reasonable, the authors suggest a few key points for optimizing identification and management of GDM.

For patients at increased risk for insulin resistance, they recommend an early screen, either the 2-hour GTT or 2-step (1-hour followed by 3-hour GTT if positive). Should patients have a positive diagnostic test before the achievement of 20 completed weeks' gestation, the authors recommend management as pregestational DM. On the contrary, the at-risk patient with an initial negative screen before 20 weeks should then be rescreened at the usual 24- to 28-week gestational age window (see **Fig. 1**).

For either at-risk patients with negative early screening or low-risk patients with no indication for early screening, the authors recommend screening with either the 1-hour GTT (followed by 3-hour GTT if positive) or 2-hour GTT for diagnosis. Patients exhibiting a negative screen may have routine pregnancy management. Patients with a positive diagnostic test (by either 2- or 3-hour GTT) should be managed as GDM in their pregnancy (see **Fig. 2**).

When GDM is identified, the authors recommend the following:

1. Glucometer for monitoring fasting and 2-hour postprandial glucose;
2. Target glycemic measures of 70 to 95 mg/dL (fasting) and less than 120 mg/dL (postprandial);
3. GDM diet;
4. Diet risk in foods with low GI; and
5. Encourage exercise (eg, aerobics, yoga, brisk walking) (see **Fig. 3**).

Provided GDM patients achieve euglycemia with diet and exercise (GDMA1), the authors recommend interval growth ultrasounds (every 4–6 weeks); delivery 39 to 41 weeks; antenatal testing upon achievement of 40 completed weeks; and, intrapartum glucose measurement every 4 hours. For patients with more than half of their glucose measurements elevated despite GDM diet (GDMA2), the authors recommend the following: initiation of glyburide, metformin, or insulin; interval growth ultrasounds every 4 weeks; antenatal testing from 32 weeks until delivery; delivery from 39 to

40 weeks; intrapartum glucose measurement every 1 to 2 hours; and initiation of insulin drip in labor if glucose is at or greater than 110 mg/dL. Last, the authors recommend following ACOG guidelines regarding an adequate discussion of risks for birth injury should EFW exceed 4500 g (see **Fig. 3**). As a good clinical practice, the authors' group exhibits caution with assisted second-stage deliveries when EFW exceeds 4250 g (ie, if spontaneous delivery cannot be facilitated by maternal expulsive efforts, the authors recommend consideration for cesarean section at this point in lieu of using either forceps or vacuum in this setting, which may facilitate an undesired outcome, shoulder dystocia).

Last, postnatal testing of GDM patients should be performed to ensure that patients who actually have DM are identified. If initially negative, women with history of GDM should be rescreened every 3 years. Warm handoffs to primary care providers with these recommendations should help facilitate better rates of screening for those at risk for DM and in turn help identify occult DM so that women receive treatment when appropriate.

REFERENCES

1. Committee on Practice Bulletins—Obstetrics. Practice bulletin no. 180 gestational diabetes mellitus. Obstet Gynecol 2017;130(1):e17–37.
2. Moyer VA, US Preventive Services Task Force. Screening for gestational diabetes mellitus: U.S. Preventive Services Task Force recommendation statement. Ann Intern Med 2014;160(6):414–20.
3. National Collaborating Centre for Women's and Children's Health. Antenatal care: routine care for the healthy pregnant woman. Appendix F economic model: screening and treatment of gestational diabetes. London: RCOG Press; 2008. Available at: https://www.ncbi.nlm.nih.gov/books/NBK51877/.
4. Farrar D, Duley L, Dowswell T, et al. Different strategies for diagnosing gestational diabetes to improve maternal and infant health. Cochrane Database Syst Rev 2017;(8):CD007122.
5. Barbour LA, McCurdy CE, Hernandez TL, et al. Cellular mechanisms for insulin resistance in normal pregnancy and gestational diabetes. Diabetes Care 2007; 30(suppl 2):S112–9.
6. Buchanan TA, Xiang AH, Page KA. Gestational diabetes mellitus: risks and management during and after pregnancy. Nat Rev Endocrinol 2012;8(11):639–49.
7. Capula C, Chiefari E, Vero A, et al. Gestational diabetes mellitus: screening and outcomes in southern Italian pregnant women. ISRN Endocrinol 2013;2013: 387495.
8. á Rogvi R, Forman JL, Damm P, et al. Women born preterm or with inappropriate weight for gestational age are at risk of subsequent gestational diabetes and pre-eclampsia. PLoS One 2012;7(3):e34001.
9. Rueda-Clausen CF, Morton JS, Davidge ST. Effects of hypoxia-induced intrauterine growth restriction on cardiopulmonary structure and function during adulthood. Cardiovasc Res 2009;81:713–22.
10. Ravlic S, Vidacek NS, Nanic L, et al. Mechanisms of fetal epigenetics that determine telomere dynamics and health span in adulthood. Mech Ageing Dev 2017. https://doi.org/10.1016/j.mad.2017.08.014.
11. Vidacek NS, Nanic L, Ravlic S, et al. Telomeres, nutrition, and longevity: can we really navigate our aging? J Gerontol A Biol Sci Med Sci 2017;73(1):39–47.
12. Eberle C, Ament C. Diabetic and metabolic programming: mechanisms altering the intrauterine milieu. ISRN Pediatr 2012;2012:975685.

13. Ravelli AC, van der Meulen JH, Michels RP, et al. Glucose tolerance in adults after prenatal exposure to famine. Lancet 1998;351:173–7.
14. Entringer S, Buss C, Wadwa PD. Prenatal stress, telomere biology, and fetal programming of health and disease risk. Sci Signal 2012;5:pt12.
15. Danilenko-Dixon DR, Van Winter JT, Nelson RL, et al. Universal versus selective gestational diabetes screening; application of 1997 American Diabetes Association recommendations. Am J Obstet Gynecol 1999;181:798.
16. Donovan L, Hartling L, Muise M, et al. Screening tests for gestational diabetes: a systematic review for the US Preventative Task Force. Ann Intern Med 2013;159:115.
17. HAPO Study Cooperative Research Group, Metzger BE, Lowe LP, Dyer AR, et al. Hyperglycemia and adverse pregnancy outcomes. N Engl J Med 2008;358:1991–2002.
18. Guariguata L, Whiting DR, Hambleton I, et al. Global estimates of diabetes prevalence for 2013 and projections for 2035. Diabetes Res Clin Pract 2014;103:137–49.
19. Beagley J, Guariguata L, Weil C, et al. Global estimates of undiagnosed diabetes in adults. Diabetes Res Clin Pract 2014;103(2):150–60.
20. Guariguata L, Linnenkamp U, Beagley J, et al. Global estimates of the prevalence of hyperglycaemia in pregnancy. Diabetes Res Clin Pract 2014;103:176–85.
21. Carpenter MW, Coustan DR. Criteria for screening tests for gestational diabetes. Am J Obstet Gynecol 1982;144:768.
22. National Diabetes Data Group. Report of the expert committee on the diagnosis and classification of diabetes mellitus. Diabetes care 1997;20(7):1183–97.
23. Cheng YW, Esakoff TF, Block-Kurbisch I, et al. Screening or diagnostic: markedly elevated glucose loading test and perinatal outcomes. J Matern Fetal Neonatal Med 2006;19:729.
24. Temming LA, Tuuli MG, Stout MJ, et al. Diagnostic ability of elevated 1-h glucose challenge test. J Perinatol 2016;36:342.
25. Vandorsten JP, Dodson WC, Espeland MA, et al. National Institutes of Health consensus development conference: diagnosing gestational diabetes mellitus. NIH Consens State Sci Statements 2013;29:1.
26. Landon MB, Spong CY, Thom E, et al, Eunice Kennedy Shriver National Institute of Child Health and Human Development Maternal-Fetal Medicine Units Network. A multicenter, randomized trial of treatment for mild gestational diabetes. N Engl J Med 2009;361:1339–48.
27. Crowther CA, Hiller JE, Moss JR, et al, Australian Carbohydrate Intolerance Study in Pregnant Women (ACHOIS) Trial Group. Effect of treatment of gestational diabetes mellitus on pregnancy outcomes. N Engl J Med 2005;352:2477–86.
28. Jovanovic-Peterson L, Peterson CM. Dietary manipulation as a primary treatment strategy for pregnancies complicated by diabetes. J Am Coll Nutr 1990;9:320–5.
29. Louie JCY, Brand-Miller JC, Moses R. Carbohydrates, glycemic index, and pregnancy outcomes in gestational diabetes. Curr Diab Rep 2013;13:6–11.
30. Marsh K, Barclay A, Colagiuiri S, et al. Glycemic index and glycemic load of carbohydrates in the diabetes diet. Curr Diab Rep 2011;11:120–7.
31. Schoenaker DA, Mishra GD, Callaway LK, et al. The role of energy, nutrients, foods, and dietary patterns in the development of gestational diabetes mellitus: a systemic review of observational studies. Diabetes Care 2016;39:16.
32. Rogozinska E, Chamillard M, Hitman GA, et al. Nutritional manipulation for the primary prevention of gestational diabetes mellitus: a meta-analysis of randomized studies. PLoS One 2015;10:e0115526.

33. Moses RG, Barker M, Winter M, et al. Can a low-glycemic index diet reduce the need for insulin in gestational diabetes mellitus? A randomized trial. Diabetes Care 2009;32:996–1000.

34. Louie JC, Markovic TP, Perera N, et al. A randomized controlled trial investigating the effects of a low-glycemic index diet on pregnancy outcomes in gestational diabetes mellitus. Diabetes Care 2011;34:2341–6.

35. Grant SM, Wolever TM, O'Connor DL, et al. Effect of a low glycemic index diet on blood glucose in women with gestational hyperglycaemia. Diabetes Res Clin Pract 2011;91:15–22.

36. White P. Pregnancy complicating diabetes. Am J Med 1949;7(5):609–15.

37. Harper LM, Tita A, Biggio JR. The Institute of Medicine guidelines for gestational weight gain after a diagnosis of gestational diabetes and pregnancy outcomes. Am J Perinatol 2015;32(3):239–46.

38. Institute of Medicine. Weight gain during pregnancy: reexamining the guidelines. Washington, DC: National Academies Press; 2009.

39. Pregnancy Weight Gain Calculator. Available at: http://www.calculator.net/pregnancy-weight-gain-calculator.html. Accessed October 1, 2017.

40. Gunderson EP. Gestational diabetes and nutritional recommendations. Curr Diab Rep 2004;4(5):377–86.

41. Elliott BD, Langer O, Schenker S, et al. Insignificant transfer of glyburide occurs across the human placenta. Am J Obstet Gynecol 1991;165(4Pt1):807–12.

42. Ko JY, Dietz PM, Conrey EJ, et al. Strategies associated with higher postpartum glucose tolerance screening rates for gestational diabetes mellitus patients. J Womens Health (Larchmt) 2013;22:681–6.

43. Itoh A, Saisho Y, Miyakoshi K, et al. Time-dependent changes in insulin requirement for maternal glycemic control during antenatal corticosteroid therapy in women with gestational diabetes: a retrospective study. Endocr J 2016;63(1):101–4.

44. Elliott BD, Schenker S, Langer O, et al. Comparative placental transport of oral hypoglycemic agents in humans: a model of human placental drug transfer. Am J Obstet Gynecol 1994;171(3):653–60.

45. Langer O, Conway DL, Berkus MD, et al. A comparison of glyburide and insulin in women with gestational diabetes mellitus. N Eng J Med 2000;343(16):1134–8.

46. Balsells M, Garcia-Patterson A, Sola I, et al. Glibenclamide, metformin, and insulin for the treatment of gestational diabetes: a systemic review and meta-analysis. BMJ 2015;350:h102.

47. Charles B, Norris R, Xiao X, et al. Population pharmacokinetics of metformin in late pregnancy. Ther Drug Monit 2006;28(1):67–72.

48. Rowan JA, Hague WM, Gao W, et al. MiG Trial Investigators. Metformin versus insulin for the treatment of gestational diabetes. N Engl J Med 2008;358(19):2003–15.

49. Rowan JA, Rush EC, Obolonkin V, et al. Metformin in gestational diabetes: the offspring follow-up (MiG TOFU); body composition at 2 years of age. Diabetes Care 2011;34(10):2279–84.

50. Witkop CT, Neale D, Wilson LM, et al. Active compared with expectant delivery management in women with gestational diabetes: a systematic review. Obstet Gynecol 2009;113:206.

51. Alberico S, Erenbourg A, Hod M, et al. Immediate delivery or expectant management in gestational diabetes at term: the GINEXMAL randomized controlled trial. BJOG 2017;124:669.

52. Gibson KS, Waters TP, Bailit JL. Maternal and neonatal outcomes in electively induced low-risk term pregnancies. Am J Obstet Gynecol 2014;211:249.e1–16.

53. ACOG committee opinion No. 579 on obstetric practice for maternal-fetal medicine. Definition of term pregnancy. Washington, DC: American College of Obstetricians and Gynecologists; 2013.

54. Feghali MN, Caritis SN, Catov JM, et al. Timing of delivery and pregnancy outcomes in women with gestational diabetes. Am J Obstet Gynecol 2016;215:243.e1.

55. Boulet SL, Alexander GR, Salihu HM, et al. Macrosomic births in the United States: determinants, outcomes, and proposed grades of risk. Am J Obstet Gynecol 2003;188:1372–8.

56. Gupta N, Kiran TU, Mulik V, et al. The incidence, risk factors and obstetric outcome in primigravid women sustaining anal sphincter tears. Acta Obstet Gynecol Scand 2003;82:736–43.

57. Zhang X, Decker A, Platt RW, et al. How big is too big? The perinatal consequences of fetal macrosomia. Am J Obstet Gynecol 2008;198:517.e1–6.

58. Grant E, Joshi GP. Glycemic control during labor and delivery: a survey of academic centers in the United States. Arch Gynecol Obstet 2012;285:305.

59. Ko JY, Dietz PM, Conrey EJ, et al. Gestational diabetes mellitus and postpartum care practices of nurse-midwives. J Midwifery Womens Health 2013;58:33–40.

60. Yee LM, Niznik MC, Simon MA. Examining the role of health literacy in optimizing the care of pregnant women with diabetes. Am J Perinatol 2016;33:1242–9.

61. Martinez NG, Charlotte MN, Yee LM. Optimizing postpartum care for the patient with gestational diabetes mellitus. Am J Obstet Gynecol 2017;217(3):314–21.

Pregestational Diabetes in Pregnancy

Ronan Sugrue, MD, MPH[a], Chloe Zera, MD, MPH[b],*

KEYWORDS

- Pregestational diabetes • Pregnancy • Pregnancy outcomes • Preconception care

KEY POINTS

- Pregestational diabetes affects 1% to 2% of pregnancies in the United States.
- Poor diabetes control is associated with both maternal and fetal adverse outcomes.
- Optimization of glucose control with intensive self-monitoring of blood glucose, lifestyle management, and pharmacologic therapy preconception and throughout pregnancy reduces risk of developing these outcomes.

INTRODUCTION

In the last 30 years, the prevalence of diabetes mellitus in women of childbearing age has grown. Much of this is attributable to the obesity epidemic, which estimates suggest will worsen over the next decade.[1] Pregestational diabetes mellitus (PDM) now affects 1% to 2% of pregnancies in the United States, and its prevalence continues to grow. Since the 1990s, PDM has increased significantly in across all age groups, ethnicities, and geographies in the United States and Canada (**Fig. 1**).[2–4] Rates of both type 1 diabetes mellitus (T1DM) and type 2 diabetes mellitus (T2DM) continue to increase,[5] of whom more than 20% are undiagnosed.[6]

Glucose Metabolism in Pregnancy

In women with normal carbohydrate metabolism, first-trimester fasting blood glucose levels are lower than at baseline due to estrogen-mediated increases in both insulin sensitivity and insulin production.[7] In the second and third trimesters, fasting blood glucose increases as hepatic glucose production increases and insulin sensitivity decreases.[8] Placental hormones, including human placental lactogen and progesterone,

Disclosure Statement: The authors have no commercial or financial conflicts of interest to disclose.
[a] Department of Obstetrics and Gynecology, Brigham and Women's Hospital, Harvard Medical School, 75 Francis Street, Boston, MA 02115, USA; [b] Division of Maternal Fetal Medicine, Brigham and Women's Hospital, Harvard Medical School, 75 Francis Street, Boston, MA 02115, USA
* Corresponding author.
E-mail address: czera@bwh.harvard.edu

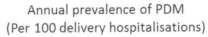

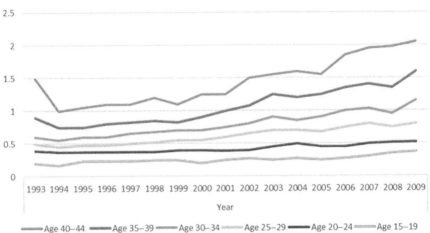

Fig. 1. Annual prevalence of pregestational diabetes in the United States. (*Adapted from* Fig. 2, Correa A, Bardenheier B, Elixhauser A, et al. Trends in prevalence of diabetes among delivery hospitalizations, United States, 1993-2009. Matern Child Health J 2015;19(3);635–42; with permission.)

also increase peripheral insulin resistance.[9] In women with normal pancreatic function, increased insulin secretion is sufficient to overcome physiologic insulin resistance and maintain normal blood glucose (**Fig. 2**).[10]

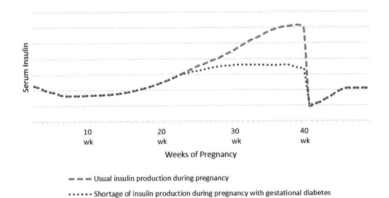

Fig. 2. Insulin requirements during pregnancy. (*Data from* Catalano PM, Tyzbir ED, Roman NM, et al. Longitudinal changes in insulin release and insulin resistance in nonobese pregnant women. Am J Obstet Gynecol 1991;165(6 Pt 1):1667–72.)

Classification

Diabetes mellitus is a syndrome of impaired glucose metabolism due to reduced or absent pancreatic insulin secretion, abnormal peripheral insulin sensitivity, or both.[11] According to the American Diabetes Association (ADA), the criteria for diagnosis of diabetes include the following[11]:

- Fasting blood glucose greater than 126 mg/dL (7.0 mmol/L)
- Two-hour postprandial glucose greater than 200 mg/dL (11.1 mmol/L) after ingestion of a 75-g glucose load
- A1c >6.5% (48 mmol/mol)
- A random plasma glucose greater than 200 mg/dL (11.1 mmol/L)

T1DM is an autoimmune condition that often develops early in life because of destruction of insulin-producing beta cells in the pancreas.[12] T2DM is characterized by late onset, increased peripheral insulin resistance, and reduced insulin sensitivity. It is associated with age, obesity, family history, and history of gestational diabetes.[13] Both mother and fetus are exposed to a wide range of risks and complications in pregnancy that are predominantly a function of glycemic control in PDM.[14] With appropriate therapy, the likelihood of these complications can be reduced to background population rates.[15]

RISKS OF PREGESTATIONAL DIABETES DURING PREGNANCY
Maternal Complications

Chronic hypertension
Chronic hypertension, defined as hypertension present before 20 weeks of gestation,[16] affects 6% to 8% of pregnant women with PDM. It is likely due to disruption of the renal-angiotensin system through reduced renal vascular compliance and glomerular sclerosis caused by diabetes.[17] The risks of hypertension include the following[18]:

- Intrauterine growth restriction (IUGR)
- Fetal demise
- Superimposed preeclampsia
- Iatrogenic preterm delivery

The goal of antihypertensive treatment in pregnancy for women with diabetes is to avoid severe range blood pressures (systolic >160 mm Hg, diastolic >105 mm/Hg). Safe antihypertensives include the following:

- Beta-blockers (eg, labetalol)
- Calcium-channel blockers (eg, nifedipine)
- Alpha-2 agonists (eg, methyldopa)

Angiotensin-converting enzyme inhibitors or angiotensin-II receptor blockers (ARBs) are contraindicated in pregnancy because of risk of fetopathy, including IUGR, fetal renal dysplasia, and oligohydramnios.[19] Although women exposed to angiotensin-converting-enzyme inhibitors or ARBs can be reassured that first-trimester use is not likely associated with congenital anomalies, switching to an antihypertensive medication compatible with pregnancy before conception is recommended.[20]

Nephropathy
Nephropathy, defined as microalbuminuria greater than 300 mg/24 hours with or without impaired renal function, occurs in 2% to 5% of pregnancies in women with PDM.[21] As the glomerular filtration rate increases during pregnancy, proteinuria often increases.[22] Women with nephropathy are at high risk for preeclampsia.[21] Approximately 50% undergo indicated preterm delivery for maternal or fetal indications, including IUGR (15%) and preeclampsia (50%).[23] Permanent deterioration in baseline kidney function during pregnancy is uncommon; however, end-stage renal disease

can occur in women with severe proteinuria in pregnancy (>3 g per 24 hours) or creatinine levels in excess of 1.5 mg/dL.[24] Aggressive antihypertensive control has been associated with better outcomes in women with nephropathy.[25]

Preeclampsia

The incidence of preeclampsia is higher in women with PDM, including 10% to 20% in those with T1DM.[26] Glycemic control in early pregnancy is associated with risk of preeclampsia.[27] Although randomized controlled trial data are lacking specifically for women with PDM, the authors recommend aspirin for preeclampsia prophylaxis from 16 weeks, consistent with US Preventive Services Task Force recommendations.[28]

Retinopathy

Diabetic retinopathy is associated with PDM and can worsen during pregnancy.[29] Factors associated with progression include duration of diabetes, presence of hypertension, and adequacy of glycemic control.[30] Although tight glycemic control has been associated with progression,[30] the benefits of glycemic control for other outcomes outweigh this risk. All women with PDM should therefore undergo thorough ophthalmic assessment early in pregnancy.[22] Women with proliferative retinopathy can be treated with laser photocoagulation during pregnancy; antivascular endothelial growth factor agents are not routinely recommended.[31]

Neuropathy

There are limited data regarding the prevalence and prognosis of neuropathy during pregnancy. Gastroparesis should be considered in women presenting with hyperemesis.[32] Diabetes-associated distal symmetric polyneuropathy may occur.[33] Multidisciplinary management of neuropathic pain may be helpful.[34]

Coronary artery disease

Coronary artery disease is uncommon in pregnancy but should be considered in symptomatic women with PDM. Women with a history of myocardial infarction should be discouraged from becoming pregnant.[35] A baseline electrocardiogram (ECG) is recommended, with consideration of echocardiogram (ECHO) as indicated.

Diabetic ketoacidosis

Diabetic ketoacidosis (DKA) is a life-threatening emergency affecting 5% to 10% of women with T1DM during pregnancy.[36] DKA remains a common first presentation in pregnant patients with undiagnosed diabetes, and distinct from non-pregnant women, can occur with mildly elevated glucose levels.[37] Women with T1DM should have specific education on DKA detection and prevention.

Fetal Complications

PDM is associated with increased risk of fetal and neonatal morbidity and mortality.[24] Known complications include congenital anomalies, abnormal fetal growth, fetal loss, birth injury, neonatal hypoglycemia, and hyperbilirubinemia.[38]

Normal fetal glucose physiology

From the time of placental formation, glucose crosses the placenta via facilitated diffusion.[39] Although the exact relationship between maternal and fetal glucose concentrations is complex, fetal glucose levels are directly related to maternal glucose levels: maternal hyperglycemia leads to fetal hyperglycemia and hyperinsulinemia.[40]

Risks to fetus in early pregnancy

Uncontrolled hyperglycemia during the first trimester affects organogenesis.[41] Spontaneous abortion and congenital malformation, of the central nervous system, cardiac, gastrointestinal, and genitourinary tract, are significantly more incident with A1c >7%, and the risk is proportional to A1c[42]: the overall risk of fetal anomalies in women with PDM is 6% to 12%.[43] A meta-analysis of 33 observational studies found no differences in incidence of major congenital malformations between mothers with T1DM and T2DM.[44]

Abnormal fetal growth

Fetal growth is determined by constitutional growth potential, genetic and epigenetic influences, and maternal characteristics, including nutritional state.[45] Maternal diabetes is associated primarily with fetal overgrowth, but also growth restriction.[46] Pedersen and colleagues[47] are credited with the hypothesis that maternal hyperglycemia drives fetal hyperinsulinemia, stimulating insulin-like growth factor receptors, resulting in excessive growth.[48] More recent understanding of fetal growth includes abnormalities in early placental oxidative stress, placental glucose, amino acid, and lipid transport.[49,50]

Amniotic fluid abnormalities

Polyhydramnios in PDM may be related to increased amniotic fluid glucose concentration or fetal polyuria.[51] Severe polyhydramnios in PDM is uncommon and should prompt consideration of other causes.[52]

Stillbirth

Stillbirth occurs in 3.1 to 5.8 per 1000 women with PDM in the United States.[53] Despite differences in underlying pathophysiology, women with T2DM do not have better perinatal outcomes than those with T1DM.[44] Risk factors for stillbirth include large for gestational age[54] and poor glycemic control.[55] Fetal acidosis is one postulated mechanism of intrauterine fetal death.[56]

Prematurity

The incidence of preterm delivery and associated neonatal risks is significantly elevated in women with PDM.[57]

MANAGEMENT OF PREGESTATIONAL DIABETES IN PREGNANCY
Preconception Counseling

Perinatal and maternal outcomes are best when glucose control is optimized before conception.[58] Women may benefit from multidisciplinary teams that include obstetrics, endocrine, and nutrition providers familiar with diabetes in pregnancy.[59] Recommended preconception measures are outlined in **Box 1**.[60–62]

Nutrition

Women with PDM should have access to a certified dietician to provide them with an individualized nutrition program. The Institute of Medicine recommends that gestational weight goals depend on maternal prepregnancy body mass index.[63] Calorie requirements in a singleton pregnancy are 300 to 350 kilocalories per day higher than prepregnancy requirements.[64] Monitoring intake of carbohydrates facilitates optimal glycemic control.[65]

Intensive Glucose Monitoring

Fasting and postprandial monitoring of blood glucose is recommended to achieve metabolic control in women with PDM.[66] Although a 2017 *Cochrane Review*

Box 1
Fundamentals of preconception care for women with pregestational diabetes mellitus

A. General measures
- Institution of a minimum of 400 μg folic acid daily to reduce risk of neural tube defects
- Monthly monitoring of A1c until stable less than 6.0%
- Effective use of contraception until pregnancy is desired or until diabetes is optimally controlled

B. Evaluation for complications of diabetes
- Urinalysis for glucose, leukocytes, nitrites, and ketones
- Urine culture test for asymptomatic bacteriuria
- A 24-hour urine collection for protein and creatinine clearance or spot albumin-creatinine ratio to assess for nephropathy
- Serum creatinine to assess for nephropathy
- HbA1c for as a measure of 6-weekly glucose control
- Thyroid-stimulating hormone for associated autoimmune thyroid dysfunction, which occurs in up to 40% of women with type 1 diabetes
- Referral for ophthalmologic assessment for retinopathy
- A baseline ECG or ECHO if prior history of chronic hypertension or ischemic heart disease

C. Education
- Counseling regarding specific maternal, fetal, and obstetric risks associated with diabetes in pregnancy, including fetal anomaly
- Effectiveness of optimizing control in reducing adverse maternal, fetal, and obstetric outcomes in pregestational diabetes
- Effective use of contraception during periods when pregnancy is not desired, or where diabetes and lifestyle are not optimized
- Understanding resources and information available for women of childbearing age through their primary care provider, obstetrician, diabetologist, or the American Diabetes Association (http://www.diabetes.org/living-with-diabetes/complications/pregnancy/)

Data from The American College of Obstetricians and Gynecologists. ACOG Committee Opinion #313: the importance of preconception care in the continuum of women's health care. Obstet Gynecol 2005;106(3):665–6; and Hanson MA, Bardsley A, De-Regil LM, et al. The International Federation of Gynecology and Obstetrics (FIGO) recommendations on adolescent, preconception, and maternal nutrition: "Think Nutrition First." Int J Gynecol Obstet 2015;131(Suppl 4):S213–53.

---

concluded there was insufficient evidence to recommend a specific glucose monitoring technique,[67] a recent randomized controlled trial suggests that women with T1DM may benefit from continuous glucose monitoring.[68] The American College of Obstetricians and Gynecologists (ACOG) and the ADA targets for women with PDM are outlined in **Box 2**.[69]

Hemoglobin A1c in Pregnancy

A1c levels decrease during pregnancy because of physiologic increased red blood cell turnover.[70] Recommended target A1c in pregnancy is less than 6% (42 mmol/mol) based on observational studies showing the lowest rate of adverse fetal outcomes in this cohort.[71] These levels should be achieved without hypoglycemia, which can increase risks to both mother and fetus.[72] Of note, A1c may not adequately capture postprandial hyperglycemia and therefore remains a secondary measure of glucose control.

Insulin Requirements Through Pregnancy

Total daily insulin requirements typically decrease in the first trimester of pregnancy.[73] Women with well-controlled diabetes in early pregnancy may experience episodes of

---

Box 2
Recommended glucose targets

- Fasting glucose concentrations ≤95 mg/dL (5.3 mmol/L)

- Preprandial glucose concentrations ≤100 mg/dL (5.6 mmol/L)

- One-hour postprandial glucose concentrations ≤140 mg/dL (7.8 mmol/L)

- Two-hour postprandial glucose concentrations ≤120 mg/dL (6.7 mmol/L)

- Mean capillary glucose 100 mg/dL (5.6 mmol/L)

- During the night, glucose levels ≥60 mg/dL (3.3 mmol/L)

Data from American Diabetes Association. Standards of medical care in diabetes–2014. Diabetes Care 2014;37(S1):S14–80.

---

hypoglycemia requiring adjustment of insulin dosage. Insulin requirements increase in the second trimester as placental hormone production begins, requiring frequent uptitration of insulin to achieve desired targets.[8] In the third trimester, insulin requirements continue to increase until plateauing near term.[74]

Insulin

The goal of insulin therapy is to achieve capillary glucose levels between 70 mg/dL and 110 mg/dL without maternal hypoglycemia. Both multiple daily injection regimens and continuous subcutaneous insulin infusion are reasonable choices in women with PDM.[75] No trials have demonstrated an optimal multiple dose injection regimen, and therefore, treatment should be individualized to optimize glycemic control.[76] Insulins commonly used in pregnancy are summarized in **Table 1**.

Basal insulin delivered as intermediate-acting or long-acting insulin suppresses hepatic gluconeogenesis in the fasting state and is necessary for women with T1DM. Neutral protamine Hagedorn is commonly used for basal dosing in pregnancy.[77] An alternative is the intermediate insulin analogue detemir (Levemir),[78] which has similar outcomes with no increased risk of hypoglycemia.[79] Although not recommended as first-line basal insulin for women initiating therapy during pregnancy, insulin glargine (Lantus) may be continued for those who benefit from once-daily basal insulin dosing.[80]

Bolus dosing of short-acting insulin analogues is usually required with meals to mimic prandial insulin secretion. Both Lispro (Humalog) and Aspart (Novolog) are safe for use in pregnancy and have been shown to normalize postprandial blood glucose better than human regular insulin in women with PDM.[81]

Table 1
Common types of insulins used

Duration of Action	Type	Derivation	Onset (h)	Peak (h)
Short	Regular	Human	0.5	2–4
	Lispro		0.25	1–2
	Aspart		0.25	1–2.5
Intermediate	Hagedorn		1–2	5–7
	Lente		1–3	4–8
Long	Glargine		1.1	5
	Detemir		1–2	5

Dosing Regimens

Insulin requirements are weight based and vary by gestational age. A typical starting dose range could be as follows[54]:

- First trimester: 0.7 to 0.8 units per kilogram per day
- Second trimester: 0.8 to 1 units per kilogram per day
- Third trimester: 0.9 to 1.2 units per kilogram per day

Regimens will typically require 50% to 60% of total daily insulin requirement given as basal insulin, with prandial requirement divided into 3 or more injections of short-acting insulin.

Oral Hypoglycemics

Many women with T2DM are on oral hypoglycemics before pregnancy; however, there are limited data on their use during pregnancy.[82] Metformin and glyburide are currently the only oral agents considered safe for use during pregnancy and are used as alternatives to therapy in women with T2DM who decline insulin.[83]

Glyburide

In small-cohort studies of women with gestational diabetes, glyburide has been found to be comparable to insulin in optimizing serum glucose control in pregnancy without evidence of significant maternal and neonatal complications.[84] However, more recent evidence has shown that concentrations in umbilical cord plasma are approximately 70% of maternal serum levels, and that use is associated with higher incidence of fetal macrosomia and neonatal hypoglycemia than metformin or insulin.[85]

Metformin

Metformin has been studied extensively in women without overt diabetes in pregnancy; however, there are limited data on use in women with PDM.[86] Metformin freely crosses the placenta but does not seem to be associated with fetal risks. Use in the first trimester is associated with a lower risk of miscarriage[87] and no increased risk of congenital malformations[88]; long-term follow-up data for exposed offspring are lacking at this time, with limited evidence suggesting possible changes in body composition in children exposed in utero.[89] In women with obesity but no diabetes, metformin is associated with reduced risk of preeclampsia[90] and lower risk of macrosomia[91]; however, these benefits have not been demonstrated in women with PDM.[92] Based on data from a randomized controlled trial of metformin for treatment of gestational diabetes in which most of the participants needed supplemental insulin, it is likely to be insufficient for glycemic control in women with T2DM.[84]

Hypoglycemia

Hypoglycemia occurs more frequently in pregnancy that at other times.[93] Patients and families should be educated on signs of and treatment of hypoglycemia. Glucagon is a peptide hormone normally secreted from pancreatic alpha cells in response to hypoglycemia, which raises the blood glucose concentration and should be made available to relatives of pregnant women on insulin for use in life-threatening hypoglycemia.[94]

Management of Diabetic Ketoacidosis

Aggressive rehydration, insulin, and electrolyte replacement as required are initial therapy. Plasma glucose and potassium levels should be rechecked frequently to avoid untreated hypoglycemia and hypokalemia.[95] If infection is a possible precipitant based on clinical presentation, empirical treatment with broad-spectrum antimicrobials is advisable.[95] The management of DKA is summarized in **Box 3**.[96]

Reported rates of fetal mortality in DKA are 10% to 35%.[97] Continuous fetal monitoring may show recurrent late decelerations with maternal acidosis,[98] but fetal acidemia is reversible with appropriate treatment of maternal acidemia.

Intrapartum Glucose Control

Maternal hyperglycemia during labor is associated with risk for neonatal hypoglycemia.[99] Data are limited on the best approach to intrapartum glycemic control; however, intravenous insulin is often needed to maintain glucose at a goal of 70 to 110 mg/dL.[100] Institutional protocols for insulin management during labor may be useful.

Fetal Monitoring

ACOG recommends antepartum fetal testing for pregnancies complicated by PDM.[61] There are limited data to guide specific test choice and frequency; however, ACOG

Box 3
Management of diabetic ketoacidosis

Laboratory assessment (every 1–2 hours)
- Arterial blood gases to quantify acidosis
- Glucose
- Electrolytes
- Ketones

Insulin
- Low-dose, intravenous
- Loading dose: 0.2 to 0.4 U/kg
- Maintenance: 2 to 10 units per hour

Fluids
- Isotonic normal saline or lactated Ringer
- 4–6 L total replacement in first 12 hours
- 1 L in first hour
- 500 mL to 1 L/h for 2 to 4 hours
- 250 mL/h until 80% replaced

Glucose
- Begin 5% dextrose in normal saline when plasma level reaches 250 mg/dL

Potassium
- If initial levels are normal or decreased, add 20 to 30 mEq/h to an intravenous solution. If levels are elevated, wait until levels decrease

Bicarbonate
- Add 1 ampule of 1 L of 0.45 normal saline if pH is <7.1

Data from American Diabetes Association. Standards of medical care in diabetes–2014. Diabetes Care 2014;37(S1):S14–80.

advises antepartum monitoring using fetal movements, biophysical profile, nonstress tests, and/or contraction stress test at appropriate intervals.[61] The authors start testing by 32 weeks and increase to twice weekly by 34 to 36 weeks.

Timing of Delivery

In the absence of compelling data to drive decision making,[101] delivery timing should be individualized based on maternal glycemic control, balancing the risk of intrauterine fetal death and ongoing fetal overgrowth with maternal and fetal morbidity associated with early delivery. Delivery in the late preterm or early term (37 weeks) may be indicated in patients with end-organ disease, persistently poor glucose control, or a previous intrauterine fetal demise.[102]

Mode of Delivery

PDM increases risk for cesarean delivery, independent of birth weight and other factors.[103] Cesarean delivery should be considered in women with diabetes and an estimated fetal weight greater than 4500 g.[104] Although no large randomized trials have been conducted in women with PDM, in one single-center study, a policy of elective cesarean delivery for an estimated fetal weight greater than 4250 g and induction of labor if greater than 90 percentile but less than 4250 g was associated with a decreased rate of shoulder dystocia and no change in cesarean delivery rate.[105]

Postpartum Care

Maternal insulin requirements

Insulin requirements decrease dramatically following the third stage of labor and placental delivery and return to prepregnancy levels over the subsequent 1 to 2 weeks.[8] Typically, insulin dosing is halved or changed to a prepregnancy dosing regimen. Particular caution should be paid to women taking insulin while breastfeeding, who may be at risk for hypoglycemia.

Breastfeeding

Breastfeeding is recommended as the standard for infant nutrition in the absence of contraindications.[106] Lactation may be of additional benefit to women with PDM because it reduces overall insulin needs.[107] It may also be associated with long-term maternal metabolic benefits.[108]

Contraception

All women of childbearing age with PDM should have access to family planning and contraceptive options to reduce the risk of future unplanned pregnancy. Although diabetes should not impact options for contraception, infant feeding and postpartum status may impact choice. Preferred postpartum contraceptive options in breastfeeding include long-acting reversible contraceptives (copper or progestin intrauterine devices, etonogestrel implants) and progestogen-only pills. Combination hormonal contraceptives may pose more risk than benefit in women with PDM because of the thromboembolic effects of estrogen and are not recommended in the immediate postpartum period.[109] Depot medroxyprogesterone acetate (DMPA) may also be associated with a higher risk for thromboembolism in mothers with PDM because of increased peripheral conversion of DMPA to peripheral estrogen than other progestogens.[110]

Postpartum transition of care

There are limited data to support specific care models for women with PDM after pregnancy; however, optimization of long-term maternal health should be a goal of all obstetric and primary care providers.[111]

SUMMARY

Diabetes is a common chronic condition in women of reproductive age. Preconception care reduces the risks associated with poor glycemic control in early pregnancy. Adverse pregnancy outcomes, including hypertensive disorders, abnormal fetal growth, traumatic delivery, and stillbirth, can be minimized with optimal glycemic control. Insulin is the preferred medication to optimize glucose control in women with T2DM, and frequent dose adjustments are needed during pregnancy. Team-based multidisciplinary care may help women achieve glycemic goals and optimize pregnancy outcomes. Postpartum care should include lactation support, counseling on contraceptive options, and transition to primary care.

REFERENCES

1. Lobstein T, Jackson-Leach R. Planning for the worst: estimates of obesity and comorbidities in school-age children in 2025. Pediatr Obes 2016;11(5):321–5.
2. Peng TY, Ehrlich SF, Crites Y, et al. Trends and racial and ethnic disparities in the prevalence of pregestational type 1 and type 2 diabetes in Northern California: 1996–2014. Am J Obstet Gynecol 2017;216(2):177.e1–8.
3. Feig DS, Hwee J, Shah BR, et al. Trends in incidence of diabetes in pregnancy and serious perinatal outcomes: a large, population-based study in Ontario, Canada, 1996-2010. Diabetes Care 2014;37(6):1590–6.
4. Correa A, Bardenheier B, Elixhauser A, et al. Trends in prevalence of diabetes among delivery hospitalizations, United States, 1993-2009. Matern Child Health J 2015;19(3):635–42.
5. Menke A, Casagrande S, Geiss L, et al. Prevalence of and trends in diabetes among adults in the United States, 1988-2012. JAMA 2015;314(10):1021–9.
6. Centers for Disease Control and Prevention. National diabetes statistics report 2017. Atlanta (GA): Centers for Disease Control and Prevention, US Department of Health and Human Services; 2017.
7. Kalhan S, Rossi K, Gruca L, et al. Glucose turnover and gluconeogenesis in human pregnancy. J Clin Invest 1997;100(7):1775–81.
8. Angueira A. New insights into gestational glucose metabolism: lessons learned from 21st century approaches. Diabetes 2015;64:327–34. American Diabetes Association.
9. Ryan EA. Hormones and insulin resistance during pregnancy. Lancet 2003; 362(9398):1777–8.
10. Catalano PM, Tyzbir ED, Roman NM, et al. Longitudinal changes in insulin release and insulin resistance in nonobese pregnant women. Am J Obstet Gynecol 1991; 165(6 Pt 1):1667–72.
11. 2. Classification and diagnosis of diabetes. Diabetes Care 2017;40(Supplement 1): S11–24.
12. Daneman D. Type 1 diabetes. Lancet 2006;367(9513):847–58.
13. Yang L, Colditz GA. Prevalence of overweight and obesity in the United States, 2007-2012. JAMA Intern Med 2015;175(8):1412–3.
14. Metzger BE, Buchanan TA, Coustan DR, et al. Summary and recommendations of the Fifth International Workshop-Conference on Gestational Diabetes Mellitus. Diabetes Care 2007;30(Suppl 2):S251–60.
15. Wahabi HA, Alzeidan RA, Bawazeer GA, et al. Preconception care for diabetic women for improving maternal and fetal outcomes: a systematic review and meta-analysis. BMC Pregnancy Childbirth 2010;10:63.

16. Sibai BM. Chronic hypertension in pregnancy. Obstet Gynecol 2002;100(2): 369–77.
17. Kattah AG, Garovic VD. The management of hypertension in pregnancy. Adv Chronic Kidney Dis 2013;20(3):229–39.
18. American College of Obstetricians and Gynecologists, Task Force on Hypertension in Pregnancy. Hypertension in pregnancy. Report of the American College of Obstetricians and Gynecologists' Task Force on Hypertension in Pregnancy. Obstet Gynecol 2013;122(5):1122–31.
19. Saji H, Yamanaka M, Hagiwara A, et al. Losartan and fetal toxic effects. Lancet 2001;357(9253):363.
20. Bateman BT, Patorno E, Desai RJ, et al. Angiotensin-converting enzyme inhibitors and the risk of congenital malformations. Obstet Gynecol 2017;129(1):174–84.
21. Damm JA, Asbjornsdottir B, Callesen NF, et al. Diabetic nephropathy and microalbuminuria in pregnant women with type 1 and type 2 diabetes: prevalence, antihypertensive strategy, and pregnancy outcome. Diabetes Care 2013; 36(11):3489–94.
22. Screening for diabetic retinopathy. San Francisco (CA): Quality of Care Secretariat, American Academy of Ophthalmology; 2014.
23. Ringholm L, Damm JA, Vestgaard M, et al. Diabetic nephropathy in women with preexisting diabetes: from pregnancy planning to breastfeeding. Curr Diab Rep 2016;16(2):12.
24. Reece EA, Leguizamon G, Homko C. Pregnancy performance and outcomes associated with diabetic nephropathy. Am J Perinatol 1998;15(7):413–21.
25. Nielsen LR, Muller C, Damm P, et al. Reduced prevalence of early preterm delivery in women with type 1 diabetes and microalbuminuria–possible effect of early antihypertensive treatment during pregnancy. Diabet Med 2006;23(4):426–31.
26. Holmes VA, Young IS, Maresh MJ, et al. The diabetes and pre-eclampsia intervention trial. Int J Gynaecol Obstet 2004;87(1):66–71.
27. Sibai BM, Caritis S, Hauth J. What we have learned about preeclampsia. Semin Perinatol 2003;27(3):239–46.
28. LeFevre ML, U.S. Preventive Services Task Force. Low-dose aspirin use for the prevention of morbidity and mortality from preeclampsia: U.S. Preventive Services Task Force recommendation statement. Ann Intern Med 2014;161(11):819–26.
29. Kaaja R, Loukovaara S. Progression of retinopathy in type 1 diabetic women during pregnancy. Curr Diabetes Rev 2007;3(2):85–93.
30. Rasmussen KL, Laugesen CS, Ringholm L, et al. Progression of diabetic retinopathy during pregnancy in women with type 2 diabetes. Diabetologia 2010; 53(6):1076–83.
31. Polizzi S, Mahajan VB. Intravitreal anti-VEGF injections in pregnancy: case series and review of literature. J Ocul Pharmacol Ther 2015;31(10):605–10.
32. Camilleri M. Diabetic gastroparesis. N Engl J Med 2007;356(8):820–9.
33. Hemachandra A, Ellis D, Lloyd CE, et al. The influence of pregnancy on IDDM complications. Diabetes Care 1995;18(7):950–4.
34. Massey EW, Guidon AC. Peripheral neuropathies in pregnancy. Continuum (Minneap Minn) 2014;20(1 Neurology of Pregnancy):100–14.
35. Roth A, Elkayam U. Acute myocardial infarction associated with pregnancy. J Am Coll Cardiol 2008;52(3):171–80.
36. Parker JA, Conway DL. Diabetic ketoacidosis in pregnancy. Obstet Gynecol Clin North Am 2007;34(3):533–43, xii.
37. Chico M, Levine SN, Lewis DF. Normoglycemic diabetic ketoacidosis in pregnancy. J Perinatol 2008;28(4):310–2.

38. Bell R, Bailey K, Cresswell T, et al. Trends in prevalence and outcomes of pregnancy in women with pre-existing type I and type II diabetes. BJOG 2008; 115(4):445–52.
39. Stanirowski PJ, Szukiewicz D, Pazura-Turowska M, et al. Expression of glucose transporter proteins in human diabetic placenta. Can J Diabetes 2017. [Epub ahead of print].
40. Combs CA, Gunderson E, Kitzmiller JL, et al. Relationship of fetal macrosomia to maternal postprandial glucose control during pregnancy. Diabetes Care 1992; 15(10):1251–7.
41. Schaefer-Graf UM, Buchanan TA, Xiang A, et al. Patterns of congenital anomalies and relationship to initial maternal fasting glucose levels in pregnancies complicated by type 2 and gestational diabetes. Am J Obstet Gynecol 2000; 182(2):313–20.
42. Balsells M, García-Patterson A, Gich I, et al. Major congenital malformations in women with gestational diabetes mellitus: a systematic review and meta-analysis. Diabetes Metab Res Rev 2012;28(3):252–7.
43. Zhao E, Zhang Y, Zeng X, et al. Association between maternal diabetes mellitus and the risk of congenital malformations: a meta-analysis of cohort studies. Drug Discov Ther 2015;9(4):274–81.
44. Balsells M, García-Patterson A, Gich I, et al. Maternal and fetal outcome in women with type 2 versus type 1 diabetes mellitus: a systematic review and metaanalysis. J Clin Endocrinol Metab 2009;94(11):4284–91.
45. Wells JCK, Chomtho S, Fewtrell MS. Programming of body composition by early growth and nutrition. Proc Nutr Soc 2007;66(3):423–34.
46. Kanda E, Matsuda Y, Makino Y, et al. Risk factors associated with altered fetal growth in patients with pregestational diabetes mellitus. J Matern Fetal Neonatal Med 2012;25(8):1390–4.
47. Pedersen O, Beck-Nielsen H, Klebe JG. Insulin receptors in the pregnant diabetic and her newborn. J Clin Endocrinol Metab 1981;53(6):1160–6.
48. Milner RD, Hill DJ. Fetal growth control: the role of insulin and related peptides. Clin Endocrinol (Oxf) 1984;21(4):415–33.
49. Schaefer-Graf UM, Graf K, Kulbacka I, et al. Maternal lipids as strong determinants of fetal environment and growth in pregnancies with gestational diabetes mellitus. Diabetes Care 2008;31(9):1858.
50. Wu G. Amino acids: metabolism, functions, and nutrition. Amino Acids 2009; 37(1):1–17.
51. Weinberg LE, Dinsmoor MJ, Silver RK. Severe hydramnios and preterm delivery in association with transient maternal diabetes insipidus. Obstet Gynecol 2010; 116(2):547–9.
52. Moore LE. Amount of polyhydramnios attributable to diabetes may be less than previously reported. World J Diabetes 2017;8(1):7–10.
53. Reddy UM, Laughon SK, Sun L, et al. Prepregnancy risk factors for antepartum stillbirth in the United States. Obstet Gynecol 2010;116(5): 1119–26.
54. Singh C, Jovanovic L. Insulin analogues in the treatment of diabetes in pregnancy. Obstet Gynecol Clin North Am 2007;34(2):275–91.
55. Lauenborg J, Mathiesen E, Ovesen P, et al. Audit on stillbirths in women with pregestational type 1 diabetes. Diabetes Care 2003;26(5):1385–9.
56. Lawn JE, Lee ACC, Kinney M, et al. Two million intrapartum-related stillbirths and neonatal deaths: where, why, and what can be done? Int J Gynaecol Obstet 2009;107(Supplement):S5–19.

57. Eidem I, Vangen S, Hanssen KF, et al. Perinatal and infant mortality in term and preterm births among women with type 1 diabetes. Diabetologia 2011;54(11): 2771–8.
58. Fischl AF, Herman WH, Sereika SM, et al. Impact of a preconception counseling program for teens with type 1 diabetes (READY-Girls) on patient-provider interaction, resource utilization, and cost. Diabetes Care 2010; 33(4):701–5.
59. Owens LA, Egan AM, Carmody L, et al. Ten years of optimizing outcomes for women with type 1 and type 2 diabetes in pregnancy-the Atlantic DIP experience. J Clin Endocrinol Metab 2016;101(4):1598–605.
60. American College of Obstetricians and Gynecologists. ACOG committee opinion number 313, September 2005. The importance of preconception care in the continuum of women's health care. Obstet Gynecol 2005;106(3): 665–6.
61. ACOG Committee on Practice Bulletins. ACOG practice bulletin. Clinical management guidelines for obstetrician-gynecologists. Number 60, March 2005. Pregestational diabetes mellitus. Obstet Gynecol 2005;105(3):675–85.
62. Hanson MA, Bardsley A, De-Regil LM, et al. The International Federation of Gynecology and Obstetrics (FIGO) recommendations on adolescent, preconception, and maternal nutrition: "Think Nutrition First". Int J Gynaecol Obstet 2015; 131(Suppl 4):S213–53.
63. Institute of Medicine and National Research Council Committee to Reexamine IOMPWG. The National Academies Collection: reports funded by National Institutes of Health. In: Rasmussen KM, Yaktine AL, editors. Weight gain during pregnancy: reexamining the guidelines. Washington, DC: National Academies Press (US) National Academy of Sciences; 2009.
64. Stuebe AM, Oken E, Gillman MW. Associations of diet and physical activity during pregnancy with risk for excessive gestational weight gain. Am J Obstet Gynecol 2009;201(1):58.e1–8.
65. Brand-Miller J, McMillan-Price J, Steinbeck K, et al. Dietary glycemic index: health implications. J Am Coll Nutr 2009;28(Suppl):446S-449S.
66. Chamberlain JJ, Rhinehart AS, Shaefer CF, et al. Diagnosis and management of diabetes: synopsis of the 2016 American Diabetes Association Standards of Medical Care in Diabetes. Ann Intern Med 2016;164(8):542–52.
67. Moy FM, Ray A, Buckley BS, et al. Techniques of monitoring blood glucose during pregnancy for women with pre-existing diabetes. Cochrane Database Syst Rev 2017;(6):CD009613.
68. Feig DS, Donovan LE, Corcoy R, et al. Continuous glucose monitoring in pregnant women with type 1 diabetes (CONCEPTT): a multicentre international randomised controlled trial. Lancet 2017;390(10110):2347–59.
69. Marathe PH, Gao HX, Close KL. American Diabetes Association Standards of Medical Care in Diabetes 2017. J Diabetes 2017;9(4):320–4.
70. Mosca A, Paleari R, Dalfra MG, et al. Reference intervals for hemoglobin A1c in pregnant women: data from an Italian multicenter study. Clin Chem 2006;52(6): 1138–43.
71. Maresh MJ, Holmes VA, Patterson CC, et al. Glycemic targets in the second and third trimester of pregnancy for women with type 1 diabetes. Diabetes Care 2015;38(1):34–42.
72. Mathiesen ER, Kinsley B, Amiel SA, et al. Maternal glycemic control and hypoglycemia in type 1 diabetic pregnancy. Diabetes Care 2007;30(4):771.

73. Jovanovic L, Knopp RH, Brown Z, et al. Declining insulin requirement in the late first trimester of diabetic pregnancy. Diabetes Care 2001;24(7):1130.

74. Buchanan TA, Metzger BE, Freinkel N, et al. Insulin sensitivity and B-cell responsiveness to glucose during late pregnancy in lean and moderately obese women with normal glucose tolerance or mild gestational diabetes. Am J Obstet Gynecol 1990;162(4):1008–14.

75. Farrar D, Tuffnell DJ, West J, et al. Continuous subcutaneous insulin infusion versus multiple daily injections of insulin for pregnant women with diabetes. Cochrane Database Syst Rev 2016;(6):CD005542.

76. O'Neill SM, Kenny LC, Khashan AS, et al. Different insulin types and regimens for pregnant women with pre-existing diabetes. Cochrane Database Syst Rev 2017;(2):CD011880.

77. Rosenstock J, Schwartz SL, Clark CM, et al. Basal insulin therapy in type 2 diabetes. Diabetes Care 2001;24(4):631.

78. Blumer I, Hadar E, Hadden DR, et al. Diabetes and pregnancy: an Endocrine Society clinical practice guideline. J Clin Endocrinol Metab 2013;98(11):4227–49.

79. Mathiesen ER, Hod M, Ivanisevic M, et al. Maternal efficacy and safety outcomes in a randomized, controlled trial comparing insulin detemir with NPH insulin in 310 pregnant women with type 1 diabetes. Diabetes Care 2012;35(10):2012–7.

80. Pollex EK, Feig DS, Lubetsky A, et al. Insulin glargine safety in pregnancy. Diabetes Care 2010;33(1):29.

81. Garcia-Dominguez M, Herranz L, Hillman N, et al. Use of insulin lispro during pregnancy in women with pregestational diabetes mellitus. Med Clin (Barc) 2011;137(13):581–6.

82. Feghali MN, Caritis SN, Catov JM, et al. Glycemic control and pregnancy outcomes in women with type 2 diabetes treated with oral hypoglycemic agents. Am J Perinatol 2017;34(7):697–704.

83. Dhulkotia JS, Ola B, Fraser R, et al. Oral hypoglycemic agents vs insulin in management of gestational diabetes: a systematic review and metaanalysis. Am J Obstet Gynecol 2010;203(5):457.e1–9.

84. Rowan JA, Hague WM, Gao W, et al. Metformin versus insulin for the treatment of gestational diabetes. N Engl J Med 2008;358(19):2003–15.

85. Camelo Castillo W, Boggess K, Sturmer T, et al. Association of adverse pregnancy outcomes with glyburide vs insulin in women with gestational diabetes. JAMA Pediatr 2015;169(5):452–8.

86. Lautatzis M-E, Goulis DG, Vrontakis M. Efficacy and safety of metformin during pregnancy in women with gestational diabetes mellitus or polycystic ovary syndrome: a systematic review. Metabolism 2013;62(11):1522–34.

87. Feng L, Lin XF, Wan ZH, et al. Efficacy of metformin on pregnancy complications in women with polycystic ovary syndrome: a meta-analysis. Gynecol Endocrinol 2015;31(11):833–9.

88. Cassina M, Dona M, Di Gianantonio E, et al. First-trimester exposure to metformin and risk of birth defects: a systematic review and meta-analysis. Hum Reprod Update 2014;20(5):656–69.

89. Rowan JA, Rush EC, Obolonkin V, et al. Metformin in gestational diabetes: the offspring follow-up (MiG TOFU): body composition at 2 years of age. Diabetes Care 2011;34(10):2279–84.

90. Syngelaki A, Nicolaides KH, Balani J, et al. Metformin versus placebo in obese pregnant women without diabetes mellitus. N Engl J Med 2016; 374(5):434–43.

91. Chiswick C, Reynolds RM, Denison F, et al. Effect of metformin on maternal and fetal outcomes in obese pregnant women (EMPOWaR): a randomised, double-blind, placebo-controlled trial. Lancet Diabetes Endocrinol 2015; 3(10):778–86.

92. Romero R, Erez O, Huttemann M, et al. Metformin, the aspirin of the 21st century: its role in gestational diabetes mellitus, prevention of preeclampsia and cancer, and the promotion of longevity. Am J Obstet Gynecol 2017;217(3): 282–302.

93. Heller S, Damm P, Mersebach H, et al. Hypoglycemia in type 1 diabetic pregnancy. Diabetes Care 2010;33(3):473.

94. Bernasko J. Intensive insulin therapy in pregnancy: strategies for successful implementation in pregestational diabetes mellitus. J Matern Fetal Neonatal Med 2007;20(2):125–32.

95. Wolfsdorf J, Craig ME, Daneman D, et al. Diabetic ketoacidosis. Pediatr Diabetes 2007;8(1):28–43.

96. Landon MB, Catalano PM, Gabbe SG. Diabetes mellitus complicating pregnancy. In: Obstetrics: normal and problem pregnancies, 2007. 2007.

97. Morrison FJR, Movassaghian M, Seely EW, et al. Fetal outcomes after diabetic ketoacidosis during pregnancy. Diabetes Care 2017;40(7):e77–9.

98. Kamalakannan D, Baskar V, Barton DM, et al. Diabetic ketoacidosis in pregnancy. Postgrad Med J 2003;79(934):454–7.

99. Kline GA, Edwards A. Antepartum and intra-partum insulin management of type 1 and type 2 diabetic women: impact on clinically significant neonatal hypoglycemia. Diabetes Res Clin Pract 2007;77(2):223–30.

100. Ryan EA, Al-Agha R. Glucose control during labor and delivery. Curr Diab Rep 2014;14(1):450.

101. Berger H, Melamed N. Timing of delivery in women with diabetes in pregnancy. Obstet Med 2014;7(1):8–16.

102. Spong CY, Mercer BM, D'Alton M, et al. Timing of indicated late-preterm and early-term birth. Obstet Gynecol 2011;118(2 Pt 1):323–33.

103. Ehrenberg HM, Durnwald CP, Catalano P, et al. The influence of obesity and diabetes on the risk of cesarean delivery. Am J Obstet Gynecol 2004;191(3): 969–74.

104. American College of Obstetricians and Gynecologists' Committee on Practice Bulletins—Obstetrics. Practice bulletin No. 173: fetal macrosomia. Obstet Gynecol 2016;128(5):e195–209.

105. Conway DL, Langer O. Elective delivery of infants with macrosomia in diabetic women: reduced shoulder dystocia versus increased cesarean deliveries. Am J Obstet Gynecol 1998;178(5):922–5.

106. ACOG Committee Opinion No. 361: breastfeeding: maternal and infant aspects. Obstet Gynecol 2007;109(2 Pt 1):479–80.

107. Gunderson EP, Crites Y, Chiang V, et al. Influence of breastfeeding during the postpartum oral glucose tolerance test on plasma glucose and insulin. Obstet Gynecol 2012;120(1):136–43.

108. Stuebe A. Associations among lactation, maternal carbohydrate metabolism, and cardiovascular health. Clin Obstet Gynecol 2015;58(4):827–39.

109. World Health Organization. Selected practice recommendations for contraceptive use. 3rd edition. 2016.

110. van Hylckama Vlieg A, Helmerhorst FM, Rosendaal FR. The risk of deep venous thrombosis associated with injectable depot–medroxyprogesterone acetate contraceptives or a levonorgestrel intrauterine device. Arterioscler Thromb Vasc Biol 2010;30:2297–300.
111. Bick D, Beake S, Chappell L, et al. Management of pregnant and postnatal women with pre-existing diabetes or cardiac disease using multi-disciplinary team models of care: a systematic review. BMC Pregnancy Childbirth 2014; 14:428.

Hypertensive Disorders in Pregnancy

Amelia L.M. Sutton, MD, PhD*, Lorie M. Harper, MD, MSCI, Alan T.N. Tita, MD, PhD

KEYWORDS

- Chronic hypertension • Gestational hypertension • Preeclampsia • Eclampsia

KEY POINTS

- Hypertensive disorders of pregnancy result in a substantial health burden, accounting for a large proportion of maternal and neonatal morbidity and mortality.
- The diagnostic criteria and classification of preeclampsia have been updated to reflect current understanding of the disease.
- Select candidates with preterm preeclampsia with severe features can be expectantly managed to decrease the risks of iatrogenic prematurity.
- Strategies to prevent preeclampsia include identification of high-risk patients and initiation of low-dose aspirin in early gestation.
- Substantial gaps in knowledge remain, including the goal blood pressures for women with chronic hypertension.

INTRODUCTION

Hypertensive disorders affect as many as 10% of all pregnancies worldwide.[1] This heterogeneous group of disorders includes chronic hypertension, gestational hypertension, preeclampsia, and preeclampsia superimposed on chronic hypertension. These disorders account for a significant proportion of perinatal morbidity and mortality. Hypertensive disorders feature among the top 6 causes of maternal mortality in the United States and are responsible for nearly 10% of all maternal deaths.[2] The incidence of preeclampsia has risen dramatically over the past few decades.[3,4] The incidence of early-onset preeclampsia, which accounts for a disproportionate degree of maternal and neonatal morbidity and mortality, has increased by greater than 140%.[5] Given the substantial health burden of hypertensive disorders in pregnancy, there is increasing interest in optimizing management of these conditions. This article summarizes the diagnosis and management of

Disclosure: The authors report no conflict of interest.
Department of Obstetrics and Gynecology, Division of Maternal-Fetal Medicine, University of Alabama at Birmingham, Women and Infants Center, 1700 6th Avenue South, Birmingham, AL 35249, USA
* Corresponding author.
E-mail address: alsutton@uabmc.edu

Obstet Gynecol Clin N Am 45 (2018) 333–347
https://doi.org/10.1016/j.ogc.2018.01.012
0889-8545/18/© 2018 Elsevier Inc. All rights reserved.

each of the disorders in the spectrum of hypertension in pregnancy and highlights recent updates in the field.

CHRONIC HYPERTENSION
Definition and Epidemiology

Hypertension is defined as either a systolic blood pressure (SBP) of 140 mm Hg or higher, a diastolic BP (DBP) of 90 mm Hg or higher, or both.[6] Chronic hypertension, by definition, is diagnosed before pregnancy or before 20 weeks' gestation and persisting after delivery.[6] Chronic hypertension is further classified as mild-to-moderate (SBP 140–159 mm Hg and/or DBP 90–109 mm Hg) or severe (SBP ≥160 mm Hg and/or DBP ≥110 mm Hg).[1] As many as 5% of pregnant women have chronic hypertension. Most of these patients will have essential hypertension but as many as 10% have secondary hypertension, with underlying endocrine or renal causes.[1] Older age at child birth and prevalence of obesity contribute to a rising prevalence of chronic hypertension during pregnancy.[3,4]

Diagnosis

Chronic hypertension is most easily diagnosed in a woman with documented prepregnancy hypertension, especially if she is already receiving antihypertensive therapy.[1] Hypertension arising in the first trimester is most likely chronic hypertension. However, a diagnostic dilemma arises in women with late prenatal care who may be normotensive during the typical nadir in the second trimester and then become hypertensive in the late second or third trimester. It is challenging to distinguish chronic hypertension from gestational hypertension and, often, preeclampsia during the pregnancy. If hypertension persists after the postpartum period (6–12 weeks), then chronic hypertension is the retrospective diagnosis. Additionally, many women with well-documented preexisting hypertension may remain normotensive without therapy throughout pregnancy.

Complications

Chronic hypertension is associated with poor outcomes in both pregnant and nonpregnant women.[6] Some complications that can occur both during and outside of pregnancy include renal failure, stroke, respiratory failure, and death.[6] However, the most significant complication of chronic hypertension is the development of superimposed preeclampsia, which develops in 20% to 40% of women with chronic hypertension.[7,8] Maternal morbidity and mortality rates are higher in patients with superimposed preeclampsia compared with women with preeclampsia in the absence of preexisting hypertension.[9] Similarly, chronic hypertension poses substantial risks to the fetus, including miscarriage, abruption, small-for-gestational age, preterm birth, and perinatal death. The perinatal mortality rate is higher in patients with superimposed preeclampsia compared with women with preeclampsia in women without chronic hypertension.[10]

Management

Women with chronic hypertension should be evaluated for evidence of end-organ damage, including a baseline serum creatinine, urine protein quantitation, and electrocardiogram. A recent study suggested that even high normal values of serum creatinine (≥0.75 mg/dL) and proteinuria (protein/creatine ratio ≥0.12) before 20 weeks' gestation are associated with an increased risk of developing preeclampsia with and without severe features.[11] If the hypertension is severe and/or long-standing, further cardiac evaluation, including an echocardiogram, may be warranted.[6] Although most cases of hypertension are primary, additional evaluation for secondary causes, such as polycystic kidney disease, hyperaldosteronism, Cushing syndrome, or renovascular disease, may be indicated by clinical findings and personal and family history.

Optimal blood pressure (BP) thresholds during pregnancy have been studied in several trials.[12–14] The benefits of tight BP control must be balanced by the effects of antihypertensives on the fetus. The Control of Hypertension in Pregnancy Study (CHIPS) randomized women with hypertension at 14 to 33 weeks to either tight (DBP <85 mm Hg) or less tight BP control (DBP <100 mm Hg).[12] Although there was a lower incidence of severe hypertension in the tight control group, there were no differences in perinatal or maternal outcomes, including the primary outcome of pregnancy loss or neonatal intensive care unit admission for at least 48 hours. A secondary analysis of the subgroup with chronic hypertension suggested an increase in small-for-gestational age infants associated with beta-blocker treatment of mild hypertension.[12] Therefore, the decision to treat mild-to-moderate hypertension in pregnancy remains a topic of debate and is the focus of an ongoing large multicenter randomized trial. Considering the available data from the CHIPS trial, as well as systematic reviews,[14] the current recommendation is that antihypertensive therapy should be initiated only in women with severe hypertension (defined as SBP ≥160 mm Hg and/or DBP ≥105 mm Hg).[13] Therapy may be discontinued in women with mild hypertension unless there are significant comorbidities.

First-line antihypertensives include labetalol, a nonselective alpha-blocker and beta-blocker; nifedipine, a calcium channel blocker; and methyldopa, an alpha2 adrenergic agonist.[1] Extensive studies have shown that methyldopa is safe during pregnancy but is less effective than beta-blockers and calcium channel blockers in preventing severe hypertension.[14] Labetalol is dosed 200 to 2400 mg per day orally in 2 to 3 divided doses. It should be avoided in patients with significant asthma and congestive heart failure.[6] Nifedipine is dosed 30 to 120 mg per day orally. Methyldopa is dosed 500 mg-3 gram per day orally in 2 to 3 divided doses. Second-line agents include thiazide diuretics. Theoretic concerns that diuretics can cause volume depletion and fetal growth restriction have not been confirmed in trials.[15] Angiotensin-converting enzyme inhibitors and angiotensin II receptor blockers have been associated with fetal abnormalities, including renal and skull anomalies, and should not be used in pregnancy.[6]

Women should be carefully monitored for the development of superimposed preeclampsia throughout pregnancy. Serial biometry is recommended given the increased risk of fetal growth restriction in patients with chronic hypertension.[1] The risk of stillbirth is 2 to 3 times higher in women with chronic hypertension compared with pregnancies not complicated by the disease[16,17]; therefore, antenatal testing should be performed in the third trimester.[1] In patients with uncomplicated disease, delivery at 38 to 39 weeks' gestation is recommended.[1]

GESTATIONAL HYPERTENSION
Definition and Epidemiology

Gestational hypertension is defined as new-onset elevated BPs after 20 weeks' gestation without proteinuria or other signs of preeclampsia.[6] The alternate diagnosis of chronic hypertension should be made if BPs do not normalize in the postpartum period. Gestational hypertension complicates 2% to 3% of pregnancies in the United States.[4,18] Approximately half of women initially diagnosed with gestational hypertension before term eventually develop preeclampsia[19]; therefore, close surveillance for worsening disease is warranted.

Diagnosis

Gestational hypertension is a diagnosis of exclusion. Specifically, chronic hypertension and preeclampsia should be ruled out during the evaluation. The diagnosis is made when there is new-onset hypertension (defined as systolic BP $\geq$140 mm Hg and/or DBP $\geq$90 mm Hg following 20 weeks' gestation) and the absence of proteinuria or the other features of preeclampsia (**Table 1**). It is often difficult to distinguish gestational hypertension from chronic hypertension, especially in women with inadequate prepregnancy care or presenting late for prenatal care (after the first trimester), so true baseline BPs are uncertain.

Complications

The most common complication of gestational hypertension is development of preeclampsia, which occurs in approximately 50% of women who are diagnosed with gestational hypertension before term.[19] Therefore, women with gestational hypertension are at risk for all of the obstetric complications associated with preeclampsia (see later discussion), including eclampsia, other central nervous system (CNS) complications, end-organ damage, fetal growth restriction, abruption, and death. The risk of adverse outcomes in gestational hypertension is considerably less than in preeclampsia unless the hypertension becomes severe, in which case outcomes are similar to preeclampsia.[20] By definition, gestational hypertension resolves in the postpartum period.[1,6] Nonetheless, women with this condition are at increased risk for developing chronic hypertension and other cardiovascular diseases, such ischemic heart disease, later in life.[21]

Management

When gestational hypertension is diagnosed at term ($\geq$37 weeks), delivery is recommended because it prevents the serious complications associated with progression

Table 1 Severe features of preeclampsia	
Severe hypertension	• SBP >160 mm Hg or • DBP >110 mm Hg • Taken on 2 occasions at least 4 h apart while on bed rest (unless antihypertensives have been administered)
CNS symptoms	• Persistent headache not relieved by analgesics • Visual changes
Pulmonary edema	• Clinically diagnosed
Thrombocytopenia	• Platelet count <100,000/mL
Renal insufficiency	• Serum creatinine >1.1 mg/dL, or • Doubling of the serum creatinine when other renal diseases have been excluded
Liver dysfunction	• Increase in liver enzymes to $\geq$ twice the upper limits of normal

Adapted from American College of Obstetrics and Gynecologists; Task Force on Hypertension in Pregnancy. Hypertension in pregnancy. Report of the American College of Obstetricians and Gynecologists' Task Force on Hypertension in Pregnancy. Obstet Gynecol 2013;122(5):1122–31; with permission.

of the disease.[1] Delivery at term is supported by a randomized trial of immediate delivery versus expectant management in patients with preeclampsia without severe features or gestational hypertension. This trial demonstrated that induction is associated with similar neonatal outcomes and a decreased risk of adverse maternal outcomes, which was a composite outcome of maternal mortality, maternal morbidity (eclampsia, hemolysis, elevated liver enzymes, and low platelets [HELLP] syndrome; pulmonary edema; thromboembolic disease; and placental abruption), progression to severe hypertension or proteinuria, and major postpartum hemorrhage (relative risk 0.71, 95% CI 0.59–0.86).[22]

When gestational hypertension is diagnosed in the preterm period, expectant management with frequent monitoring for signs of worsening disease is recommended.[1] Management is similar to preterm preeclampsia without severe features (see later discussion), with at least weekly maternal visits for assessment of symptoms and BP measurement, twice weekly antenatal testing, weekly measurement of amniotic fluid volume, and monitoring of fetal growth.[1] Delivery should be planned at 37 weeks. An induction of labor is preferred, with cesarean delivery for the typical obstetric indications.

PREECLAMPSIA-ECLAMPSIA
Definition and Epidemiology

Preeclampsia is defined as new-onset hypertension after 20 weeks of gestation and proteinuria and/or evidence of end-organ compromise, including CNS symptoms (headache and/or visual changes), pulmonary edema, thrombocytopenia, renal insufficiency, or liver dysfunction.[1] HELLP syndrome is a variant of preeclampsia, with severe features, and is not specifically characterized as a separate entity by the American College of Obstetrics and Gynecologists (ACOG).[1] Preeclampsia complicates 2% to 8% of pregnancies worldwide.[23] Most cases arise in the late preterm and term periods. Preeclampsia diagnosed before 34 weeks' gestation complicates only 0.3% to 0.4% of all pregnancies.[24] There has been a marked increase in hypertensive disorders of pregnancy over the last several years, with a 143% increase in incidence of early-onset disease from 1990 to 2010.[5] Eclampsia is new-onset generalized seizures in a woman with preeclampsia. It remains a rare condition, with an estimated incidence of 5 to 8 per 10,000 and has decreased over time.[25]

The multiple risk factors for preeclampsia include primiparity, age 40 years or greater, chronic hypertension, obesity, renal disease, pregestational diabetes, lupus, thrombophilia, multifetal gestation, in vitro fertilization, history of preeclampsia in prior pregnancy, or family history of preeclampsia.[6] Attention has been devoted to developing tools that predict preeclampsia, including uterine artery Doppler ultrasounds and serum and/or urine biomarkers, or a combination. Current evidence has not shown a benefit of these tools in predicting preeclampsia compared with known risk factors.[1]

Diagnosis

Patients with preeclampsia present with a wide range of symptoms and signs.[6] Most women are asymptomatic at the onset of the disease, so frequent prenatal visits are warranted as pregnancy progresses. A recent US Preventive Task Force (USPTF) statement endorsed the standard practice of screening for preeclampsia with BP measurements throughout pregnancy.[26,27] The task force did not endorse concomitant urinalysis for protein; however, this remains routine in most obstetric practices.

Symptoms are often an indicator of more severe disease and reflect the underlying microvascular insult that leads to diminished perfusion. The CNS symptoms include persistent headache, visual changes, altered mental status, or seizures (ie, eclampsia). Symptoms of liver dysfunction include abdominal pain localized to the right upper quadrant and/or epigastrium and nausea and vomiting. Severe generalized abdominal pain or tetanic contractions with or without vaginal bleeding is likely due to placental abruption.

The diagnosis of preeclampsia requires new-onset hypertension (defined as systolic BP $\geq$140 mm Hg and/or DBP $\geq$90 mm Hg after 20 weeks' gestation) and proteinuria, or CNS symptoms, pulmonary edema, thrombocytopenia, renal insufficiency, or liver dysfunction.[1] That proteinuria is not essential for the diagnosis represents a shift in the diagnostic criteria and highlights the variable natural history of the disease.[1] However, in most cases, the diagnosis of preeclampsia will be based on the presence of hypertension and proteinuria. Depending on the BP and the presence of specific symptoms, signs, and laboratory findings, preeclampsia is classified as with or without severe features (see **Table 1**).[1] Of note, severe proteinuria (>5 g/24 hour urine specimen) is no longer denoted a severe feature of preeclampsia because perinatal outcomes do not correlate with the degree of proteinuria.[1] Fetal growth restriction is also not considered a severe feature.[1]

The diagnosis of HELLP syndrome requires confirmation of hemolysis (on blood smear, an indirect hyperbilirubinemia, low serum haptoglobin, or markedly elevated lactate dehydrogenase) in conjunction with both thrombocytopenia (platelet count <100,000/mm) and elevated liver enzymes (AST [aspartate amniotransferase] or ALT [alanine aminotransferase] greater than twice the upper limit of normal).[28] As indicated previously, HELLP syndrome is thought to be a variant of preeclampsia with severe features and, thus, is managed similarly.

Complications

Preeclampsia can result in a wide spectrum of complications in multiple organ systems owing to associated microangiopathy, vasoconstriction, and malperfusion.[6] One of the most striking complications is, of course, eclampsia, which is a generalized tonic-clonic seizure due to encephalopathy from underperfusion of the brain.[6] Other CNS complications include cortical blindness, hemorrhagic stroke, and posterior reversible encephalopathy syndrome. Visual impairment can also result from retinopathy, retinal detachment, or cortical blindness, which typically resolves following delivery.[29] Liver dysfunction can rarely progress to fulminant hepatic failure. Thrombocytopenia can lead to excessive bleeding, including postpartum hemorrhage, complications with regional anesthesia, and hepatic subcapsular hematomas and rupture. Renal impairment may evolve into severe acute kidney injury, leading to electrolyte abnormalities.

Fetal complications, due to uteroplacental underperfusion, include growth restriction, oligohydramnios, and placental abruption.[6] Placental abruption often triggers disseminated intravascular coagulopathy (DIC), a consumptive process that can cause massive hemorrhage.[6] Unfortunately, these complications can result in the death of the mother, fetus, or both, unless recognized and treated promptly.

Although, by definition, preeclampsia resolves in the postpartum period, women remain at risk for the development of chronic medical conditions later in life.[21] A preeclamptic pregnancy increases the risk of cardiovascular complications, such as hypertension and ischemic heart disease, cerebrovascular disease, diabetes, renal disease, and thromboembolism.[21] The American Heart Association and American Stroke Association have highlighted these strong associations in their recent guidelines that urge providers to fully query pregnancy history in assessing a woman's risk for cardiovascular and cerebrovascular disease.[30]

Management

Antepartum

The only cure for preeclampsia is delivery of the fetus and placenta. Once the diagnosis is established, delivery should be expedited in term ($\geq$37 weeks) gestations in both preeclampsia with and without severe features.[1] Although delivery averts the maternal complications of the disease, preterm gestations are subjected to iatrogenic prematurity and its sequelae. Thus, optimal management of preterm preeclampsia involves careful navigation of the maternal-fetal conflict that plagues the obstetrician. The recommended standard of care has evolved from delivery soon after diagnosis to expectant management in preterm preeclampsia with severe features.[1] Some studies have shown that expectant management of preterm preeclampsia results in improved neonatal outcomes without a significant increased risk of adverse maternal outcomes, even in the setting of severe features meeting specific selection criteria.[31–34] Although there is a small increased risk of stillbirth associated with expectant management, this is balanced by decreased risks of neonatal death, complications of prematurity, and cerebral palsy.[31] Furthermore, there is no significant increase in maternal morbidity associated with expectant management in the absence of specific contraindications.[31] Therefore, the current recommendation in the United States is to delay delivery in patients with early-onset preeclampsia if the maternal and fetal status remains stable (**Table 2**).[35]

In the absence of severe features, expectant management includes frequent monitoring of maternal and fetal status for progression of the disease, with delivery planned for 37 weeks. The choice of inpatient versus outpatient management should be individualized based on the clinical presentation, medical comorbidities, and patient reliability because neither approach has been demonstrated to improve

Table 2 Indications for delivery during expectant management	
Maternal Indications	**Fetal Indications**
Recurrent severe hypertension	Gestational age of 34[0/7] wk
Recurrent symptoms	Growth restriction <5%
Renal insufficiency (defined in **Table 1**)	Persistent oligohydramnios (greatest vertical
Thrombocytopenia or HELLP syndrome	pocket <2 cm)
Pulmonary edema	BPP of 4/10 or less on at least 2 occasions 6 h
Eclampsia	apart
Suspected placental abruption	Reversed end-diastolic flow on umbilical
Labor or rupture of membranes	artery Doppler ultrasound studies
	Recurrent variable or late decelerations
	Fetal death

Abbreviation: BPP, biophysical profile.

Data from American College of Obstetrics and Gynecologists; Task Force on Hypertension in Pregnancy. Hypertension in pregnancy. Report of the American College of Obstetricians and Gynecologists' Task Force on Hypertension in Pregnancy. Obstet Gynecol 2013;122(5):1122–31.

maternal or perinatal morbidity.[36] The ACOG recommends at least weekly maternal evaluations with assessment for symptoms and BP measurement.[1] Laboratory evaluations may also be performed, with complete blood count, creatinine, and transaminases, although the yield seems to be low.[37] Serial monitoring of the degree of proteinuria is not recommended after the diagnosis is established because worsening proteinuria is expected, it does not seem to affect outcomes, and does not alter management.[38] There is a paucity of data to guide other management. Twice weekly or weekly antenatal testing and amniotic fluid volume and fetal growth assessed every 3 to 4 weeks with ultrasound and fetal movement counts daily by the patient are recommended.[6]

If there are severe features in the late preterm period ($34^{0/7}$ to $36^{6/7}$ weeks' gestation), delivery should occur after maternal stabilization.[6] Administration of antenatal corticosteroids is now recommended up to $36^{6/7}$ weeks' gestation but delivery should not be delayed to complete the course.[39,40]

Before $34^{0/7}$ weeks' gestation, severe preeclampsia may be expectantly managed if strict criteria are met.[1] Immediate contraindications to expectant management include eclampsia, pulmonary edema, DIC, uncontrolled severe hypertension, nonviable fetus, abnormal fetal testing, placenta abruption, or fetal demise. Delivery should occur once maternal status is stable. Additional contraindications to expectant management include persistent symptoms, HELLP or partial HELLP syndrome, severe fetal growth restriction, severe oligohydramnios, reversed enddiastolic flow on umbilical artery Doppler ultrasounds, progressive labor, rupture of membranes, or significant renal impairment. Delivery should be initiated 48 hours after the first corticosteroid dose.[1] If the patient does not have the listed contraindications, expectant management may be continued with the patient as an inpatient at an appropriate facility, with daily assessment of maternal and fetal status and antihypertensive treatment. Delivery should be undertaken for the following indications: after $34^{0/7}$ weeks is achieved, if contraindications to expectant management develop, if there is abnormal maternal or fetal testing; or if labor or rupture of membranes occurs.[1]

Intrapartum

Induction of labor is preferred and cesarean delivery is reserved for the usual obstetric indications. Although it is common practice to deliver preterm patients with unfavorable cervices via cesarean, recent studies have shown that the success rate for inductions is greater than 60% in patients less than 34 weeks.[41]

Parenteral magnesium sulfate is the treatment of choice for prophylaxis against eclampsia in preeclampsia with severe features.[6] The Magpie [MAGnesium sulphate for Prevention of Eclampsia] randomized trial of magnesium versus placebo in 10,000 women with preeclampsia demonstrated the efficacy of magnesium sulfate in the prevention of eclampsia.[42] An additional benefit of magnesium sulfate is its neuroprotective effects in the preterm (<32 weeks') fetus, with a decreased risk of cerebral palsy.[43,44]

Although magnesium sulfate is routinely administered to patients with preeclampsia without severe features, the evidence supporting this practice is limited. Randomized trials examining magnesium sulfate in patients without severe features were underpowered, precluding a firm conclusion regarding its efficacy.[45,46] A decision analysis concluded that the decision to treat women with preeclampsia with magnesium sulfate or not was equivocal in terms of maternal and neonatal outcomes.[47] Therefore, the ACOG does not currently recommend routine intrapartum administration of magnesium sulfate to women with preeclampsia without severe features.[1] However, scrupulous surveillance for progression of the disease is warranted throughout labor so that therapy may be initiated expeditiously.

Magnesium sulfate is typically administered as a 4 to 6 g loading dose over 15 to 30 minutes followed by 2 g per hour maintenance dose.[6] The infusion should be continued until 24 hours following delivery. The therapeutic range of magnesium is 4 to 6 mEq/L.[6] Above this level, magnesium toxicity may be apparent. The first sign is diminished deep tendon reflexes (10 mEq/L), followed by respiratory paralysis (10 mEq/L), and cardiac arrest (>25 mEq/L).[6] Magnesium toxicity is treated with discontinuation of the infusion and administration of intravenous calcium gluconate (10 mL of a 10% solution). Although magnesium toxicity can be life-threatening, in a patient with normal renal function and adequate urine output, routine serum monitoring of magnesium levels is not warranted.[6] Most hospitals have a protocol of careful measurement of urine output and assessment of deep tendon reflexes to detect the early stages of magnesium toxicity. In patients with renal insufficiency (serum creatinine >1.0 mg/dL) and/or diminished urine output, the serum magnesium level should be monitored for the duration of the therapy and the magnesium sulfate dose can be empirically decreased. A bolus and no maintenance therapy, or a decreased maintenance dose of 1 g per hour, are options for patients with significant impairment in renal clearance.[6]

The first-line treatment of eclampsia is magnesium, which is superior to other anticonvulsants, such as phenytoin or benzodiazepines.[48] Magnesium should be continued for at least 24 hours after the last seizure activity.[1] If a woman develops eclampsia while receiving a magnesium infusion, another anticonvulsant, such as a benzodiazepine or a barbiturate, can be used to break the seizure.[6] If anticonvulsant therapy proves ineffective, general anesthesia may be necessary.[6] Care should be taken prevent trauma, protect the airway, and maintain oxygenation during the seizure. Prompt delivery is necessary following maternal stabilization.[1]

Intrapartum antihypertensives are indicated for BPs persistently greater than 160 mm Hg systolic and/or greater than 105 to 110 mm Hg diastolic.[6] There are limited data to guide choice of any medication compared with another. Parenteral labetalol, a mixed alpha-adrenergic and beta-adrenergic antagonist,[1] is contraindicated in the setting of asthma, congestive heart failure, or other significant cardiac disease. The initial dose should be 10 to 20 mg, followed by 20 to 80 mg every 20 to 30 minutes to a maximum dose of 300 mg in 24 hours.[6] Hydralazine, a direct vasodilator, may be administered intravenously or intramuscularly. The starting dose is 5 mg, followed by 5 to 10 mg every 20 to 40 minutes.[6] Adverse effects include tachycardia, headache, and maternal hypotension leading to abnormal fetal heart rate tracings. Finally, nifedipine, a calcium channel blocker, may be used. The starting dose is 10 to 20 mg orally, with repeat doses in 30 minutes then every 2 to 6 hours as needed.[6] Adverse effects include tachycardia and headache. The theoretic risk of potentiating the cardiorespiratory and other effects of magnesium sulfate remains to be proven; women receiving both nifedipine and magnesium should be monitored.[6]

Postpartum

Because approximately a third of eclamptic seizures occur postpartum, seizure prophylaxis with magnesium sulfate or alternate anticonvulsant should be continued for at least 24 hours after delivery.[6] Persistent hypertension (>150 mm Hg systolic and/or >100 mm Hg diastolic) should be treated with oral antihypertensives.[6] Often, the therapy can be tapered or discontinued after the first few weeks after BPs normalize. The ACOG suggests that women with gestational hypertension or preeclampsia receive BP monitoring up to 72 hours postpartum and again 7 to 10 days after delivery, or sooner with symptoms.[1] Because preeclampsia and eclampsia can occur up to 4 weeks postpartum, all women should be educated on warning signs and evaluated promptly for potential hypertensive complications.

Prevention

Intense interest in identifying strategies to prevent preeclampsia in women at increased risk for the condition has yielded limited positive results. Trials of antioxidant treatment with vitamins C and E failed to show any benefit.[9,49] In a large US study, calcium supplementation was not effective[50] but did reduce the incidence of preeclampsia in settings with low calcium intake.[51] In a large meta-analysis, conflicting data regarding the potential benefit of aspirin in the prevention of preeclampsia[52–54] revealed a small but significant (17%) reduction in preeclampsia in women treated with aspirin.[55] In these studies, lower doses (60–81 mg) of aspirin were used. One randomized trial of more than 1700 women at high risk of preeclampsia, in which 150 mg of aspirin was compared with placebo,[56] showed aspirin was associated with a 62% reduction in the risk of preterm preeclampsia. Higher doses of aspirin may be more effective in the prevention of preeclampsia in high-risk patients. The USPTF recommends low-dose aspirin therapy for prevention of preeclampsia if the patient has 1 high-risk factor or 2 or more moderate-risk factors (**Table 3**).[57]

PREECLAMPSIA SUPERIMPOSED ON CHRONIC HYPERTENSION
Definition and Epidemiology

Superimposed preeclampsia is the development of preeclampsia in women with preexisting chronic hypertension and is the hypertensive disorder associated with the highest risk of adverse outcomes. This condition develops in as many as 40% of women with chronic hypertension.[7,8]

Table 3
US Preventive Services Task Force risk factors for preeclampsia

High-Risk Factors	Moderate-Risk Factors
History of preeclampsia, especially associated with adverse outcome	Nulliparity
Multifetal gestation	Obesity
Chronic hypertension	Family history of preeclampsia (mother or sister)
Pregestational diabetes	Demographic characteristics (African American or low socioeconomic status)
Renal disease	Age ≥35 y
Autoimmune disease	Personal history factors (ie, low birthweight infant, previous adverse pregnancy outcome, >10 y pregnancy interval)

Recommend low-dose aspirin started after 12 weeks for patient with 1 high-risk factor or greater than 2 moderate risk factors.

Adapted from LeFevre ML, U.S. Preventive Services Task Force. Low-dose aspirin use for the prevention of morbidity and mortality from preeclampsia: U.S. Preventive Services Task Force recommendation statement. Ann Intern Med 2014;161(11):821; with permission.

Diagnosis

Distinguishing superimposed preeclampsia from the physiologic increase in BP that occurs in the third trimester is a diagnostic challenge. The ACOG recommends erring on the side of overdiagnosis of superimposed preeclampsia, given the high possibility of adverse perinatal outcomes if the condition is misclassified.[1] Superimposed preeclampsia is suspected when

1. BP suddenly increases in a patient with well-controlled BP, either on or off antihypertensives
2. There is new-onset proteinuria or sudden worsening of proteinuria in a patient with baseline proteinuria.

Superimposed preeclampsia with severe features is diagnosed the same way as preeclampsia with severe features (see **Table 1**).[1]

Complications

The same range of complications is associated with superimposed preeclampsia and preeclampsia. However, the risks are higher in superimposed preeclampsia. For example, the perinatal mortality rate is higher in patients with superimposed preeclampsia compared with women with preeclampsia in women without chronic hypertension.[10]

Management

The management principles of superimposed preeclampsia are similar to those of preeclampsia (see previous discussion). For preterm superimposed preeclampsia, the disease should be characterized as with or without severe features. Patients with preterm superimposed preeclampsia without severe features are candidates for expectant management.[1] They should be monitored frequently for development of severe features and delivered at 37 weeks' gestation if the maternal-fetal status remains stable. Antenatal corticosteroids should be administered up to $36^{6/7}$ weeks.[39,40] Patents with preterm superimposed preeclampsia with severe features should be managed similarly to preterm preeclampsia with severe features, with careful consideration of expectant management in appropriate patients and delivery by $34^{0/7}$ weeks' gestation.[1] BP goals for superimposed preeclampsia are similar to those of preeclampsia, with antihypertensive treatment indicated for SBP greater than or equal to 160 mm Hg or DBP greater than or equal to 105 mm Hg.[1]

SUMMARY

Although there have been great advancements in the diagnosis and management of the hypertensive disorders of pregnancy, these conditions account for a substantial proportion of maternal and perinatal morbidity and mortality in the United States and worldwide. Updates to management guidelines have focused on improved diagnosis of preeclampsia, expectant management of select candidates with preterm preeclampsia, and prevention of preeclampsia in high-risk women. However, further research is needed to combat the rising incidence of hypertension in pregnancy and to further refine management strategies that improve maternal and neonatal health.

REFERENCES

1. American College of Obstetrics and Gynecologists Task Force on Hypertension in Pregnancy. Hypertension in pregnancy. Report of the American College of

Obstetricians and Gynecologists' Task Force on Hypertension in Pregnancy. Obstet Gynecol 2013;122(5):1122–31.

2. Creanga AA, Berg CJ, Syverson C, et al. Pregnancy-related mortality in the United States, 2006-2010. Obstet Gynecol 2015;125(1):5–12.

3. Ananth CV, Keyes KM, Wapner RJ. Pre-eclampsia rates in the United States, 1980-2010: age-period-cohort analysis. BMJ 2013;347:f6564.

4. Wallis AB, Saftlas AF, Hsia J, et al. Secular trends in the rates of preeclampsia, eclampsia, and gestational hypertension, United States, 1987-2004. Am J Hypertens 2008;21(5):521–6.

5. Shih T, Peneva D, Xu X, et al. The rising burden of preeclampsia in the United States impacts both maternal and child health. Am J Perinatol 2016;33(4): 329–38.

6. Markham K, Funai EF. Pregnancy-related hypertension. In: Creasy RK, Resnik R, Iams JD, et al, editors. Creasy and Resnik's maternal-fetal medicine. 7th edition. Philadephia: Elsevier; 2015. p. 756–81.

7. Sibai BM, Lindheimer M, Hauth J, et al. Risk factors for preeclampsia, abruptio placentae, and adverse neonatal outcomes among women with chronic hypertension. National Institute of Child Health and Human Development Network of Maternal-Fetal Medicine Units. N Engl J Med 1998;339(10): 667–71.

8. Ferrer RL, Sibai BM, Mulrow CD, et al. Management of mild chronic hypertension during pregnancy: a review. Obstet Gynecol 2000;96(5 Pt 2):849–60.

9. Rumbold A, Duley L, Crowther CA, et al. Antioxidants for preventing preeclampsia. Cochrane Database Syst Rev 2008;(1):CD004227.

10. Lin CC, Lindheimer MD, River P, et al. Fetal outcome in hypertensive disorders of pregnancy. Am J Obstet Gynecol 1982;142(3):255–60.

11. Kuper SG, Tita AT, Youngstrom ML, et al. Baseline renal function tests and adverse outcomes in pregnant patients with chronic hypertension. Obstet Gynecol 2016;128(1):93–103.

12. Magee LA, von Dadelszen P, Rey E, et al. Less-tight versus tight control of hypertension in pregnancy. N Engl J Med 2015;372(5):407–17.

13. SMFM Publications Committee. SMFM statement: benefit of antihypertensive therapy for mild-to-moderate chronic hypertension during pregnancy remains uncertain. Am J Obstet Gynecol 2015;213(1):3–4.

14. Abalos E, Duley L, Steyn DW. Antihypertensive drug therapy for mild to moderate hypertension during pregnancy. Cochrane Database Syst Rev 2014;(2):CD002252.

15. Churchill D, Beevers GD, Meher S, et al. Diuretics for preventing pre-eclampsia. Cochrane Database Syst Rev 2007;(1):CD004451.

16. Bateman BT, Bansil P, Hernandez-Diaz S, et al. Prevalence, trends, and outcomes of chronic hypertension: a nationwide sample of delivery admissions. Am J Obstet Gynecol 2012;206(2):134.e1-8.

17. Reddy UM, Laughon SK, Sun L, et al. Prepregnancy risk factors for antepartum stillbirth in the United States. Obstet Gynecol 2010;116(5):1119–26.

18. Hutcheon JA, Lisonkova S, Joseph KS. Epidemiology of pre-eclampsia and the other hypertensive disorders of pregnancy. Best Pract Res Clin Obstet Gynaecol 2011;25(4):391–403.

19. Report of the National High Blood Pressure Education Program Working Group on High Blood Pressure in pregnancy. Am J Obstet Gynecol 2000;183(1): S1–22.

20. Buchbinder A, Sibai BM, Caritis S, et al. Adverse perinatal outcomes are significantly higher in severe gestational hypertension than in mild preeclampsia. Am J Obstet Gynecol 2002;186(1):66–71.

21. Williams D. Long-term complications of preeclampsia. Semin Nephrol 2011; 31(1):111–22.

22. Koopmans CM, Bijlenga D, Groen H, et al. Induction of labour versus expectant monitoring for gestational hypertension or mild pre-eclampsia after 36 weeks' gestation (HYPITAT): a multicentre, open-label randomised controlled trial. Lancet 2009;374(9694):979–88.

23. Duley L. The global impact of pre-eclampsia and eclampsia. Semin Perinatol 2009;33(3):130–7.

24. Lisonkova S, Joseph KS. Incidence of preeclampsia: risk factors and outcomes associated with early- versus late-onset disease. Am J Obstet Gynecol 2013; 209(6):544.e1-12.

25. Fong A, Chau CT, Pan D, et al. Clinical morbidities, trends, and demographics of eclampsia: a population-based study. Am J Obstet Gynecol 2013;209(3): 229.e1-7.

26. US Preventive Services Task Force, Bibbins-Domingo K, Grossman DC, et al. Screening for preeclampsia: US Preventive Services Task Force Recommendation Statement. JAMA 2017;317(16):1661–7.

27. Henderson JT, Thompson JH, Burda BU, et al. Preeclampsia screening: evidence report and systematic review for the US Preventive Services Task Force. JAMA 2017;317(16):1668–83.

28. Sibai BM. Diagnosis, controversies, and management of the syndrome of hemolysis, elevated liver enzymes, and low platelet count. Obstet Gynecol 2004;103(5 Pt 1):981–91.

29. Abu Samra K. The eye and visual system in the preeclampsia/eclampsia syndrome: what to expect? Saudi J Ophthalmol 2013;27(1):51–3.

30. Bushnell C, McCullough LD, Awad IA, et al. Guidelines for the prevention of stroke in women: a statement for healthcare professionals from the American Heart Association/American Stroke Association. Stroke 2014;45(5):1545–88.

31. Churchill D, Duley L, Thornton JG, et al. Interventionist versus expectant care for severe pre-eclampsia between 24 and 34 weeks' gestation. Cochrane Database Syst Rev 2013;(7):CD003106.

32. Odendaal HJ, Pattinson RC, Bam R, et al. Aggressive or expectant management for patients with severe preeclampsia between 28-34 weeks' gestation: a randomized controlled trial. Obstet Gynecol 1990;76(6):1070–5.

33. Sibai BM, Mercer BM, Schiff E, et al. Aggressive versus expectant management of severe preeclampsia at 28 to 32 weeks' gestation: a randomized controlled trial. Am J Obstet Gynecol 1994;171(3):818–22.

34. GRIT Study Group. A randomised trial of timed delivery for the compromised preterm fetus: short term outcomes and Bayesian interpretation. BJOG 2003;110(1): 27–32.

35. Publications Committee, Society for Maternal-Fetal Medicine, Sibai BM. Evaluation and management of severe preeclampsia before 34 weeks' gestation. Am J Obstet Gynecol 2011;205(3):191–8.

36. Schoen CN, Moreno SC, Saccone G, et al. Outpatient versus inpatient management for superimposed preeclampsia without severe features: a retrospective, multicenter study. J Matern Fetal Neonatal Med 2017;1–7.

37. Cantu J, Clifton RG, Roberts JM, et al. Laboratory abnormalities in pregnancy-associated hypertension: frequency and association with pregnancy outcomes. Obstet Gynecol 2014;124(5):933–40.

38. Schiff E, Friedman SA, Kao L, et al. The importance of urinary protein excretion during conservative management of severe preeclampsia. Am J Obstet Gynecol 1996;175(5):1313–6.

39. Gyamfi-Bannerman C, Thom EA, Blackwell SC, et al. Antenatal Betamethasone for women at risk for late preterm delivery. N Engl J Med 2016;374(14):1311–20.

40. Society for Maternal-Fetal Medicine (SMFM) Publications Committee. Implementation of the use of antenatal corticosteroids in the late preterm birth period in women at risk for preterm delivery. Am J Obstet Gynecol 2016;215(2):B13–5.

41. Sievert RA, Kuper SG, Jauk VC, et al. Predictors of vaginal delivery in medically indicated early preterm induction of labor. Am J Obstet Gynecol 2017;217(3):375.e1-7.

42. Altman D, Carroli G, Duley L, et al. Do women with pre-eclampsia, and their babies, benefit from magnesium sulphate? The Magpie trial: a randomised placebo-controlled trial. Lancet 2002;359(9321):1877–90.

43. Rouse DJ, Hirtz DG, Thom E, et al. A randomized, controlled trial of magnesium sulfate for the prevention of cerebral palsy. N Engl J Med 2008;359(9):895–905.

44. Nguyen TM, Crowther CA, Wilkinson D, et al. Magnesium sulphate for women at term for neuroprotection of the fetus. Cochrane Database Syst Rev 2013;(2):CD009395.

45. Livingston JC, Livingston LW, Ramsey R, et al. Magnesium sulfate in women with mild preeclampsia: a randomized controlled trial. Obstet Gynecol 2003;101(2):217–20.

46. Witlin AG, Friedman SA, Sibai BM. The effect of magnesium sulfate therapy on the duration of labor in women with mild preeclampsia at term: a randomized, double-blind, placebo-controlled trial. Am J Obstet Gynecol 1997;176(3):623–7.

47. Cahill AG, Macones GA, Odibo AO, et al. Magnesium for seizure prophylaxis in patients with mild preeclampsia. Obstet Gynecol 2007;110(3):601–7.

48. Which anticonvulsant for women with eclampsia? Evidence from the Collaborative Eclampsia Trial. Lancet 1995;345(8963):1455–63.

49. Roberts JM, Myatt L, Spong CY, et al. Vitamins C and E to prevent complications of pregnancy-associated hypertension. N Engl J Med 2010;362(14):1282–91.

50. Levine RJ, Hauth JC, Curet LB, et al. Trial of calcium to prevent preeclampsia. N Engl J Med 1997;337(2):69–76.

51. Hofmeyr GJ, Lawrie TA, Atallah AN, et al. Calcium supplementation during pregnancy for preventing hypertensive disorders and related problems. Cochrane Database Syst Rev 2014;(6):CD001059.

52. Wallenburg HC, Dekker GA, Makovitz JW, et al. Low-dose aspirin prevents pregnancy-induced hypertension and pre-eclampsia in angiotensin-sensitive primigravidae. Lancet 1986;1(8471):1–3.

53. Schiff E, Peleg E, Goldenberg M, et al. The use of aspirin to prevent pregnancy-induced hypertension and lower the ratio of thromboxane A2 to prostacyclin in relatively high risk pregnancies. N Engl J Med 1989;321(6):351–6.

54. Caritis S, Sibai B, Hauth J, et al. Low-dose aspirin to prevent preeclampsia in women at high risk. National Institute of Child Health and Human Development Network of Maternal-Fetal Medicine Units. N Engl J Med 1998;338(11):701–5.

55. Duley L, Henderson-Smart DJ, Meher S, et al. Antiplatelet agents for preventing pre-eclampsia and its complications. Cochrane Database Syst Rev 2007;(2):CD004659.

56. Rolnik DL, Wright D, Poon LC, et al. Aspirin versus placebo in pregnancies at high risk for preterm preeclampsia. N Engl J Med 2017;377(7):613–22.
57. LeFevre ML, U.S. Preventive Services Task Force. Low-dose aspirin use for the prevention of morbidity and mortality from preeclampsia: U.S. Preventive Services Task Force recommendation statement. Ann Intern Med 2014;161(11): 819–26.

Seizures in Pregnancy

Kassie J. Bollig, MD[a], Daniel L. Jackson, MD, MS[b],*

KEYWORDS

- Seizure • Eclampsia • Epilepsy • Pregnancy • Antiepileptic drug

KEY POINTS

- Seizures during pregnancy pose significant maternal and fetal risks.
- The initial evaluation of seizures involves detailed clinical and physical examination histories, seizure classification, laboratory studies, and imaging interpretation.
- The management of epilepsy among women of reproductive age is complex and involves unique considerations during the preconception, antepartum, intrapartum, and postpartum periods.
- The management of the acute seizure during pregnancy should follow a predetermined algorithm with the presumptive diagnosis of eclampsia until proven otherwise.

INTRODUCTION: BACKGROUND AND EPIDEMIOLOGY

Seizures are the most common major neurologic complication encountered in pregnancy with a prevalence of in the United States of 1.2%.[1] Nearly one-half million women with epilepsy are of reproductive age and between 0.5% and 1.0% of all pregnancies occur among women with epilepsy.[2,3]

The etiology of seizures covers a wide range of diseases, vascular insults, infectious sequelae, malignant processes, metabolic derangements, toxic insults, primary central nervous system dysfunction, and more.[4,5] In pregnancy, eclampsia represents a unique consideration among possible causes of seizure. Although epileptic seizures are the most common, it is crucial to accurately determine the underlying cause of seizures in pregnancy to provide appropriate therapy.[4]

Epilepsy

Women with epilepsy who become pregnant are at a substantially increased risk of adverse outcomes, including preeclampsia, preterm labor, stillbirth, cesarean delivery, and a more than 10-fold increased risk of death.[6] The majority of maternal deaths

Disclosure Statement: None.
a Department of Obstetrics, Gynecology and Women's Health, University of Missouri, 500 North Keene Street, Suite 400, Columbia, MO 65201, USA; b Department of Obstetrics, Gynecology and Women's Health, University of Missouri School of Medicine, 500 North Keene Street, Suite 406, Columbia, MO 65201, USA
* Corresponding author.
E-mail address: jacksondl@health.missouri.edu

Obstet Gynecol Clin N Am 45 (2018) 349–367
https://doi.org/10.1016/j.ogc.2018.02.001
0889-8545/18/© 2018 Elsevier Inc. All rights reserved.

obgyn.theclinics.com

are related to poor seizure control. As such, achieving control of maternal epilepsy is the primary concern in the management of pregnant women with an underlying seizure disorder.[3] This goal is complicated by the risk of potential congenital malformations owing to the use of antiepileptic therapy.[7–11]

DEFINITION AND CLASSIFICATION
Definition

Conceptually, an epileptic seizure is defined as "a transient occurrence of signs and/or symptoms owing to abnormal excessive or synchronous neuronal activity in the brain."[12] The clinical application of this definition is difficult, because it is often not possible to prove the presence of "abnormal excessive or synchronous neuronal activity." In addition, some seizures that are confirmed electrographically do not demonstrate detectable signs or symptoms.[13] To combat this issue, 3 separate operational definitions of epilepsy have been developed by the International League Against Epilepsy that can be more reasonably applied to the clinical setting:

1. At least 2 unprovoked seizures occurring greater than 24 hours apart,
2. One unprovoked seizure and the probability of further seizures similar to the general recurrence risk ($\geq$60%) after 2 unprovoked seizures, occurring over the next 10 years, and
3. Diagnosis of an epilepsy syndrome.[13,14]

Awareness of and recognition by providers that epilepsy represents a diverse array of brain diseases sharing the common presentation of seizure is critical. It is important for those providing pregnancy care to work closely with a neurologist to improve understanding of an individual's disease. This responsibility not only bears weighty implications for treatment, but also gives insight into predicting the character of the seizure disorder throughout pregnancy.[15,16] The resolution of epilepsy may be determined by a neurologist in the setting of women who have remained seizure free for the last 10 years, with the last 5 years off antiseizure medication, or individuals who were diagnosed with a childhood epilepsy syndrome who are now in adulthood.[14]

Classification System

The classification of epilepsy type greatly influences clinical management. In 2017, the International League Against Epilepsy developed a new classification system allowing for diagnosis at 3 levels according to the range of resources that may be available (Fig. 1).[17] In areas of resource-poor settings, diagnosis may be limited to level 1, whereas in settings of high diagnostic capabilities, a seizure can be considered among all levels of diagnosis.[17] Important changes include:

1. Extinction of the terms partial and complex, and instead only describing the presence of awareness;
2. The addition of a motor and nonmotor classification of focal seizures; and
3. The addition of a combined focal and generalized seizure category, and an unknown seizure type category.

Owing to the significant treatment implications, the International League Against Epilepsy also added 6 etiology subgroups to be considered among all levels of diagnosis. These subgroups are genetic, structural, metabolic, immune, infectious, and unknown.[17]

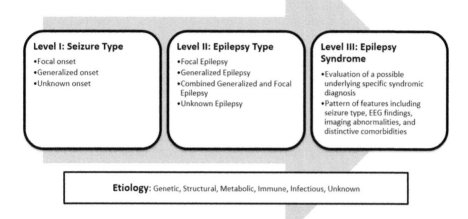

Fig. 1. The 2017 International League Against Epilepsy seizure classification system. EEG, electroencephalograph. (*Data from* Scheffer IE, Berkovic S, Capovilla G, et al. ILAE classification of the epilepsies: position paper of the ILAE commission for classification and terminology. Epilepsia 2017;58(4):512–21.)

INITIAL EVALUATION

The path toward diagnosis of a first seizure in a pregnant patient begins with a thorough history and physical examination. Although not always feasible, a detailed description of the event is helpful in both classifying the event as a seizure and to rule out differential diagnoses. This description includes possible triggers, behaviors, and postictal symptoms, if present. Attempts should also be made to uncover past episodes and underlying risk factors such as medications, poisonings, medical comorbidities, or genetic predispositions.[4,13] In patients suffering from a true epileptic event, the physical examination is typically normal, but it can be a critical component when there is concern for central nervous system bleeding, infarction, or infection. A thorough neurologic examination is important to evaluate upper or lower motor neuron signs and lateralizing lesions.[13]

Adjuvant laboratory tests and imaging are obligatory elements of the evaluation of a seizure to examine triggering factors and guide next steps in management.[18] Although not routinely recommended, the American Academy of Neurology (AAN) and the American Epilepsy Society state that blood counts, blood glucose, electrolyte panels, urinary analysis for protein, lumbar puncture, and toxicology studies may be helpful based on the clinical circumstances.[18] These 2 groups do advise routine electroencephalographic (EEG) and brain imaging with computed tomography (CT) scans or MRI as a part of the initial evaluation.[18] EEG is important for diagnosing the subtype of seizure, influencing therapy choice, and to predict seizure recurrence.[13,18] Between 8% and 50% of patients presenting with a first seizure will have a positive EEG demonstrating epileptiform abnormalities.[18] However, nearly 50% of patients who are clinically diagnosed with a seizure may have a normal EEG.[18] As such, a normal EEG does not rule out the diagnosis of epileptic seizures. EEGs performed in the first 24 hours after a seizure or serial EEGs may prove to better aid in diagnosis and be more likely to demonstrate epileptiform abnormalities.[13] with regard to imaging, CT scanning is more commonly used in the acute workup of seizure owing to its quick availability compared with MRI.[4] Importantly, MRI is more sensitive for minor abnormalities common in focal and recurrent, unprovoked seizures.[13,18] Both CT scanning and MRI may diagnose an underlying brain tumor, stroke, infection, or other structural lesion.[4,18] Regarding the safety of CT scans in pregnancy, women should be made aware that the American College of Radiology states that the developing preembryo, embryo, or fetus is not at risk after receiving radiation exposure from a single diagnostic radiographic procedure.[19] During standard CT scanning of the head, the fetus is exposed to less than 1 rad of ionizing radiation.[19] An increase in fetal anomalies or pregnancy loss is not demonstrated in radiologic exposures of less than 5 rad.[20]

Throughout the initial evaluation, a broad differential diagnosis is appropriate **(Fig. 2)**.[4,21,22] Neurovascular causes, cardiac causes, and metabolic conditions are

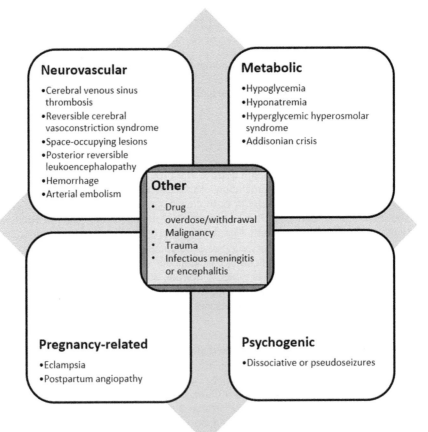

Fig. 2. Differential diagnosis of acute seizure. BP, blood pressure; CI, contraindication; DBP, diastolic blood pressure; EEG, electroencephalograph; HR, heart rate; ICU, intensive care unit; IM, intramuscular; IV, intravenous; OB, obstetrics; Pulse ox, pulse oxygenation; SBP, systolic blood pressure. (*Data from* Refs.[4,21,22])

all important considerations for first presentation of seizures in pregnancy.[4,21,22] Perhaps one of the most difficult diagnoses is that of psychogenic nonepileptic seizures, also called dissociative seizures or pseudoseizures, which are characterized by drug-resistant attacks.[13,22]

In addition to these differential diagnoses, the evaluation of seizure in pregnancy should begin with a consideration for eclampsia. Preeclampsia is defined as hypertension caused by pregnancy with the addition of end-organ involvement (proteinuria, thrombocytopenia, abnormal liver enzymes, elevated creatinine, or neurologic symptoms).[20] Eclampsia is defined as tonic–clonic seizures in the setting of preeclampsia.[20] Preeclampsia is generally seen in the later one-half of gestation and is more common with underlying chronic hypertension, diabetes, autoimmune disease (lupus), multiple gestation, and extremes of maternal age. Preeclampsia and eclampsia can occasionally be seen in early pregnancy in the setting of higher order multiple gestation, molar pregnancy, and severe maternal renal disease.[23,24] Unique to the initial evaluation of seizure in pregnancy is the consideration of fetal well-being. The management of women in whom preeclampsia and epilepsy are both potential etiologies of seizures of unknown etiology is discussed elsewhere in this article.

PRECONCEPTION COUNSELING AND MANAGEMENT

Preconception counseling is of utmost importance for all women of childbearing age who have epilepsy. Because many pregnancies are unplanned and changes initiated before conception and early in pregnancy can decrease adverse outcomes, the best time to begin preconception counseling is at disease diagnosis and the initiation of the first antiepileptic drug (AED).[15] Epilepsy is not a contraindication to pregnancy. Although the risk of fetal malformations is about double the risk of that in a nonepileptic woman, the absolute risk is still low, with a greater than 90% chance that she will have an uneventful pregnancy and a normal child.[15,25] If known risk factors exist for epilepsy inheritance, or if there is significant anxiety surrounding the possible inheritance of seizures, genetic counseling should be provided.[26] Components of preconception counseling include a discussion of contraception, maternal and fetal risks in pregnancy, selection and management of AEDs, and folate supplementation.

Contraception

Owing to induction of the hepatic cytochrome P-450 system, contraceptive failures in women taking oral contraceptives are increased if they are concomitantly taking AEDs.[27] Many of the most common AEDs fall into this category, including phenytoin, phenobarbital, carbamazepine, primidone, topiramate, oxcarbazepine, and to a lesser extent lamotrigine. As a result, the World Health Organization recommends that women choose long-acting reversible contraceptives such as the copper or levonorgestrel intrauterine devices and etonogestrel implants owing to their higher efficacy and lower drug interactions with AEDs.[27]

Maternal and Fetal Risks

Data regarding the effect of epilepsy during pregnancy on the mother and fetus are limited. A 2009 review by the AAN was not able to determine if an increased incidence of preeclampsia or gestational hypertension was present in women with epilepsy,[28] and they also concluded that preterm labor was only found to be increased in women who also smoked.[28] Many reports contained low case numbers, lack of adequate control groups, diversity among study methods, and absence of the influences of contributing social factors such as smoking and alcohol consumption.[15] In recent years, however, larger population-based cohort studies and metaanalyses have shed light on relationships between maternal and fetal health and epilepsy (**Table 1**).[6,9–11,29–36]

Maternal complications

A population-based cohort study of 69,000 pregnant women with epilepsy were examined from 2007 to 2011[6] and a metaanalysis examining studies from January 1990 to January 2015 have provided risk estimates regarding maternal and fetal outcomes.[29] Among pregnant women with epilepsy compared with the general population, there is an increased risk of complications such as cesarean delivery (odds ratio [OR], 2.5), gestational hypertension (OR, 1.3), preeclampsia (OR, 1.6), antepartum hemorrhage (OR, 1.4), postpartum hemorrhage (OR, 1.8), preterm labor (OR, 1.5), and, most strikingly, maternal death with an overall adjusted OR of 11.5.[6] Results from the metaanalysis yielded additional findings of increased maternal risks of spontaneous miscarriage (OR, 1.5), preterm birth (OR, 1.16), and induction of labor (OR, 1.6).[29] Many of these risks were also cited in studies in Norway, Iceland, Canada, and Sweden, including the risks of preterm labor,[30] preeclampsia,[30–32] postpartum hemorrhage,[32,33] induction of labor,[31,34] and cesarean delivery.[30,32,35]

The increased risk of maternal mortality deserves requires further study.[3,6,15] Possible explanations include a higher percentage of contributing comorbidities, the overall increase of pregnancy-related life-threatening complications, an increase in seizure-related complications such as sudden unexpected death in epilepsy and status epilepticus, and a greater rate of depression and anxiety in these women.[37,38] The risk of mortality in pregnant women with epilepsy may be as high as 1 in 1000, a nearly 10-fold increase compared with women without epilepsy. The majority of these deaths are due to sudden unexpected death in epilepsy, which in turn is related to poor seizure control, highlighting the importance of continuing clinically indicated antiepileptic treatment throughout pregnancy and delivery.[3] The risk of developing status epilepticus is reported as 0% to 1.8%.[28]

Fetal complications

It is difficult to separate whether maternal epilepsy itself, or the effects of AED therapy, is to blame for many of the fetal and neonatal risks associated with these pregnancies. Studies still lack consistency regarding increased risk of perinatal death or stillbirth.[10,28,29] Women with epilepsy are more likely to have an infant who is small for gestational age[6,28] and with 1-minute Apgar scores of less than 7.[28] In addition, the

---

Table 1
Maternal and fetal complications in pregnancies affected by epilepsy

Maternal Complications	Fetal Complications
• Spontaneous miscarriage	• Small for gestational age
• Preterm labor	• 1-minute Apgar <7
• Preterm birth	• Perinatal death or stillbirth
• Antepartum hemorrhage	• Congenital malformations owing to AED use
• Gestational hypertension	• Adverse behavioral developmental and cognitive outcomes
• Preeclampsia	owing to AED use
• Induction of labor	
• Cesarean delivery	
• Postpartum hemorrhage	
• Maternal death	

Abbreviation: AED, antiepileptic drug.
Data from Refs.[6,9–11,29–36]

risk of spontaneous abortion in women taking AEDs is slightly increased compared with those not using medication.[39]

Current research suggests that fetal complications in epilepsy are related to the teratogenicity of AED rather than epilepsy itself.[7] The overall risk of fetal congenital malformations in women on anticonvulsant therapy ranges from 4% to 9% and depends greatly on the exact AED prescribed.[7] The overall risk for major congenital malformations is approximately 2.2% for carbamazepine, 3.2% for lamotrigine, 3.7% for phenytoin, and 6.2% for valproate.[8] Of all the AEDs, valproate has been shown to most consistently demonstrate a higher risk of congenital malformations as well as being associated with adverse behavioral developmental and cognitive outcomes.[15,36] In addition, polytherapy increased the overall risk of major congenital anomaly from 3.5% to 4.0% to 6% to 8% in 2 separate studies.[7,8] Common congenital malformations associated with specific AEDs are shown in **Table 2**.[4,15,25] Currently, the most commonly prescribed AEDs for women of reproductive age are lamotrigine and levetiracetam.[40] Women with epilepsy who have had a previous child with a congenital malformation have an increased risk of 16.8 per 100 births of having another child with a malformation.[41] In assessing the risk posed by antiepileptic therapy, it is important to recall that the baseline rate of fetal malformations in the general population is around 3%.[42,43]

Selection and Management of Antiepileptic Drugs

In epileptic women desiring pregnancy, a thorough history regarding the accuracy of seizure diagnosis, subtype, duration, frequency of seizure, and anticonvulsant use is essential. Most women with epilepsy will require continuing AED therapy. It is reasonable to wean AED therapy in patients who have been seizure free for 2 to 4 years.[15]

Table 2
Teratogenicity of antiepileptic drugs

Drug (Brand Name)	Rate of Teratogenicity (%)	Major Congenital Anomalies
Phenytoin (Dilantin)	0.7–7.0	Fetal hydantoin syndrome (cleft palate, hypoplasia of nails and distal phalanges), IUGR, cardiac malformations, NTDs, hypospadias
Carbamazepine (Tegretol)	2–6	Orofacial clefts, cardiac
Valproic Acid (Depakote)	4–14	Neural tube defects, orofacial clefts, Fetal valproate syndrome (limb abnormalities, cardiac malformations, fetal growth restriction, facial dysmorphology), polydactyly, craniosynostosis, hypospadias, poor cognitive and behavioral outcomes
Lamotrigine (lamictal)	2–5	Cleft lip and/or cleft palate
Levetiracetam (Keppra)	0–2	Nonspecific
Topiramate (Topamax)	3–4	Cleft lip and/or palate
Gabapentin (Neurotin)	0–6	Nonspecific
Phenobarbital	1–6	Cardiac malformations, oral clefts, poor cognitive outcomes

Abbreviations: IUGR, intrauterine growth restriction; NTD, neural tube defect.
Data from Refs.[4,15,25]

Because the frequency of seizure recurrence is greatest during the period immediately after the discontinuation of therapy, an attempt to wean anticonvulsant medication should ideally take place in the 9 to 12 months before attempting pregnancy.[28] During pregnancy, 20% to 30% of women will experience an increase in seizure frequency,[44] but those who are seizure free for at least 9 months before conception have an 84% to 92% likelihood to remain seizure free throughout pregnancy.[28] Overall, monotherapy is preferred over polytherapy owing to its lower risk for congenital malformations.[15,45] Similarly, a lower dose of anticonvulsant is preferred to a higher dose.[11] The teratogenic potential should also be considered with an attempt to avoid valproate and phenytoin if possible, with special efforts to avoid both valproate and carbamazepine in a patient with a family history of neural tube defects.[46] In an established pregnancy, it is generally best to continue an effective AED, even if teratogenic. The window for teratogenic effect is generally before the recognition of pregnancy; changing the regimen exposes the fetus to additional drug effects, and a change in therapy may precipitate seizures.[47]

Folate Supplementation

For all women of childbearing age, preconception folic acid supplementation of 0.4 mg/d is recommended to decrease the risk of neural tube defects in case of pregnancy.[46] Decreased first trimester maternal serum levels of folic acid in women with epilepsy are associated with an increased risk of congenital malformations.[48] Moreover, some AEDs decrease folic acid levels.[49] In women with epilepsy, the recommended dose of folic acid supplementation varies across guidelines. The 2009 AAN and American Epilepsy Society guidelines concluded that evidence was insufficient to determine whether a dose higher than 0.4 mg offers greater protection for women with epilepsy.[50] The American College of Obstetricians and Gynecologists, however, recommend 4 mg of folic acid daily for women at an increased risk of having a fetus with neural tube defects, including women on AEDs.[46] Higher doses of folate are not recommended because a dosage of more than 5 mg/d may be associated with delayed psychomotor development in offspring.[51]

ANTEPARTUM MANAGEMENT
Anticonvulsant Drug Monitoring

The main goal of pregnancy management is seizure prevention. Treatment for pregnancy complications that affect AED efficacy, such as nausea and vomiting, should be provided, stimuli causing seizures avoided, and medication compliance stressed.[52] As discussed, basic AED management principles include using monotherapy at the lowest effective dose as possible and avoidance of teratogenic AEDs.[15,45] Increased renal clearance, liver metabolism, and volume of distribution as well as decreased plasma protein binding and gastrointestinal absorption can affect anticonvulsant efficacy.[15,25] Recent AAN guidelines suggest that pregnancy produces a significant enough increase in clearance and decrease in the concentration of lamotrigine, phenytoin, carbamazepine, levetiracetam, and oxcarbazepine to warrant monitoring of plasma levels throughout pregnancy.[50] To identify the serum level that adequately controls seizures for the individual patient, measurement of a trough value of total and free concentrations of each AED should be performed before pregnancy or as early as possible in the first trimester.[25] This value can serve as a reference throughout the course of pregnancy. Some investigators suggest testing at weeks 5 to 6, week 10, and then once a trimester[53] Others suggest monthly monitoring.[15,25] As pregnancy progresses, the dose of AED should be increased for women who experience an increase in seizure frequency or a decrease in the free level of the anticonvulsant drug of 30% or more.[25]

Vitamin K

Evidence regarding antenatal maternal administration of vitamin K is weak at best.[50] Historically, small studies suggested that mothers taking anticonvulsants with hepatic enzyme inducing properties (termed enzyme-inducing AEDs) may cross the placenta and cause degradation of vitamin K in the fetus, leading to hemorrhagic complications.[54–56] These enzyme-inducing AEDs included phenobarbital, phenytoin, carbamazepine, primidone, topiramate, eslicarbazepine, and oxcarbazepine. Indeed, infants of mothers taking AEDs have decreased levels of factors II, VII, IX, and X and normal values of factors V and VIII and fibrinogen,[54–56] a pattern indicative of vitamin K deficiency.[25] In 1993, a small case control study demonstrated increased vitamin K found in cord blood in women with epilepsy on AEDs and receiving vitamin K during the last month of pregnancy compared with mothers without supplementation.[57] Based on this study, some physicians routinely prescribe 10 mg/d of oral vitamin K to mothers on AEDs during the last month of pregnancy. Subsequent research has cast doubt on this practice. In 2002, an epidemiologic study examined 662 pregnancies of mothers taking AEDs without concomitant vitamin K supplementation and found no increase in bleeding complications in neonates.[58] All neonates received 1 mg vitamin K at birth, as is now standard practice.[58] Moreover, the AAN guidelines state that the evidence is insufficient to recommend for or against the practice of peripartum maternal vitamin K supplementation.[50] In the case that AED use does induce vitamin K deficiency in the neonate, routine vitamin K administration at birth seems sufficient to combat any adverse effects.[58]

Antepartum Testing

As in any pregnancy, early and accurate gestational dating is essential in the setting of epilepsy. According to the American College of Obstetricians and Gynecologists and the Society of Maternal Fetal Medicine guidelines, regardless of aneuploidy screening, an ultrasound examination at 11 to 14 weeks is recommended to confirm dates and screen for neural tube defects.[59–61] In cases of anencephaly, this approach provides the mother the option of terminating the pregnancy during the first trimester when this procedure is safest. In cases where termination is not pursued, early knowledge of a malformation can provide information important for later pregnancy planning. Because many centers may not be staffed with sonographers skilled in detailed first trimester ultrasound abnormalities, the first opportunity for screening for neural tube defects and other open defects may be approximately 15 to 22 weeks of gestation in the form of serum maternal alpha-fetoprotein.[62] At 18 to 22 weeks of gestation, women should undergo a detailed anatomic ultrasound examination to screen for neural tube defects as well as other malformations, such as cleft lip and palate, or heart anomalies with a maternal fetal medicine subspecialist.[59–61] When serum screening is combined with ultrasound examination, the detection rate of neural tube defects is between 94% and 100%.[63] Because fetal heart malformations are more common in women taking AEDs, a fetal echocardiogram is recommended between 18 and 22 weeks of gestation.[64] Antenatal testing is often performed empirically in women with epilepsy, although data are conflicting. Some authors have reported an increased risk of fetal growth restriction in epilepsy,[65] although others have not.[66] At this time, existing data are not sufficient to recommend definitively for or against ultrasound monitoring for fetal growth restriction in women with epilepsy. Studies are also conflicting in terms of the increased risk of stillbirth in the setting of epilepsy[6,27–29,66] and, as such, there are insufficient data to recommend for or against antenatal testing in the setting of epilepsy in the absence of other comorbid medical conditions or fetal anomalies. In the setting of epilepsy complicated by fetal anomalies or other maternal conditions associated with stillbirth, antenatal testing is recommended.[67]

INTRAPARTUM CARE
Route of Delivery

Although epidemiologic data describe an increased risk of induction of labor[31,34] and cesarean delivery[30,32,35] for women with epilepsy, indications for the mode and timing of delivery in these women should follow routine obstetric practice. Cesarean delivery is not indicated simply for maternal epilepsy or AED use, except when seizures occur frequently during labor, when they are precipitated by physical activity, or when patients cannot cooperate during labor because of neurologic disorder or mental abnormality.[68] The vast majority of women will have successful vaginal deliveries.[69] There are no restrictions regarding regional anesthesia in the setting of epilepsy.[5,15,70] Regional anesthesia aids in decreasing stress levels, a known seizure precipitant, and reduces the risk for emergency general anesthesia induction when refractory seizures necessitate urgent delivery.[15,16] If general anesthesia becomes necessary, pethidine and ketamine should be avoided owing to their ability to lower seizure threshold, and sevoflurane should be avoided owing to its epileptogenic potential.[71]

Management of the Acute Seizure During Labor

Epileptic seizure

Women who have been on AEDs throughout pregnancy should continue during labor. Sudden cessation of anticonvulsant therapy or missed doses during a long labor course will predispose the patient to an acute seizure.[25] Overall, the risk of seizures during labor in women with epilepsy is 3.5% or less; these seizures are most likely to occur in women who had seizures during their pregnancy.[72,73] Other risk factors for seizures in labor include insomnia, pain, fatigue, and dehydration.[16] Women with recent convulsive seizures, recent seizures after stress or sleep deprivation, or a history of seizures in a previous labor may benefit from the use of a prophylactic benzodiazepine during labor.[16,74] Status epilepticus, which can be fatal to both the patient and her offspring, occurs in 0% to 1.8% of pregnancies in women with epilepsy.[28] In a small series of 29 patients, a total of 9 mothers and 14 fetuses died during or after an episode of status epilepticus.[75] A combination of fetal and maternal hypoxia and acidosis as well as changes in placental blood flow have been proposed as potential etiologies of maternal and fetal death in the setting of status epilepticus.[16,76,77]

Eclamptic seizure

Women with severe preeclampsia are at highest risk for developing eclampsia. In women with severe preeclampsia not receiving antiseizure prophylaxis, eclampsia occurs in 2% to 3% of cases compared with 0.6% of women with mild preeclampsia.[78] Owing to the increasing prevalence of hypertension disorders in pregnancy,[79] it is necessary to briefly discuss preeclampsia and eclamptic seizure. Risk factors for the development of preeclampsia include but are not limited to chronic hypertension, preeclampsia in a previous pregnancy, extremes of maternal age, renal disease, vascular disease, autoimmune disease, diabetes mellitus, and multifetal gestation.[80] A systematic review of more than 21,000 women with eclampsia demonstrated the most common preceding signs and symptoms of eclampsia are hypertension, headache, visual disturbances, right upper quadrant or epigastric pain, and ankle clonus.[81] Occurring most commonly during the intrapartum and postpartum periods, maternal eclamptic seizure is most frequently manifested by generalized tonic–clonic seizures.[80]

Initial management considerations

As soon as a seizure (epileptic or eclamptic) is clinically recognized, the patient's medical stability should be assessed. Respiratory and circulatory status should be evaluated first, with supportive therapy such as oxygen or mechanical ventilation started if appropriate. Suctioning of secretions can be performed and maternal repositioning to the side should occur to increase blood supply to the placenta.[15] A seizure episode that occurs for the first time during pregnancy should be treated as eclampsia until proven otherwise.[15,25] The management principles specific to eclampsia include the use of magnesium sulfate for seizure control and antihypertensive agents to decrease stroke risk.[82–84] It is prudent to initiate intravenous or intramuscular magnesium sulfate if there is any suspicion for eclampsia. The superiority of magnesium sulfate as compared with phenytoin for eclamptic seizure management in terms of both prophylaxis and prevention of further seizure activity is well-established.[78,84,85] If seizures persist despite magnesium administration, benzodiazepines such as diazepam or lorazepam are a common choice for second-line therapy.[82] In this scenario, clinical suspicion for an underlying etiology beyond eclampsia would be increased. Importantly, the initial empiric treatment with benzodiazepines in the setting of a suspected eclamptic seizure should be avoided. The unnecessary addition of benzodiazepines coupled with the expected postictal state of the patient can obtund the patient and make it more difficult to protect the airway. Magnesium sulfate is absolutely contraindicated in patients with myasthenia gravis and, in patients with severe renal dysfunction, the dose should be adjusted or an alternative agent such as phenytoin used.[27,84,85] In a patient with known epilepsy, preeclampsia remains a likely cause of seizure. Management of epileptic and eclamptic seizure is summarized in **Fig. 3.**[82–84,86]

At the time of initial presentation, it may not be possible to differentiate between epileptic and eclamptic seizure. Although eclampsia is more common in the setting of hypertension, proteinuria, and patient report of headache, an eclamptic seizure can occur in a patient with only mild hypertension, no proteinuria, and no neurologic symptoms.[5,23,24] In addition, if the patient is unresponsive and records or family members are unavailable, it may not be possible to evaluate these factors.

Fetal heart rate monitoring

Maternal seizure activity is associated with uterine hypertonus and fetal bradycardia that, if present, can be treated with terbutaline by rapidly relaxing the uterus and improving fetal oxygenation.[16] Continuous fetal monitoring should be instituted if the fetus is at a viable gestational age. During or immediately after the seizure, fetal heart tracing abnormalities are common. Specifically, maternal hypoxemia may result in a loss of variability and a category II fetal tracing.[5] With prolonged maternal hypoxemia, fetal bradycardia and a category III fetal heart tracing may occur.[5] Fortunately, these findings typically resolve in 3 to 10 minutes.[5] However, the presence of fetal tachycardia and absent variability or sinusoidal pattern may suggest placental abruption and fetal anemia. In this case, preparations should be made to provide appropriate management of neonatal hypovolemia and maternal peripartum hemorrhage.[5] Management should focus on improving maternal oxygenation through treatment and prevention of future seizures and positioning and oxygen as noted.

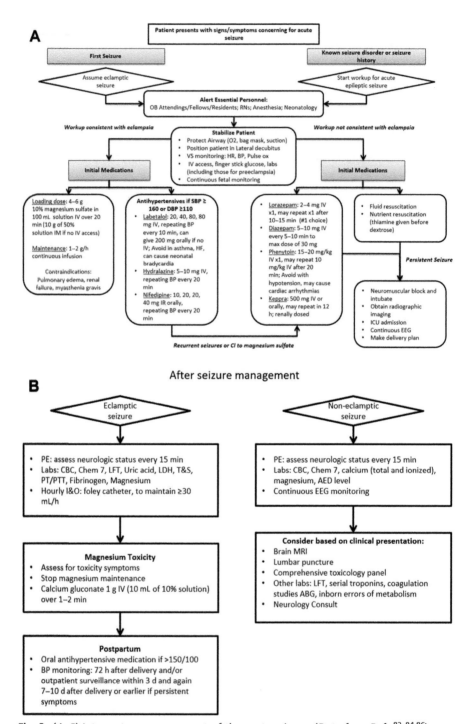

Fig. 3. (*A, B*) Intrapartum management of the acute seizure. (*Data from* Refs.[82–84,86])

Delivery

Although eclampsia is an indication for delivery at all gestational ages,[24] eclamptic seizure, even with fetal bradycardia, does not mandate immediate cesarean delivery.[5] To the contrary, attempting to transport an actively seizing patient to the operating room without controlling her seizures can compromise care and is generally discouraged.[5] Instead, further attempts at maternal and fetal stabilization, including the use of anticonvulsants, oxygen, antihypertensives, uterotonics, and maternal repositioning are recommended. However, if category III fetal heart tracing persists for 10 to 15 minutes despite resuscitative efforts, this may be a sign of placental abruption and immediate delivery should be considered.[5,15,16,80] In addition, women without improvement within 10 to 20 minutes of therapy initiation may benefit from an evaluation by a neurologist for consideration of other etiologies such as subarachnoid hemorrhage.[15] The time frame in which delivery should be undertaken is ultimately individualized in the setting of maternal seizure. Owing to the potential for administration of multiple benzodiazepines and AEDs, the neonatal care team should be notified of the potential for neonatal central nervous system depression.[16]

POSTPARTUM MANAGEMENT
Antiepileptic Drug Management

After delivery, active AED management is important, because the clearance and metabolism of these medications rapidly reverts to prepregnancy parameters. Most AED drug levels increase and plateau by 10 weeks postpartum,[87] but others, such as lamotrigine, increase rapidly, usually within 10 to 14 days.[4] If the dose was increased during gestation, the anticonvulsant dose should be tapered to that of prepregnancy levels or slightly higher over approximately 3 weeks. Changes in lamotrigine serum levels in particular increase quickly within the first week and dose reductions on postpartum days 3, 7, and 10 may be needed to prevent toxicity.[15,88] Above all, it is important that AED therapy is continued postpartum and that all mothers are monitored for signs of toxicity as dose alterations are made.

Safety in the Postpartum Period

The same vigilance over the antepartum and intrapartum safety of women with epilepsy should continue into the postpartum period because the 3-day peripartum period is the time of maximal seizure exacerbation.[89] All new mothers with epilepsy should be counseled on the importance of therapy compliance, signs of postpartum depression, and prevention of seizure triggers such lack of sleep and increased stress.[4,15] To prevent sleep deprivation, family members may need to help with night feedings to allow 6 to 8 hours of uninterrupted sleep. To counteract the likely increase in stress levels new mothers are bound to experience, AED dosage may need to be tapered to levels just above prepregnancy levels.[15] Further safety prevention measures that should be emphasized to the mother and family incorporate steps to protect the newborn in case of maternal seizure.[15] These measures include bathing the infant only when another caregiver is present, changing diapers on the floor instead of a changing table, using a stroller instead of a carrier that straps onto the mother, and avoiding stairs when possible.[4,15]

Breastfeeding

The benefits of breastfeeding are well-established.[90] All AEDs are measurable in breast milk in varying concentrations, but most experts agree that AED use does not preclude breastfeeding.[53,91] The NEAD (Neurodevelopmental Effects of Antiepileptic Drugs) study examined the cognitive outcomes of infants exposed to carbamazepine, lamotrigine, phenytoin, and valproate. Investigators found no differences at 3 years of age in children exposed to all AEDs combined and for each individual AED group, but at 6 years the breastfed infants were found to have higher IQs and language scores than the infants of mothers who did not breastfeed.[92,93] Additional studies have demonstrated that the small amount of AED present in breast milk is eliminated with ingestion and not measurable in the neonatal plasma and supported the conclusion of the NEAD study that exposure to AED in breast milk does not seem to impede central nervous system development of the offspring.[94–97] Although not all confounding factors may have been accounted for in these studies and further prospective studies on AED exposure through breast milk are necessary, studies thus far are reassuring and support that benefits of breastfeeding while taking AED likely outweigh risks.

SUMMARY

Seizures remain among the most serious complications encountered in pregnancy. Both maternal and fetal risks associated with seizure management demand the need for comprehensive and standardized care both at time of initial diagnosis of a seizure disorder and throughout pregnancy. Counseling provided during the preconception, antepartum, intrapartum, and postpartum periods is essential in providing patient-centered care and to limit adverse pregnancy outcomes.

REFERENCES

1. Zack M, Kobau R. National and state estimates of the numbers of adults and children with active epilepsy — United States, 2015. MMWR Morb Mortal Wkly Rep 2017;66:821–5.
2. Harden C, Meador K, Pennell P, et al. Practice parameter update: management issues for women with epilepsy—focus on pregnancy (an evidence-based review): teratogenesis and perinatal outcomes: report of the Quality Standards Subcommittee and Therapeutics and Technology Assessment Subcommittee of the American Academy of Neurology and American Epilepsy Society. Neurology 2009;73(2):133–41.
3. Edey S, Moran N, Nashef L. SUDEP and epilepsy-related mortality in pregnancy. Epilepsia 2014;55(7):e72–4.
4. Hart L, Sibai B. Seizures in pregnancy: epilepsy, eclampsia, and stroke. Semin Perinatol 2013;37:207–24.
5. Sibai BM. Diagnosis, prevention, and management of eclampsia. Obstet Gynecol 2005;105(2):402.
6. MacDonald S, Bateman B, McElrath T, et al. Mortality and morbidity during delivery hospitalization among pregnant women with epilepsy in the United States. JAMA Neurol 2015;72:981–8.
7. Holmes L, Harvey E, Coull B, et al. The teratogenicity of anticonvulsant drugs. N Engl J Med 2001;344(15):1132.
8. Marrow J, Russell A, Guthrie E, et al. Malformation risks of antiepileptic drugs in pregnancy: a prospective study from the UK epilepsy and pregnancy register. J Neurol Neurosurg Psychiatry 2006;77(2):193–8.
9. Meador K, Pennell P, Harden C, et al. Pregnancy registries in epilepsy: a consensus statement on health outcomes. Neurology 2008;71(14):1109.
10. Hernandez-Diaz S, Werler M, Walker A. Folic acid antagonists during pregnancy and the risk of birth defects. N Engl J Med 2000;343(22):1608.

11. Tomson T, Battino D, Bonizzoni E, et al. Dose-dependent risk of malformations with antiepileptic drugs: an analysis of data from the EURAP epilepsy and pregnancy registry. Lancet Neurol 2011;10(7):609.

12. Fisher R, van Emde Boas W, Blume W, et al. Epileptic seizures and epilepsy: definitions proposed by the International League Against Epilepsy (ILAE) and the International Bureau for Epilepsy (IBE). Epilepsia 2005;46:470–2.

13. Moeller JJ, Hirsch LJ. Diagnosis and classification of seizures and epilepsy. In: Winn RH, editor. Youmans and Winn neurological Surgery. 7th edition. Philadelphia: Elsevier; 2017. p. 388–95.

14. Fisher R, Acevedo C, Arzimanoglou A, et al. ILAE official report: a practical clinical definition of epilepsy. Epilepsia 2014;55:475–82.

15. Gerard EE, Samuels P. Neurologic disorders in pregnancy. In: Gabbe SG, editor. Obstetrics: normal and problem pregnancies. 7th edition. Philadelphia: Elsevier; 2017. p. 1030–56.

16. Epilepsy in Pregnancy. In: Royal College of Obstetricians & Gynaecologists Greentop Guideline No. 68. 2016. Available at: https://www.rcog.org.uk/globalassets/documents/guidelines/green-top-guidelines/gtg68_epilepsy.pdf. Accessed August 15, 2017.

17. Scheffer I, Berkovic S, Capovilla G, et al. ILAE classification of the epilepsies: position paper of the ILAE commission for classification and terminology. Epilepsia 2017;58:512.

18. Krumholz A, Wiebe S, Gronseth G, et al. Practice Parameter: evaluating an apparent unprovoked first seizure in adults (an evidence-based review): report of the Quality Standards Subcommittee of the American Academy of Neurology and the American Epilepsy Society. Neurology 2007;69(21):1996–2007.

19. ACOG Committee on Obstetric Practice. ACOG Committee Opinion. Number 299, September 2004. Guidelines for diagnostic imaging during pregnancy. Obstet Gynecol 2004;104(3):647–51.

20. Establishing the diagnosis for preeclampsia and eclampsia. In: hypertension in pregnancy. 2013. Available at: https://www.acog.org/Resources-And-Publications/Task-Force-and-Work-Group-Reports/Hypertension-in-Pregnancy. Accessed November 13, 2017.

21. Beach R, Kaplan P. Seizures in pregnancy: diagnosis and management. Int Rev Neurobiol 2008;83:259–71.

22. Reuber M, Baker G, Gill R, et al. Failure to recognize psychogenic nonepileptic seizures may cause death. Neurology 2004;62:834–5.

23. Prediction of preeclampsia. In: hypertension in pregnancy. 2013. Available at: https://www.acog.org/Resources-And-Publications/Task-Force-and-Work-Group-Reports/Hypertension-in-Pregnancy. Accessed November 13, 2017.

24. Management of preeclampsia and HELLP syndrome. In: hypertension in pregnancy. 2013. Available at: https://www.acog.org/Resources-And-Publications/Task-Force-and-Work-Group-Reports/Hypertension-in-Pregnancy. Accessed November 13, 2017.

25. Aminoff MJ, Douglas VC. Neurologic disorders. In: Creasy RK, Resnik R, Iams JD, editors. Creasy & Resnik's maternal-fetal medicine: principles and practice. 7th edition. Philadelphia: Elsevier; 2014. p. 1100–3.

26. Shostak S, Ottman R. Ethical, legal, and social dimensions of epilepsy genetics. Epilepsia 2006;47:1595–602.

27. Curtis K, Tepper N, Jatlaoui T, et al. U.S. medical eligibility criteria for contraceptive use, 2016. MMWR Recomm Rep 2016;65(3):1.

28. Harden C, Hopp J, Ting T, et al. Practice parameter update: management issues for women with epilepsy–focus on pregnancy (an evidence-based review): obstetrical complications and change in seizure frequency: report of the Quality Standards Subcommittee and Therapeutics and Technology Assessment Subcommittee of the American Academy of Neurology and American Epilepsy Society. Neurology 2009;73(2):126–32.

29. Viale L, Allotey J, Cheong-See F, et al. Epilepsy in pregnancy and reproductive outcomes: a systematic review and meta-analysis. Lancet 2015;386(10006): 1845.

30. Borthen I, Eide M, Veiby G, et al. Complications during pregnancy in women with epilepsy: population-based cohort study. BJOG 2009;116(13):1736–42.

31. Borthen I, Eide M, Daltveit A, et al. Obstetric outcome in women with epilepsy: a hospital-based, retrospective study. BJOG 2011;118(8):956–65.

32. Pilo C, Wide K, Winbladh B. Pregnancy, delivery, and neonatal complications after treatment with antiepileptic drugs. Acta Obstet Gynecol Scand 2006;85:643.

33. Borthen I, Eide M, Daltveit A, et al. Delivery outcome of women with epilepsy: a population-based cohort study. BJOG 2010;117(12):1537–43.

34. Richmond J, Krishnamoorthy P, Andermann E, et al. Epilepsy and pregnancy: an obstetric perspective. Am J Obstet Gynecol 2004;190:371.

35. Olafsson E, Hallgrimsson J, Hauser W, et al. Pregnancies of women with epilepsy: a population-based study in Iceland. Epilepsia 1998;39:887.

36. Bromley R, Weston J, Adab N, et al. Treatment for epilepsy in pregnancy: neurodevelopmental outcomes in the child. Cochrane Database Syst Rev 2014;(10):CD010236.

37. Bjork M, Veiby G, Reiter S, et al. Depression and anxiety in women with epilepsy during pregnancy and after delivery: a prospective population-based cohort study on frequency, risk factors, medication, and prognosis. Epilepsia 2015; 56(1):28.

38. Turner K, Piazzini A, Franza A, et al. Epilepsy and postpartum depression. Epilepsia 2009;50(1):24.

39. Bech B, Kjaersgaard M, Pedersen H. Use of antiepileptic drugs during pregnancy and risk of spontaneous abortion and stillbirth: population based cohort study. BMJ 2014;349:g5159.

40. Wen X, Meador K, Martzema A. Antiepileptic drug use by pregnant women enrolled in Florida Medicaid. Neurology 2015;84(9):944–50.

41. Campbell E, Kennedy F, Russell A, et al. Malformation risks of antiepileptic drug monotherapies in pregnancy: updated results from the UK and Ireland epilepsy and pregnancy registers. J Neurol Neurosurg Psychiatry 2014;85:1029–34.

42. Hoyert DL, Mathews TJ, Menacker F, et al. Annual summary of vital statistics: 2004. Pediatrics 2006;117:168–83.

43. Yoon PW, Olney RS, Khoury MJ, et al. Contributions of birth defects and genetic diseases to pediatric hospitalizations: a population-based study. Arch Pediatr Adolesc Med 1997;151:1096–103.

44. Mawer G, Briggs M, Baker G, et al. Pregnancy with epilepsy: obstetric and neonatal outcome of a controlled study. Seizure 2010;19(2):112.

45. Buhimschi C, Weiner C. Medication in pregnancy and lactation: part 1. Teratology. Obstet Gynecol 2009;113:166.

46. Cheschier N. ACOG practice bulletin. Neural tube defects. Number 44, July 2003. Int J Gynaecol Obstet 2003;83(1):123–33.

47. Practice Parameter. management issues for women with epilepsy. Report of the quality standards subcommittee of the American Academy of Neurology. Neurology 1998;51(4):944.

48. Kjaer D, Horvath-Puhó E, Christensen J, et al. Antiepileptic drug use, folic acid supplementation, and congenital abnormalities: a population-based case-control study. BJOG 2008;115(1):98–103.

49. Linnebank M, Moskau S, Semmler A, et al. Antiepileptic drugs interact with folate and vitamin B12 serum levels. Ann Neurol 2011;69(2):352–9.

50. Harden C, Pennell P, Koppel B, et al. Practice parameter update: management issues for women with epilepsy–focus on pregnancy (an evidence-based review): vitamin K, folic acid, blood levels, and breastfeeding: report of the Quality Standards Subcommittee and Therapeutics and Technology Assessment Subcommittee of the American Academy of Neurology and American Epilepsy Society. Neurology 2009;73(2):142.

51. Valera-Gran D, García de la Hera M, Navarrete-Muñoz E, et al. Folic acid supplements during pregnancy and child psychomotor development after the first year of life. JAMA Pediatr 2014;168(11):e142611.

52. Neurologic disorders. In: Fried A, Boyle PJ, editors. Williams obstetrics. 24th edition. Philadelphia: McGraw-Hill Education; 2014. p. 1189–91.

53. Munshi A, Munshi S. Neurological diseases. In: Malhotra N, Puri R, Malhotra J, editors. Donald school manual of practical problems in obstetrics. 1st edition. New Delhi (India): Jaypee Brothers Medical Publishers (P) Ltd; 2012. p. 281–3.

54. Yerby M. Problems and management of the pregnant woman with epilepsy. Epilepsia 1987;28(Suppl 3):S29.

55. Bleyer W, Skinner A. Fatal neonatal hemorrhage after maternal anticonvulsant therapy. JAMA 1976;235:626.

56. Mountain K, Hirsh J, Gallus A. Neonatal coagulation defect due to anticonvulsant drug treatment in pregnancy. Lancet 1970;1(7641):265.

57. Cornelissen M, Steegers-Theunissen R, Kollee L, et al. Supplementation of vitamin K in pregnant women receiving anticonvulsant therapy prevents neonatal vitamin K deficiency. Am J Obstet Gynecol 1993;168:884.

58. Kaaja E, Kaaja R, Matila R, et al. Enzyme-inducing antiepileptic drugs in pregnancy and the risk of bleeding in the neonate. Neurology 2002;58(4):549.

59. Committee on Practice Bulletins—Obstetrics and the American Institute of Ultrasound in Medicine. ACOG practice bulletin No. 175. Ultrasound in pregnancy. Obstet Gynecol 2016;128(6):241–56.

60. Wax J, Minkoff H, Johnson A, et al. Consensus report on the detailed fetal anatomic ultrasound examination: indications, components, and qualifications. J Ultrasound Med 2014;33:189–95.

61. Reddy U, Abuhamad A, Levine D, et al. Fetal imaging: executive summary of a Joint Eunice Kennedy Shriver National Institute of Child Health and Human Development, Society for Maternal-Fetal Medicine, American Institute of Ultrasound in Medicine, American College of Obstetricians and Gynecologists, American College of Radiology, Society for Pediatric Radiology, and Society of Radiologists in Ultrasound Fetal Imaging Workshop. Obstet Gynecol 2014; 123(5):1070–82.

62. Committee on Practice Bulletins—Obstetrics, Committee on Genetics, and the Society for Maternal-Fetal Medicine. ACOG practice bulletin No. 163. Screening for fetal aneuploidy. Obstet Gynecol 2016;127(5):e123–37.

63. Nadel A, Green J, Holmes L, et al. Absence of need for amniocentesis in patients with elevated levels of maternal serum alpha-fetoprotein and normal ultrasonographic examinations. N Engl J Med 1990;323(9):557.

64. AIUM Practice parameter for the performance of fetal echocardiography. In: AIUM resource guidelines. 2013. Available at: http://www.aium.org/resources/guidelines/fetalEcho.pdf. Accessed August 15, 2017.

65. Viinikainen K, Heinonen S, Eriksson K, et al. Community-based, prospective, controlled study of obstetric and neonatal outcome of 179 pregnancies in women with epilepsy. Epilepsia 2006;47(1):186–92.

66. McPherson J, Harper L, Odibo A, et al. Maternal seizure disorder and risk of adverse pregnancy outcomes. Am J Obstet Gynecol 2013;208(5):378.e1-5.

67. ACOG practice bulletin No. 145. Antepartum fetal surveillance. Obstet Gynecol 2014;124(1):182–92.

68. Tomson T, Hiilesmaa V. Epilepsy in pregnancy. BMJ 2007;335:769–73.

69. Hiilesmaa V. Pregnancy and birth in women with epilepsy. Neurology 1992;42(4 Suppl 5):8.

70. Sibai B. Diagnosis and management of gestational hypertension and preeclampsia. Obstet Gynecol 2003;102:181–92.

71. Kuczkowski K. Seizures on emergence from sevoflurane anaesthesia for Caesarean section in a healthy parturient. Anaesthesia 2002;57:1234–5.

72. Battino D, Tomson T, Bonizzoni E, et al. Seizure control and treatment changes in pregnancy: observations from the EURAP epilepsy pregnancy registry. Epilepsia 2013;54(9):1621–7.

73. EURAP Study Group. Seizure control and treatment in pregnancy: observations from the EURAP epilepsy pregnancy registry. Neurology 2006;66:354–60.

74. Kevat D, Mackillop L. Neurological diseases in pregnancy. J R Coll Physicians Edinb 2013;43:49–58.

75. Pennell P. Pregnancy in the woman with epilepsy: maternal and fetal outcomes. Semin Neurol 2002;22(3):299–308.

76. Sveberg L, Svalheim S, Taubøll E. The impact of seizures on pregnancy and delivery. Seizure 2015;28:35–8.

77. Teramo K, Hiilesmaa V, Bardy A, et al. Fetal heart rate during a maternal grand mal epileptic seizure. J Perinat Med 1979;7(1):3–6.

78. Sibai BM. Magnesium sulfate prophylaxis in preeclampsia: lessons learned from recent trials. Am J Obstet Gynecol 2004;190(6):1520.

79. Wallis A, Saftlas A, Hsia J, et al. Secular trends in the rates of preeclampsia, eclampsia, and gestational hypertension, United States, 1987-2004. Am J Hypertens 2008;21:521–6.

80. Markham KB, Edmund FF. Pregnancy-related hypertension. In: Creasy RK, Resnik R, Iams JD, editors. Creasy & Resnik's maternal-fetal medicine: principles and practice. 7th edition. Philadelphia: Elsevier; 2014. p. 756–80.

81. Berhan Y, Berhan A. Should magnesium sulfate be administered to women with mild pre-eclampsia? A systematic review of published reports on eclampsia. J Obstet Gynaecol Res 2015;41(6):831.

82. Key elements for the management of hypertensive crisis in pregnancy (In-Patient). In: optimizing protocols in obstetrics. 2013. Available at: http://www.ilpqc.org/docs/htn/Recognition/ACOGDII(NY)KeyElementsManagementHypertensiveCrisisPregnancy.pdf. Accessed September 25, 2017.

83. Committee on Obstetric Practice. ACOG Committee Opinion. Emergent therapy for acute-onset, severe hypertension during pregnancy and the postpartum period number 692. Obstet Gynecol 2017;129(4):e90–5.

84. Eclampsia checklist. In ACOG safe motherhood initiative. 2017. Available at: https://www.acog.org/-/media/Districts/District-II/Public/SMI/v2/sm02a170713EclampsiacheckRev072017.pdf?dmc=1&ts=20170928T0147570258. Accessed September 25, 2017.

85. Lucas MJ, Leveno KJ, Cunningham FG. A comparison of magnesium sulfate with phenytoin for the prevention of eclampsia. N Engl J Med 1995;333:201.

86. Brophy B, Bell R, Claassen J, et al. Guidelines for the evaluation and management of status epilepticus. Neurocrit Care 2012;17(1):3–23.

87. Pennell P. Antiepileptic drugs during pregnancy: what is known and which AEDs seem to be safest? Epilepsia 2008;49(Suppl 9):43–55.

88. Pennell P, Peng L, Newport D, et al. Lamotrigine in pregnancy: clearance, therapeutic drug monitoring, and seizure frequency. Neurology 2008;70(22 Pt 2):2130.

89. Thomas S, Syam U, Devi JS. Predictors of seizures during pregnancy in women with epilepsy. Epilepsia 2012;53:e85–8.

90. Ip S, Chung M, Raman G, et al. A summary of the Agency for Healthcare Research and Quality's evidence report on breastfeeding in developed countries. Breastfeed Med 2009;4(suppl 1):S17–30.

91. Crawford P. Best practice guidelines for the management of women with epilepsy. Epilepsia 2005;46(suppl9):117–24.

92. Meador K. Breastfeeding and antiepileptic drugs. JAMA 2014;311(17):1797–8.

93. Meador K, Baker G, Browning N, et al. Effects of breastfeeding in children of women taking antiepileptic drugs. Neurology 2010;75(22):1954–60.

94. Veiby G, Engelsen B, Gilhus N. Early child development and exposure to antiepileptic drugs prenatally and through breastfeeding: a prospective cohort study on children of women with epilepsy. JAMA Neurol 2013;70(11):1367–74.

95. Johannessen S, Helde G, Brodtkorb E. Levetiracetam concentrations in serum and in breast milk at birth and during lactation. Epilepsia 2005;46(5):775–7.

96. Ohman I, Vitols S, Luef G, et al. Topiramate kinetics during delivery, lactation, and in the neonate: preliminary observations. Epilepsia 2002;43(10):1157–60.

97. Ohman I, Vitols S, Tomson T. Pharmacokinetics of gabapentin during delivery, in the neonatal period, and lactation: does a fetal accumulation occur during pregnancy? Epilepsia 2005;46(10):1621–4.

Infections in Pregnancy and the Role of Vaccines

Kimberly B. Fortner, MD[a],*, Claudia Nieuwoudt, MD[b], Callie F. Reeder, MD[b], Geeta K. Swamy, MD[c]

KEYWORDS

- Influenza • Pertussis • Zika • Influenza vaccine • Tdap vaccine
- Maternal vaccination

KEY POINTS

- The Advisory Committee of Immunization Practices recommends administration of tetanus toxoid, reduced diphtheria toxoid, and acellular pertussis with each pregnancy and inactivated influenza vaccine in influenza season.
- There are other vaccines that may (or should) be used in pregnancy under certain circumstances.
- As women's health providers, we have come a long way in the arena of maternal vaccination, and continued research is paramount.

INTRODUCTION

Infectious disease remains a major cause of mortality worldwide, but before the advent of modern medicine, was the leading cause of mortality in the United States.[1] The 3 leading causes of death reported in 1900 in America were pneumonia, tuberculosis, and diphtheria, causing one-third of all deaths.[1] Between 1900 and 2000, the life expectancy for a person born in the United States increased from 47.3 to 76.8 years[1] with decreased mortality attributed in part to advances in vaccinology.[2] Avoidance of

Conflicts of Interest: G.K. Swamy is on a Data and Safety Monitoring Board for a GlaxoSmithKline-funded respiratory syncytial virus (RSV) vaccine study in pregnant women. She has received research funding for studies of group B streptococcus vaccine in pregnant women produced by Novartis and for RSV vaccine in pregnant women produced by Novavax. K.B. Fortner has received research funding for studies of group B streptococcus vaccine in pregnant women produced by Novartis and for RSV and cytomegalovirus surveillance among pregnant women and their infants by Pfizer and Regeneron. The remaining authors have no conflicts of interest to declare.
^a Department of Obstetrics and Gynecology, Maternal-Fetal Medicine, University of Tennessee Medical Center, 1924 Alcoa Highway, Box 96, Knoxville, TN 37919, USA; ^b Department of Obstetrics and Gynecology, University of Tennessee Medical Center, 1924 Alcoa Highway, Box U27, Knoxville, TN 37920, USA; ^c Department of Obstetrics and Gynecology, Obstetrics Clinical Research, Duke University Medical System, Durham, NC, USA
* Corresponding author.
E-mail address: kfortner@utmck.edu

millions of deaths are attributed to expanded coverage of measles, polio, and, more recently, pneumococcal vaccines.[2]

At present, 17 vaccine-preventable diseases are covered by 14 routine vaccines, 2 of which are recommended during most pregnancies.[3] Starting in 1997, the Centers for Disease Control and Prevention's (CDC) Advisory Committee of Immunization Practices (ACIP) recommended annual vaccination against influenza in all women pregnant during influenza season.[4] In October of 2012, the tetanus–diphtheria–acellular pertussis vaccine was recommended in pregnancy in response to increased rates of pertussis infection.[5,6] Pregnant women are at risk for infection just as their nongravid counterparts and, in some cases, may have more significant morbidity and mortality than their peers.[7,8] This review outlines the following:

1. Maternal immunization and types of immunizations,
2. Immunizations recommended during pregnancy,
3. Conditional vaccines to be considered,
4. Research frontiers in immunization, and
5. The role of obstetrician/gynecologists as vaccinators.

MATERNAL IMMUNIZATION BENEFITS

Maternal immunization is a purposeful, successful strategy to prevent or mitigate the severity of infections in pregnant women and their newborn infants. The prevention of illness during pregnancy impacts the health care system 2-fold by keeping the mother–infant dyad intact and healthy.[9] For example, flu vaccinated pregnant women seem to have longer pregnancies with larger neonates.[10,11] Pregnancy, by virtue of innate physiologic changes, increases a woman's susceptibility to illness.[7] Ensuing flu seasons have revealed that infected pregnant women have higher rates of hospitalization, cardiopulmonary complications, and death compared with the general public.[8,12,13] Pregnancy increases a woman's exposure to the health care system and to a provider with whom she can build a relationship, giving time for education, planning, vaccine administration, and follow-up.[9] The majority of pregnant women report visits to their obstetric provider more than 6 times during pregnancy, allowing many opportunities to discuss and give vaccines.[12] Immunization in pregnancy also seems to have maternal, neonatal, and obstetric benefit, with several studies showing improved birth outcomes.[10,14]

Types of Vaccines

Pregnancy modulates the baseline immune response in a protective effort to diminish an inflammatory reaction to the fetus.[7] A shift occurs from T-helper cells, which produce cytokines that facilitate pregnancy loss, to T-helper 2 cells, which render and permit fetal antigen tolerance.[7] This modulatory effect diminishes maternal protection, yielding gravid women vulnerable compared with their nongravid counterparts as evidenced by the 1918, 1959, and 2009 pandemic flu seasons.[15–17] In the 2009 pandemic, pregnant women were 4 times more likely to be hospitalized secondary to flu-related complications and represented 5% of flu-related mortalities despite only representing 1% of the US population.[16] Thus, vaccination can help to combat the disproportionate representation of pregnant women in morbidity and mortality statistics.

Vaccines are categorized into 2 basic groups: inactivated or live attenuated (Table 1). Inactivated vaccines consist of a component of the infectious pathogen rendered incapable of causing clinical disease. For example, the tetanus vaccine contains the tetanus toxoid, which is produced by *Clostridium tetani*. As such, the pathogen is not introduced, but produces a humoral immune response to the toxoid, conferring immunity. Other types of components used in vaccines include whole

Table 1
Inactivated and live attenuated vaccines

Inactivated Vaccines

Indicated in Pregnancy		Indicated in Pregnant Women with Risk Factors		Contraindicated, Limited Data in Pregnancy
Influenza	One dose of inactivated vaccine during flu season during any gestational age	Hepatitis A	2 scheduled doses	Typhoid
Tetanus, diphtheria, pertussis	1 dose Tdap after 20 wk, preferably 27–36 wk	Hepatitis B	3 scheduled doses	Human papilloma virus
		Pneumococcal (PPSV23)	1 dose	Japanese encephalitis
		Meningococcal (MPSV4)	1 dose	
		Yellow fever	1 dose	
		Cholera	1 dose after exposure	
		Anthrax	3 schedules doses after exposure	
		Polio	1 dose	
		Rabies	3 scheduled doses	

Live Attenuated Vaccines

Contraindicated in Pregnancy		Contraindicated in Pregnancy with Specific Postpartum Indication	
Vaccinia	Oral polio	Mumps, measles, rubella	1 dose postpartum if rubella nonimmune or equivocal
Rotavirus	Oral typhoid	Varicella	1 dose postpartum if varicella nonimmune
Intranasal Influenza	Bacille Calmette-Guerin		

Abbreviations: MPSV4, tetravalent polysaccharide-protein vaccine; PPSV23, 23-serotype polysaccharide vaccine; Tdap, tetanus toxoid, reduced diphtheria toxoid, and acellular pertussis.

cell virus and bacteria, fractional protein-based subunits (such as with tetanus), and fractional polysaccharide-based subunits.[18] Inactivated vaccines tend to require multiple booster doses because antibody levels wane over time.[18] Currently available inactivated vaccines are listed in **Table 1**. All available inactivated vaccines are not recommended in pregnancy, but can be administered when considering exposure to the vaccine versus exposure to the infection and associated morbidity/mortality.

Live attenuated vaccines are living organisms modified so as to not produce fulminant disease. Attenuated vaccines generate an immune response sufficient to approximate exposure to the intended infection.[19] Live attenuated vaccines are widely accepted. The remote potential to cause clinical infection exists; however, disease is usually mild when compared with natural infection. Live attenuated vaccines are contraindicated in pregnancy owing to the theoretic risk of perinatal infection via vertical transmission. Inadvertent administration of a live attenuated influenza vaccine during pregnancy has not been associated with adverse pregnancy outcomes to date.[20] Currently administered live attenuated vaccines are listed in **Table 1**.[18]

VACCINES RECOMMENDED IN PREGNANCY OR POSTPARTUM

Currently, there are 2 recommended vaccines for administration during pregnancy:

1. Inactivated influenza and
2. Tetanus toxoid, reduced diphtheria toxoid, and acellular pertussis (Tdap).[3,6]

Although this next section reviews current vaccines indicated before, during, and after pregnancy, data are evolving and providers should consult regularly updated sources referencing maternal immunization guidelines.

Influenza Vaccine

The influenza vaccine is the longest studied vaccine administered in pregnancy and has no demonstrated safety concerns since its recommendation in 1997.[4] For decades, the CDC has recommended that all pregnant women be immunized during the flu season.[3,4,21] Influenza is an upper respiratory illness occurring in a temporal pattern from December to March in the northern hemisphere.[18] The seasonal influenza epidemic generally causes milder disease, but higher rates of hospitalization are still seen in pregnant women.[22,23] During the H1N1 pandemic, multiple fetal complications occurred in women with infection, including higher rates of spontaneous abortion, fetal demise, neonatal death, preterm delivery, and low birth weight.[8,24,25]

A single dose of the seasonal inactivated influenza vaccine given in pregnancy achieves the following:

- Sufficient maternal seroconversion and seroprotection.[26]
- Mitigation of maternal illness.[18,27]
- Decreased risk for poor obstetric outcomes.[10,27–29]
- Lowered rates of influenza-like illness among newborns.[29,30]

Maternal vaccination benefits are from reduced disease prevalence and mitigated illness.[18] Multiple studies continue to demonstrate maternal benefit to vaccination, including a Norwegian population-based study of gravid women that reported a 70% decrease in influenza illness among immunized mothers.[27] A prospective trial of 340 Bangladeshi pregnant women randomized to trivalent inactivated influenza vaccine or the pneumococcal vaccine demonstrated a 36% reduction of respiratory illness among women who received the influenza vaccine.[29] Madhi and colleagues[28] reported 2 double-blind, randomized, placebo-controlled trials of trivalent influenza vaccine in South Africa in pregnant women with and without a diagnosis of human immunodeficiency virus. Influenza vaccine was immunogenic in both human immunodeficiency virus–infected and –uninfected pregnant women and provided reduction in confirmed influenza in both groups.

Fetal and neonatal benefits of maternal influenza vaccination include a decreased risk of spontaneous abortion, intrauterine fetal demise, neonatal death, preterm birth, and low birth weight.[10,29] A large Swedish cohort study of 18,000 patients showed that influenza vaccination significantly decreased the risk of intrauterine fetal demise during the H1N1 pandemic of 2009.[24] The efficacy of influenza vaccination to decrease poor fetal outcomes was further demonstrated by a European cohort study of 117,000 mother–infant pairs with significantly decreased risk of intrauterine fetal demise among immunized mothers.[27] The Bangladeshi study previously described investigated neonatal outcomes as well and found a 29% decrease in respiratory illness and a 63% decrease in laboratory-confirmed influenza in newborns up to 6 months of age born to mothers receiving the influenza vaccination as opposed to the pneumococcal vaccine.[29] A US matched case-control study showed that maternal influenza immunization was 91.5% effective in preventing infant hospitalization for influenza in the first 6 months of life.[30] Influenza vaccination benefits the mother, the fetus, and the infant, and should be administered as soon as available during the flu season for every pregnancy, without delay.

Tetanus Toxoid, Reduced Diphtheria Toxoid, and Acellular Pertussis Vaccine

Vaccination against tetanus, pertussis, and diphtheria starts at 2 months of age in the United States, with booster vaccinations given across the lifespan and exposure-related incidents.[31] Young infants are at greatest risk for severe respiratory disease and death.[32] Children less than 3 months of age have the greatest burden of hospitalization and infants less than 1 month of age have the highest mortality.[32–34] There are 8 vaccines currently licensed against tetanus, diphtheria, and pertussis.

Pertussis infections declined for decades; however, owing to waning immunity and increasing susceptible hosts, cases are again on the rise.[35] During pregnancy, it is recommended that the Tdap vaccine is administered, which includes only Adacel,[36] produced by Sanofi Pasteur, and Boostrix,[37] produced by GlaxoSmithKline Biologicals. Both vaccines contain a dose of tetanus toxoid, a reduced amount of diphtheria toxoid (compared with DTaP), and several acellular pertussis antigens; Adacel[36] contains 4 (inactivated pertussis toxin, filamentous hemagglutinin, pertactin, and fimbrae types 2 and 3), whereas Boostrix[37] does not contain fimbrae types 2 and 3.[38]

Maternal pertussis vaccination between 27 and 36 weeks of gestational was initiated in the United States in 2012 because of increasing annual pertussis incidence.[21,39] Previous efforts to protect the neonate involved Tdap administration in the postpartum period in an effort to cocoon the neonate against infection; however, this proved to be ineffective given the inability to vaccinate all contacts and did not prevent infantile pertussis.[40,41] Halasa and colleagues[42] conducted a randomized clinical trial in infants to assess effectiveness of pertussis vaccination at birth by evaluating serial antibody responses for the first few months of life. Although well-tolerated, subsequent immune responses to pertussis and other vaccine antigens were suppressed among vaccinated infants when compared with control children. Passive immunity via maternal immunization was recognized as an ideal way to target transplacental immunoglobulin G (IgG) antibody transfer during the third trimester.[43] An observational study by Gall and colleagues[44] demonstrated high concentrations of anti-pertussis antibodies in infant cord blood among mothers vaccinated with Tdap during pregnancy. In 2011 and 2012, ACIP concluded that available data did not suggest any association of Tdap administration during pregnancy with adverse maternal or infant outcomes.[45,46] Motivated by the need to combat the resurgence of pertussis and its grave impact on young infants, ACIP recommended Tdap administration to all pregnant women, regardless of history of prior Tdap receipt. This shift in recommendations was supported by a recent cohort study in California that compared neonatal outcomes in nearly 43,000 mothers vaccinated between 27 to 36 weeks gestation to around 32,000 mothers vaccinated within 14 days post-partum. Antetnatal Tdap vaccination proved 85% more effective in preventing pertussis in neonates less than 8 weeks of age.[47] Research in timing and efficacy of Tdap remains ongoing, and data remain supportive of the 2012 ACIP change in recommendations.

Tetanus Vaccine

In reviewing maternal infections, and successes with vaccine preventable illness, maternal tetanus remains an important example. Tetanus that occurs during pregnancy or within 6 weeks postpartum is termed, "maternal tetanus," while tetanus that occurs within the first 28 days of life is termed, "neonatal tetanus".[18] Disease from tetanus is particularly serious in newborn babies and their mothers when infants are not protected by passive immunity. Neonatal infection occurs when the unhealed umbilical cord stump is cut with an unsterile instrument,[18] and is mostly fatal. Neonatal tetanus can be prevented by immunizing women of reproductive age and can be safely given during pregnancy. The Maternal and Neonatal Tetanus Elimination (MNTE) initiative is aimed at reducing maternal and neonatal tetanus (MNT) to levels low enough that the disease is no longer a major public health problem. MNTE initiative consists of administration of 2 initial doses of tetanus toxoid (TT) 1 month apart followed by a third dose 6 months later in pregnancy and another dose for each subsequent pregnancy culminating in 5 total doses. Through MNTE efforts, and WHO efforts to improve perinatal hygienic habits, attributable neonatal deaths, there has been a 96% reduction from the late 1980s.[48] While monumental progress has been made, by the end of June 2017, 16 countries still have not eliminated neonatal disease.[49]

Measles, Mumps, Rubella Vaccine

Measles, mumps and rubella are acute preventable viral infections that can cause serious disease and complications. Owing to successful vaccination, measles, rubella, congenital rubella syndrome (CRS), and mumps are now rare in the United States.[50] Measles is a paramyxovirus that presents with fever, cough, coryza, conjunctivitis, exanthem and severe complications include encephalitis.[18] Measles in pregnancy is associated with preterm birth, low birthweight and spontaneous abortions.[51,52] Mumps is another paramyxovirus presenting with flu-like illness and bilateral parotitis and is associated with spontaneous abortion.[18,52] Rubella is a togavirus presenting with nonspecific symptoms such as lymphadenopathy, arthralgias, fever and rash. Rubella infection during pregnancy, especially during the first trimester, can lead to severe fetal effects.[18,51] During the last rubella epidemic in 1964 to 1965, nearly 12.5 million rubella infections lead to 11,250 spontaneous or therapeutic abortions, 2100 neonatal deaths and 20,000 infants with congenital rubella syndrome.[53] The CDC recommends measles, mumps, rubella (MMR) vaccine as a 2-dose vaccine schedule for children starting ages 12 to 15 months with second dose ages 4 to 6 years of age followed by a young adult booster.[31,50]

As a live attenuated vaccine, MMR administration should be avoided during pregnancy given the theoretic risk for live vaccines to adversely impact mother or fetus exists despite insufficient data.[54] In women vaccinated just before or inadvertently during pregnancy, no cases of congenital rubella syndrome or outcomes attributed to measles are reported.[55] Termination of pregnancy is not recommended solely on the theoretic risk for embryopathy.[18,50] Establishing immunity before pregnancy is ideal in women of childbearing age given maternal morbidity and adverse fetal outcomes from rubella and measles infections. Women receiving the MMR vaccine should be advised to delay conception until 4 weeks after vaccination.[18,50]

Following initiation of universal MMR vaccination programs, a dramatic decline in rubella cases was noted. From 2004 to 2012, 79 cases of rubella and 6 cases of congenital rubella syndrome were documented. The cases were associated with either an unknown source or occurred in individuals who came to the US already infected.[53] Rubella immunity should be screened for in routine prenatal laboratory panels and any woman lacking immunity should be vaccinated immediately postpartum. The vaccine can be given safely in breastfeeding patients. Although rubella virus is excreted in breast milk, only seroconversion without serious infection has been reported in breastfed infants.[56]

Varicella Vaccine

Maternal varicella infection can lead to adverse pregnancy and infant outcomes, such as congenital varicella syndrome (CVS), with highest transmission risk occurring with first or second trimester infection.[57] CVS is characterized by limb hypoplasia, cutaneous lesions, neurologic abnormalities and structural eye damage, and has mortality rates around 30% in the first few months of life.[57] Maternal infection immediately before or after delivery can result in neonatal varicella, leading to severe neonatal infection or death.[57,58] Varicella immunoglobulin (VZIG) should be administered to all infants born to nonimmune mothers who develop varicella 5 days before 2 days after delivery.

The prevention of varicella and congenital complications begins with establishing immunity before pregnancy. Maternal report of prior infection is highly predictive of varicella zoster virus IgG antibodies, and the presence of antibodies confers long-term immunity.[59,60] Without a history or documentation of infection, serologic testing is recommended in all women of childbearing age.[18,54] Women who do not exhibit immunity should be advised to avoid contact with infected individuals until they are not infectious and should be vaccinated immediately postpartum.[61] The varicella vaccine, first introduced in 1995, is a live attenuated vaccine that has been successful in reducing both hospitalizations and deaths attributable to varicella illness.[60] Breastfeeding is not a contraindication to vaccination.[62] After vaccination, women should be advised to avoid conceiving for 1 month.[60,61] If a woman is inadvertently vaccinated during pregnancy, she should be advised of theoretic risk to the fetus, but this risk is not considered a reason to terminate a pregnancy.[60]

VACCINES RECOMMENDED IN PREGNANCY AND POSTPARTUM IN SPECIAL CIRCUMSTANCES
Hepatitis A

Epidemic jaundice was first described by Hippocrates in the 5th century BCE, and was not recognized as distinct from hepatitis B until the 1940s.[18] Hepatitis A virus is an RNA picornavirus endemic in many developing countries. With humans as the only known reservoirs, the potential for eradication exists with universal vaccination.[18] Illness from hepatitis A virus is common in travelers, and spreads by the fecal–oral route from close contact with another infected individual or contaminated beverage or food.[63] Illness is usually self-limiting, and includes fever, nausea, abdominal pain, and jaundice.[18] Hepatitis A vaccination was first available in 1995 as inactivated virus and now is available from 3 manufacturers (**Table 2**). Hepatitis A vaccine is

Table 2
Provisional vaccines, available formulations, and indications

Infection Prevented	Vaccines Formulations Available	Risk Factor/Special Circumstance	Data Regarding Pregnancy Use
Hepatitis A	Havrix (GlaxoSmithKline Biologicals)[a] Vaqta (Merck and Co)[a] Twinrix (GlaxoSmithKline Biologicals)[a]	• Travel to developing countries • Men having sex with men • Exposure to individuals with HAV infection • Individuals receiving clotting factor concentrates • Exposure to biologic specimens	Reviews from VAERS did not find any pattern of pregnancy-specific outcomes.
Hepatitis B	Single antigen Recombivax HB (Merck and Co)[a] Engerix-B (GlaxoSmithKline Biologicals)[a] Combination vaccine Twinrix (GlaxoSmithKline Biologicals)[a]	• Pregnant women with ≥1 sexual partners in the past 6 mo • Household or sexual contact with known HBV-positive individual • Ongoing intravenous drug use • Health care and public safety workers with risk for exposure to blood or blood-contaminated body fluids • End-stage renal disease • Diabetes • International travelers • Adults with chronic liver disease, including, but not limited to, HCV infection • Pregnant women evaluated or treated for a sexually transmitted infection	Using PubMed, Scopus, VAERS, and VAMPSS, no safety concerns reported during pregnancy[67]

Streptococcus pneumoniae	Pneumovax 23-valent polysaccharide vaccine licensed (PPSV23) (Merck and Co)[a] Prevnar 13 pneumococcal conjugate vaccine PCV13 (Wyeth/Pfizer)	• Functional or anatomic asplenia (eg, from sickle cell disease or splenectomy) • Chronic heart or lung disease (asthma, obstructive lung disease, cardiomyopathy, etc) • Alcoholism or other chronic liver disease • Diabetes • Immunosuppression or malignancy (HIV infection, leukemia, lymphoma, Hodgkin disease, multiple myeloma, generalized malignancy) • Chronic renal failure, nephrotic syndrome, or other conditions associated with immunosuppression (eg, organ or bone marrow transplantation) • Those receiving immunosuppressive chemotherapy, including long-term corticosteroids • CSF leak or cochlear implants	Systematic review[71] and randomized trial[70] reported no maternal or fetal safety concerns
Neisseria meningitidis	Meningococcal conjugate vaccines Menactra (Sanofi Pasteur, Inc),[a] MenACWY (contains meningococcal A, C, W, and Y polysaccharides) Menveo (Novartis),[a] MenACWY Meningococcal polysaccharide vaccine (MPSV4) Menomune (Sanofi Pasteur, Inc)	Adolescents 11–18 y and at-risk individuals 2–55 y • College freshmen • Military • Travelers in endemic countries • Functional asplenia or complement deficiencies • Microbiologists exposed to the organism frequently	Reviews with both MPSV4[67] and meningococcal conjugate vaccine MenACWY-D (Menactra)[74] did not identify any maternal or fetal safety concerns

Abbreviations: CSF, cerebrospinal fluid; HAV, hepatitis A virus; HBV, hepatitis B virus; HCV, hepatitis C virus; HIV, human immunodeficiency virus; MPSV4, tetravalent polysaccharide-protein vaccine; PPSV23, 23-serotype polysaccharide vaccine; VAERS, Vaccine Adverse Event Reporting System; VAMPSS, Vaccines and Medications in Pregnancy Surveillance System.
[a] Available without preservative, thimerisol free.

recommended for young children routinely and for certain groups with increased risk for hepatitis A virus exposure.[31] See **Table 2** for conditional indications. The ACIP recommends that the hepatitis A vaccine should be considered for women at increased risk for infection.[3,21] Although data evaluating safety of hepatitis A vaccination during pregnancy are not robust, a review of the Vaccine Adverse Event Reporting System database reports from 1996 to 2013 did not find any concerning pattern of pregnancy specific outcomes among pregnant women or their infants who received single or combination hepatitis A vaccination.[64]

Hepatitis B

Hepatitis B was recognized as "serum hepatitis" by the 20th century.[18] Hepatitis B virus (HBV) is a DNA virus of the Hepadnaviridae family with humans as the only known host.[18] HBV infection can be self-limiting or lead to chronic carrier state. In the United States, the most important routes of transmission are perinatal or sexual transmission with an infected person.[18] Mucosal or parental exposures can transmit infection with highest titers of virus found in blood and serous fluids. A 3-dose vaccine series of recombinant HBV DNA provides indefinite immunity in most individuals and is currently started at birth as part of CDC recommended childhood vaccination schedule.[31,65] See **Table 2** for vaccine formulations.

Knowing a woman's HBV status is important during pregnancy owing to the increased chance for the development of chronic disease after perinatal acquisition.[13] Mother-to-child transmission is highly efficient. Mothers who are positive for both HBV surface antigen and hepatitis B e antigen have a 70% to 90% of mother to child transmission if postexposure prophylaxis is not initiated[18] thus prompting routine screening for HBV surface antigen in pregnancy.[66] Neonates born from seropositive mothers are treated with HB immunoglobulin and newborn vaccination initiated.[18,31,66] Unvaccinated pregnant women with risk factors for seroconversion in pregnancy should be counseled that the vaccine is highly effective in preventing maternal infection and, therefore, fetal infection.[54] Individuals at risk are specified in **Table 2**. Further, when the 3-part HBV vaccine series has been given during pregnancy, no safety concerns have been reported.[67] Although not routinely given during pregnancy, initiating or completing the 3-dose HBV vaccine series should be considered among women at risk for HBV infection.

Pneumococcal Vaccine

Streptococcus pneumoniae, a gram-positive, lancet-shaped bacteria initially discovered by Pasteur, has multiple serotypes, but 10 account for more than one-half of invasive disease worldwide.[18] Pneumococcal infection is typically in the form of pneumonia, bacteremia, or meningitis.[18] Pneumonia is the most common pneumococcal disease in adults leading to approximately 400,000 hospitalizations annually with a case fatality rate of 5% to 7%.[18] During pregnancy, the incidence of pneumonia is just less than 5%, but the most common single pathogen is *S pneumoniae*.[68] Pregnancy-associated pneumonia has higher rates of hospitalization, acute respiratory distress syndrome, cardiorespiratory failure, and death owing in part to maternal physiologic changes in respiratory physiology and cell-mediated immunity.[68] Adriani and colleagues[69] reported 31 cases of pneumococcal meningitis during pregnancy, but with a maternal mortality rate of 28% and a 37% incidence of miscarriage, stillbirth, or neonatal death.

The prevention of pneumococcal disease is indicated among children and adults with chronic medical conditions. The CDC recommends the 23-serotype polysaccharide vaccine (PPSV23) be given to adults with risk factors (see **Table 2**).[3,31] Both systematic review and randomized trial of PPSV23 given in pregnancy reported no maternal or fetal safety concerns.[67,70] A Cochrane review evaluating maternal pneumococcal vaccination for infant protection from illness did not find sufficient evidence for reduction of infant illness.[71] Current data are not sufficient to recommend universal pneumococcal vaccination in pregnancy, but its use should be considered in pneumococcal-naïve women with the comorbidities described in **Table 2**.[13]

Meningococcal Vaccine

Meningococcal disease is caused by the gram-negative, encapsulated diplococci, *Neisseria meningitidis*. Illness is typically characterized by fever, meningitis, sepsis, and can have serious sequelae despite antibiotics, including severe cognitive impairment, hearing loss, seizures, and learning disabilities; between 10% and 14% cases are fatal.[72,73]

The ACIP recommends vaccination for adolescents aged 11 to 18 years and individuals age 2 to 55 years who are at increased risk for meningococcal disease (see **Table 2**).[3,21] Similarly, pregnant women may be among those with potential exposure, and who may benefit from conditional immunization.[13,18] Both tetravalent meningococcal conjugate vaccine (MenACWY) and tetravalent polysaccharide-protein vaccine (MPSV4) exist and are both inactivated vaccines (see **Table 2**). The Vaccine Adverse Event Reporting System database reports were reviewed between 2005 and 2011. Although pregnant women were excluded from prelicensure trials, they made up 1% of reports following the tetravalent meningococcal conjugate vaccine, MenACWY-D (Menactra) and review of these data did not reveal any unusual or unexpected pattern of pregnancy-associated or neonatal events.[74] Reviews evaluating vaccination during pregnancy with both MPSV4[67] and meningococcal conjugate vaccine MenACWY-D (Menactra)[74] did not identify any maternal or fetal safety concerns. Thus, previously unvaccinated women who are at risk should be vaccinated.[13,18,54]

VACCINES CURRENTLY UNDER INVESTIGATION

Historically, vaccine trials have excluded patients based on pregnancy status. Obstetric providers face barriers and challenges to the current vaccine recommendations in pregnancy.[9] Nevertheless, as data continue to demonstrate both safety and benefits to maternal immunization, opportunities for expansion exist. Currently explored vaccines for use in pregnancy include the prevention of Zika, group B streptococcus (GBS), respiratory syncytial virus (RSV), and CMV.

Zika Vaccine

Zika virus is a flavivirus, closely related to dengue and chikungunya,[75] and requires vector transmission. Zika virus and infection from Zika seem to have a far greater impact on the fetus than on the mother.[76] Evidence now correlates Zika virus infection during pregnancy with fetal death, growth restriction, and a spectrum of central nervous system abnormalities.[77]

Prevention and testing for Zika virus in pregnancy continue to be a challenge, both in laboratory techniques and in the role of clinical practice, making vaccine investigation invaluable. Testing for Zika virus currently uses IgM, a nucleic acid test, and a plaque reduction neutralization test. Cross-reactivity of Zika with other flaviviruses and duration of Zika virus IgM antibody presence makes testing and interpretation of timing of infection difficult.[78]

Zika testing algorithms are constantly changing as updated scientific study provides new information. For the most recent guidelines, the provider should confirm recommended testing with the CDC, American College of Obstetricians and Gynecologists, or local public health authorities (information is also available at: https://www.cdc.gov/zika/index.html and https://www.acog.org/About-ACOG/ACOG-Departments/Zika-Virus).[79] Zika testing recommendations at the time of publication include the following:

- Pregnant women with exposure during the current gestation with symptoms of Zika virus illness,[78] should have Zika testing performed as soon as possible up through 12 weeks from symptom onset with: nucleic acid test (serum and urine) and Zika virus IgM (serum).[80]
- Pregnant women with exposure during the current gestation without symptoms and in the absence of ongoing exposure, are not routinely recommended to have Zika virus testing.
- Pregnant women with ongoing Zika exposure should be offered Zika virus nucleic acid test (serum and urine) 3 times during their pregnancy, with a note that IgM is no longer recommended given prolonged persistence.[79]

Testing algorithm changes are in response to the decreasing prevalence of Zika virus disease[76,79] and recent data indicating an extended presence of Zika virus IgM antibodies, raising the concern for increased numbers of false positive-results.[78,81] No specific treatment for adults or pregnant women with Zika virus infection is recommended other than management of symptomatic relief via rest, adequate hydration, and use of antipyretics (preferably acetaminophen as opposed to aspirins). Pregnant women are recommended to avoid travel to locations experiencing Zika outbreaks.[80]

Primary prevention seems to be the best strategy, and could provide sustainable protection. Vaccines are already in existence for the prevention of other flaviviruses, such as Japanese encephalitis and yellow fever, suggesting that the prevention of Zika virus is both safe and feasible.[82] Both industry and the National Institute of Allergy and Infectious Diseases are working on several candidate vaccines.[83] One DNA-based vaccine, VRC 705, entered a phase I clinical trial in August 2016 and launched a phase II clinical trial in March 2017 enrolling healthy nonpregnant volunteers (clinicaltrials.gov: NCT03110770). Another purified inactivated Zika vaccine, ZPIV, was developed by Walter Reed Army Institute of Research,[84] and is similar to vaccines for Japanese encephalitis and dengue. Phase I trials have begun at various clinical sites in the United States and Puerto Rico (clinicaltrials.gov: NCT02963909, NCT03008122). Third, a live-attenuated vaccine candidate offering protection against Zika and dengue virus infections is currently being evaluated in phase III study in Brazil. Several messenger RNA vaccines by GlaxoSmithKline and Moderna/Valera (clinicaltrials.gov: NCT03014089) are being evaluated as well; several other vaccines are in preclinical testing.

Group B Streptococcus Vaccine

Despite screening and intrapartum prophylaxis, GBS remains the leading cause of invasive infection in the first 90 days of neonatal life causing sepsis and meningitis.[85] Intrapartum antibiotic use has reduced the incidence of early-onset GBS infection (first 7 days of life), but has had no impact on late-onset disease (from the first week of life through 3 months).[85] Late-onset disease occurs too early in life for the neonate to mount an effective immune response and is untouched by current prevention strategies, making maternal immunization an ideal strategy.[86] Phase I and II trials of a trivalent GBS vaccine (CRM197-conjugated capsular polysaccharides of GBS serotypes Ia, Ib, and III) have been performed in more than 600 nonpregnant and more than 500 pregnant women in 4 countries (NCT01193920, NCT01446289, NCT02046148).[86] Several trials are ongoing, but are aimed to assess optimal dose, immunogenicity, placental transfer, and other variables. Candidate vaccines seems to be well-tolerated and immunogenic.[86]

Respiratory Syncytial Virus Vaccine

RSV is a seasonal respiratory virus with naturally induced waning immunity, meaning that an individual can be repeatedly infected during their lifespan.[87] In the United States, 25% to 40% of infants and young children will develop pneumonia or bronchiolitis with their first RSV infection.[87] Premature and very young infants, as well as those with cardiopulmonary disease have a greater chance of developing more severe disease and requiring hospitalization.[87] Prevention of RSV during early life is currently accomplished with the use of an effective but costly monoclonal antibody given as monthly injections during RSV season. The administration of the medication is currently restricted to a subset of neonates likely to experience the most complications from illness.[87] A recombinant RSV vaccine is currently in phase II clinical trials in nonpregnant women with plans for a phase I trial in pregnancy underway.[88] A phase III randomized trial by Novavax is ongoing to evaluate a candidate RSV vaccine in third trimester of pregnancy examining the incidence of RSV in infants through 90 days of life (clinicaltrials.gov: NCT02624947).

Cytomegalovirus Vaccine

Congenital CMV is the most common viral infection of the fetus.[89] CMV can be transmitted from mother to fetus, but the precise mechanism of transplacental infection remains unclear. Fetal infection may follow maternal primary or recurrent infection, exposure to contaminated genital tract secretions during delivery, or breastfeeding.[28,90,91] Further, maternal testing for primary and non primary CMV infection remains challenging (**Figure 1**). Most data suggest symptomatic neonatal infection occurs more frequently among children born to mothers with primary CMV infection during pregnancy[89,91,92]; however, recent international data propose similar rates of symptomatic neonatal infection after maternal primary and nonprimary infections.[93] There are no current well-established methods to prevent congenital CMV transmission. Owing to the large number of infants affected by CMV and the associated economic burden (estimated educational and medical costs of affected children is approximately 1.9 billion per year[94]), the Institute of Medicine deemed the development of maternal vaccine to be of the highest priority.[94] Despite 40 years of research to develop a vaccine, success remains a challenge. Previous development of the Towne live attenuated vaccine found the vaccine incapable of eliciting wild type–like immunity.[95] Further development was targeted toward CMV glycoproteins because glycoprotein B-directed antibodies are invariantly present in CMV seropositive individuals, are capable of viral neutralization, and this protein is relatively conserved among different viral strains.[96]

With these mentioned targets in attempts to develop a vaccine, there are multiple trials recently completed or active in CMV vaccine development. Per a review by Schleiss,[95] many different approaches are being explored, including recombinant protein vaccines targeted to immunodominant envelope glycoprotein, CMV glycoprotein B. Challenges remain in vaccine development, including many questions regarding the vaccine's effect on fetal transmission.[97] Because congenital CMV infection can occur in reactivation or recurrent infection, the question arises: Will a vaccine augment the immune response?[94] Still, the substantial disabilities children experience owing to CMV infection demands a vaccine.

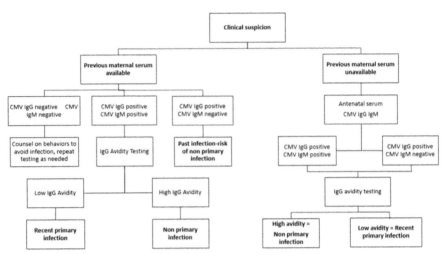

Fig. 1. Cytomegalovirus (CMV) testing algorithm to evaluate for maternal infection. Ig, immunoglobulin. Note: lower CMV IgG avidity is correlated with more recently occurring infection.

ROLE OF OBSTETRICIANS AS VACCINATORS

Support from numerous advisory committees and professional societies (eg, the ACIP, American College of Obstetricians and Gynecologists, American Academy of Family Physicians, American Academy of Pediatrics, and the National Vaccine Advisory Committee) has contributed to the increased uptake of vaccines during pregnancy in the United States. Numerous studies repeatedly report that provider recommendation is the greatest predictor of pregnant women accepting either influenza or pertussis vaccination.[9,12] Women's health providers face challenges with vaccination, including ordering, storage, handling, liability concerns, and vaccine tracking.[9,12] Given groups who delay recommended immunization schedules or refuse vaccines altogether, obstetrics/gynecology providers may encounter difficulty providing coverage. It is also difficult to estimate the appropriate supply and demand for each of the vaccines. Accomplishing maternal immunization remains critical because vaccine acceptance during pregnancy may lead to positive attitudes toward immunization in general, which may prompt greater vaccine awareness and acceptance, for themselves and their children.[12]

SUMMARY

Vaccines are an effective way to prevent many infectious diseases posing maternal and neonatal risks. Some vaccines are specifically recommended during pregnancy or immediately postpartum, and have demonstrated efficacy in either maternal or neonatal illness prevention or both. As women's health providers, we have come a long way in the arena of maternal vaccination, specifically with the tetanus, influenza, and Tdap vaccines. Further, the initiation of multiple novel vaccine studies conducted under US Food and Drug Administration regulation with direct indication for use during pregnancy for disease prevention (GBS and RSV) is unprecedented. New information may change vaccine recommendations over time; consequently, information should be confirmed periodically, and several websites are available containing current guidance (**Table 3**). Delayed successes in the arena of maternal vaccination are multifactorial. As providers, we may lack the ability to stock vaccines in our offices, have inadequate time to educate and vaccinate, or feel

Table 3
Resources for current guidance on vaccines during pregnancy

Sponsoring Organization	Title	Website
ACOG	Immunization for women; immunization information for OB-GYNS and their patients	http://www.immunizationforwomen.org/
CDC	Vaccines and Immunizations	https://www.cdc.gov/vaccines/index.html
	Pregnancy and Vaccination; Maternal Vaccines: Part of a Healthy Pregnancy	https://www.cdc.gov/vaccines/pregnancy/pregnant-women/index.html
CDC's ACIP	ACIP Immunization Schedules	https://www.cdc.gov/vaccines/acip/index.html https://www.cdc.gov/vaccines/schedules/hcp/adult.html

Abbreviations: ACIP, Advisory Committee for Immunization Practices; ACOG, American College of Obstetricians and Gynecologists; CDC, Centers for Disease Control and Prevention; OB-GYN, obstetrician-gynecologist.

inadequate to report vaccine tracking or adverse events. However, volumes of research continue to support the safety and efficacy of maternal immunizations, making our efforts worthwhile. The ability to successfully implement maternal immunization and reduce maternal infections relies on provider awareness, recommendations, and patient education regarding dual health benefits for mother and fetus. Success also depends on continued collaborative relationships between professional organizations, providers, patients, and regulatory agencies.[9]

REFERENCES

1. Centers for Disease Control and Prevention (CDC). Achievements in public health, 1990-1999: control of infectious disease. MMWR Morb Mortal Wkly Rep 1999;48(29):621–9.
2. Centers for Disease Control and Prevention (CDC). Ten great public health achievements–worldwide, 2001-2010. MMWR Morb Mortal Wkly Rep 2011; 60(24):814–8.
3. Centers for Disease Control and Prevention (CDC): Recommended adult immunization schedule. 2017. Available at: https://www.cdc.gov/vaccines/schedules/hcp/imz/adult.html. Accessed September 15, 2017.
4. Prevention and control of influenza: recommendations of the Advisory Committee on Immunization Practices (ACIP). MMWR Recomm Rep 1997; 46(RR-9):1–25.
5. Centers for Disease Control and Prevention (CDC). 2012 final pertussis surveillance report. 2013. Available at: http://www.cdc.gov/pertussis/downloads/pertuss-surv-report-2012.pdf. Accessed September 15, 2017.
6. ACOG committee opinion no. 566: update on immunization and pregnancy: tetanus, diphtheria, and pertussis vaccination. Obstet Gynecol 2013;121(6): 1411–4.
7. Raghupathy R. Th1-type immunity is incompatible with successful pregnancy. Immunol Today 1997;18(10):478–82.
8. Rasmussen SA, Jamieson DJ, Uyeki TM. Effects of influenza on pregnant women and infants. Am J Obstet Gynecol 2012;207(3 Suppl):S3–8.

9. Beigi RH, Fortner KB, Munoz FM, et al. Maternal immunization: opportunities for scientific advancement. Clin Infect Dis 2014;59(Suppl 7):S408–14.

10. Bratton KN, Wardle MT, Orenstein WA, et al. Maternal influenza immunization and birth outcomes of stillbirth and spontaneous abortion: a systematic review and meta-analysis. Clin Infect Dis 2015;60(5):e11–9.

11. Steinhoff MC, Omer SB, Roy E, et al. Neonatal outcomes after influenza immunization during pregnancy: a randomized controlled trial. CMAJ 2012;184(6): 645–53.

12. National Vaccine Advisory Committee. The National Vaccine Advisory Committee: reducing patient and provider barriers to maternal immunizations: approved by the National Vaccine Advisory Committee on June 11, 2014. Public Health Rep 2015;130(1):10–42.

13. Swamy GK, Beigi RH. Maternal benefits of immunization during pregnancy. Vaccine 2015;33(47):6436–40.

14. Fell DB, Platt RW, Lanes A, et al. Fetal death and preterm birth associated with maternal influenza vaccination: systematic review. BJOG 2015;122(1):17–26.

15. Freeman DW, Barno A. Deaths from Asian influenza associated with pregnancy. Am J Obstet Gynecol 1959;78:1172–5.

16. Jamieson DJ, Honein MA, Rasmussen SA, et al. H1N1 2009 influenza virus infection during pregnancy in the USA. Lancet 2009;374(9688):451–8.

17. Harris JW. Influenza occurring in pregnant women, a statistical study of thirteen hundred and fifty cases. JAMA 1919;72:978–80.

18. Centers for Disease Control and Prevention. Epidemiology and prevention of vaccine-preventable diseases. In: Hamborsky J, Kroger A, Wolfe S, editors. 13th edition. Washington D.C.: Public Health Foundation, 2015.

19. Plotkin S, Orenstein W, Dffit P, et al. Vaccines. 7th edition. Philadelphia: Saunders; 2017.

20. Toback SL, Beigi R, Tennis P, et al. Maternal outcomes among pregnant women receiving live attenuated influenza vaccine. Influenza Other Respir Viruses 2012; 6(1):44–51.

21. Centers for Disease Control and Prevention (CDC). Guidelines for vaccinating pregnant women. 2017. Available at: https://www.cdc.gov/vaccines/pregnancy/hcp/guidelines.html. Accessed September 20, 2017.

22. Dodds L, McNeil SA, Fell DB, et al. Impact of influenza exposure on rates of hospital admissions and physician visits because of respiratory illness among pregnant women. CMAJ 2007;176(4):463–8.

23. Neuzil KM, Reed GW, Mitchel EF, et al. Impact of influenza on acute cardiopulmonary hospitalizations in pregnant women. Am J Epidemiol 1998;148(11): 1094–102.

24. Kallen B, Olausson PO. Vaccination against H1N1 influenza with Pandemrix((R)) during pregnancy and delivery outcome: a Swedish register study. BJOG 2012; 119(13):1583–90.

25. Louie JK, Acosta M, Jamieson DJ, et al, California Pandemic (H1N1) Working Group. Severe 2009 H1N1 influenza in pregnant and postpartum women in California. N Engl J Med 2010;362(1):27–35.

26. Schlaudecker EP, McNeal MM, Dodd CN, et al. Pregnancy modifies the antibody response to trivalent influenza immunization. J Infect Dis 2012;206(11):1670–3.

27. Haberg SE, Trogstad L, Gunnes N, et al. Risk of fetal death after pandemic influenza virus infection or vaccination. N Engl J Med 2013;368(4):333–40.

28. Madhi SA, Cutland CL, Kuwanda L, et al. Influenza vaccination of pregnant women and protection of their infants. N Engl J Med 2014;371(10):918–31.

29. Zaman K, Roy E, Arifeen SE, et al. Effectiveness of maternal influenza immunization in mothers and infants. N Engl J Med 2008;359(15):1555–64.

30. Benowitz I, Esposito DB, Gracey KD, et al. Influenza vaccine given to pregnant women reduces hospitalization due to influenza in their infants. Clin Infect Dis 2010;51(12):1355–61.

31. Centers for Disease Control and Prevention (CDC): recommended immunization schedule for children and adolescents. 2017. Available at: https://www.cdc.gov/vaccines/schedules/hcp/imz/child-adolescent.html. Accessed November 29, 2017.

32. Nieves DJ, Singh J, Ashouri N, et al. Clinical and laboratory features of pertussis in infants at the onset of a California epidemic. J Pediatr 2011;159(6):1044–6.

33. Centers for Disease Control and Prevention (CDC). Pertussis–United States, 1997-2000. MMWR Morb Mortal Wkly Rep 2002;51(4):73–6.

34. Centers for Disease Control and Prevention (CDC). Pertussis deaths–United States, 2000. MMWR Morb Mortal Wkly Rep 2002;51(28):616–8.

35. Centers for Disease Control and Prevention (CDC). Pertussis (whooping cough): surveillance and reporting. 2017. Available at: https://www.cdc.gov/pertussis/surv-reporting.html. Accessed September 14, 2017.

36. US Food and Drug Administration (FDA). Tetanus toxoid, reduced diphtheria toxoid and acellular pertussis vaccine, adsorbed. Adacel Package Insert. 2015. Available at: http://www.fda.gov/downloads/biologicsbloodvaccines/vaccines/approvedproducts/ucm142764.pdf. Accessed April 25 2016.

37. US Food and Drug Administration (FDA). Tetanus toxoid, reduced diphtheria toxoid and acellular pertussis vaccine, adsorbed. Boostrix Package Insert. 2016. Available at: http://www.fda.gov/downloads/BiologicsBloodVaccines/UCM152842.pdf. Accessed April 29 2016.

38. Centers for Disease Control and Prevention (CDC). Vaccines and preventable diseases, vaccines by disease, about diphtheria, tetanus, and pertussis vaccines. 2016. Available at: https://www.cdc.gov/vaccines/vpd/dtap-tdap-td/hcp/about-vaccine.html. Accessed September 14, 2017.

39. Advisory Committee on Immunization Practices (ACIP). Updated recommendations for use of tetanus toxoid, reduced diphtheria toxoid, and acellular pertussis vaccine (Tdap) in pregnant women — Advisory Committee on Immunization Practices (ACIP). 2012. Available at: http://www.cdc.gov/mmwr/preview/mmwrhtml/mm6207a4.htm. Accessed May 10, 2017.

40. Kretsinger K, Broder KR, Cortese MM, et al. Preventing tetanus, diphtheria, and pertussis among adults: use of tetanus toxoid, reduced diphtheria toxoid and acellular pertussis vaccine recommendations of the Advisory Committee on Immunization Practices (ACIP) and recommendation of ACIP, supported by the Healthcare Infection Control Practices Advisory Committee (HICPAC), for use of Tdap among health-care personnel. MMWR Recomm Rep 2006;55(RR-17):1–37.

41. Steiner B, Swamy GK, Walter EB. Engaging expectant parents to receive Tdap vaccination. Am J Perinatol 2014;31(5):407–12.

42. Halasa NB, O'Shea A, Shi JR, et al. Poor immune responses to a birth dose of diphtheria, tetanus, and acellular pertussis vaccine. J Pediatr 2008;153(3):327–32.

43. Malek A, Sager R, Kuhn P, et al. Evolution of maternofetal transport of immunoglobulins during human pregnancy. Am J Reprod Immunol 1996;36(5):248–55.

44. Gall SA, Myers J, Pichichero M. Maternal immunization with tetanus-diphtheria-pertussis vaccine: effect on maternal and neonatal serum antibody levels. Am J Obstet Gynecol 2011;204(4):334.e1-5.

45. Centers for Disease Control and Prevention (CDC). Updated recommendations for use of tetanus toxoid, reduced diphtheria toxoid and acellular pertussis (Tdap) vaccine from the Advisory Committee on Immunization Practices, 2010. MMWR Morb Mortal Wkly Rep 2011;60(1):13-5.

46. Centers for Disease Control and Prevention (CDC). Updated recommendations for use of tetanus toxoid, reduced diphtheria toxoid, and acellular pertussis vaccine (Tdap) in pregnant women–Advisory Committee on Immunization Practices (ACIP), 2012. MMWR Morb Mortal Wkly Rep 2013;62(7):131-5.

47. Winter K, Nickell S, Powell M, et al. Effectiveness of prenatal versus postpartum tetanus, diphtheria, and acellular pertussis vaccination in preventing infant pertussis. Clin Infect Dis 2017;64(1):3-8.

48. World Health Organization (WHO). Maternal and neonatal tetanus elimination (MNTE). 2017. Available at: http://www.who.int/immunization/diseases/MNTE_initiative/en/. Accessed August 3, 2017.

49. Blencowe H, Lawn J, Vandelaer J, et al. Tetanus toxoid immunization to reduce mortality from neonatal tetanus. Int J Epidemiol 2010;39(Suppl 1):i102-9.

50. McLean HQ, Fiebelkorn AP, Temte JL, et al, Centers for Disease Control and Prevention (CDC). Prevention of measles, rubella, congenital rubella syndrome, and mumps, 2013: summary recommendations of the Advisory Committee on Immunization Practices (ACIP). MMWR Recomm Rep 2013;62(RR-04):1-34.

51. Siegel M, Fuerst HT. Low birth weight and maternal virus diseases. A prospective study of rubella, measles, mumps, chickenpox, and hepatitis. JAMA 1966;197(9): 680-4.

52. Siegel M, Fuerst HT, Peress NS. Comparative fetal mortality in maternal virus diseases. A prospective study on rubella, measles, mumps, chicken pox and hepatitis. N Engl J Med 1966;274(14):768-71.

53. Centers for Disease Control and Prevention (CDC). Three cases of congenital rubella syndrome in the postelimination era–Maryland, Alabama, and Illinois, 2012. MMWR Morb Mortal Wkly Rep 2013;62(12):226-9.

54. Swamy GK, Heine RP. Vaccinations for pregnant women. Obstet Gynecol 2015; 125(1):212-26.

55. Centers for Disease Control and Prevention (CDC). Revised ACIP recommendation for avoiding pregnancy after receiving a rubella-containing vaccine. MMWR Morb Mortal Wkly Rep 2001;50(49):1117.

56. Watson JC, Hadler SC, Dykewicz CA, et al. Measles, mumps, and rubella–vaccine use and strategies for elimination of measles, rubella, and congenital rubella syndrome and control of mumps: recommendations of the Advisory Committee on Immunization Practices (ACIP). MMWR Recomm Rep 1998;47(RR-8):1-57.

57. Lamont RF, Sobel JD, Carrington D, et al. Varicella-zoster virus (chickenpox) infection in pregnancy. BJOG 2011;118(10):1155-62.

58. Brunell PA. Fetal and neonatal varicella-zoster infections. Semin Perinatol 1983; 7(1):47-56.

59. Watson B, Civen R, Reynolds M, et al. Validity of self-reported varicella disease history in pregnant women attending prenatal clinics. Public Health Rep 2007; 122(4):499-506.

60. Marin M, Guris D, Chaves SS, et al. Prevention of varicella: recommendations of the Advisory Committee on Immunization Practices (ACIP). MMWR Recomm Rep 2007;56(RR-4):1-40.

61. Kroger AT, DJ, Vázquez M. General best practice guidelines for immunization. Best practices guidance of the Advisory Committee on Immunization Practices (ACIP). 2017. Available at: https://www.cdc.gov/vaccines/hcp/acip-recs/general-recs/downloads/general-recs.pdf. Accessed September 17, 2017.

62. Bohlke K, Galil K, Jackson LA, et al. Postpartum varicella vaccination: is the vaccine virus excreted in breast milk? Obstet Gynecol 2003;102(5 Pt 1):970–7.

63. Advisory Committee on Immunization Practices (ACIP), Fiore AE, Wasley A, Bell BP. Prevention of hepatitis A through active or passive immunization: recommendations of the Advisory Committee on Immunization Practices (ACIP). MMWR Recomm Rep 2006;55(RR-7):1–23.

64. Moro PL, Museru OI, Niu M, et al. Reports to the vaccine adverse event reporting system after hepatitis A and hepatitis AB vaccines in pregnant women. Am J Obstet Gynecol 2014;210(6):561.e1-6.

65. Mast EE, Weinbaum CM, Fiore AE, et al. A comprehensive immunization strategy to eliminate transmission of hepatitis B virus infection in the United States: recommendations of the Advisory Committee on Immunization Practices (ACIP) Part II: immunization of adults. MMWR Recomm Rep 2006;55(RR-16):1–33 [quiz: CE1–4].

66. American College of Obstetricians and Gynecologists (ACOG). ACOG practice bulletin no. 86: viral hepatitis in pregnancy. Obstet Gynecol 2007;110(4):941–56.

67. Makris MC, Polyzos KA, Mavros MN, et al. Safety of hepatitis B, pneumococcal polysaccharide and meningococcal polysaccharide vaccines in pregnancy: a systematic review. Drug Saf 2012;35(1):1–14.

68. Sheffield JS, Cunningham FG. Community-acquired pneumonia in pregnancy. Obstet Gynecol 2009;114(4):915–22.

69. Adriani KS, Brouwer MC, van der Ende A, et al. Bacterial meningitis in pregnancy: report of six cases and review of the literature. Clin Microbiol Infect 2012;18(4):345–51.

70. Munoz FM, Bond NH, Maccato M, et al. Safety and immunogenicity of tetanus diphtheria and acellular pertussis (Tdap) immunization during pregnancy in mothers and infants: a randomized clinical trial. JAMA 2014;311(17):1760–9.

71. Chaithongwongwatthana S, Yamasmit W, Limpongsanurak S, et al. Pneumococcal vaccination during pregnancy for preventing infant infection. Cochrane Database Syst Rev 2015;(1):CD004903.

72. Rosenstein NE, Perkins BA, Stephens DS, et al. Meningococcal disease. N Engl J Med 2001;344(18):1378–88.

73. Thigpen MC, Whitney CG, Messonnier NE, et al. Bacterial meningitis in the United States, 1998-2007. N Engl J Med 2011;364(21):2016–25.

74. Zheteyeva Y, Moro PL, Yue X, et al. Safety of meningococcal polysaccharide-protein conjugate vaccine in pregnancy: a review of the Vaccine Adverse Event Reporting System. Am J Obstet Gynecol 2013;208(6):478.e1-6.

75. Lanciotti RS, Kosoy OL, Laven JJ, et al. Genetic and serologic properties of Zika virus associated with an epidemic, Yap State, Micronesia, 2007. Emerg Infect Dis 2008;14(8):1232–9.

76. Meaney-Delman D, Hills SL, Williams C, et al. Zika virus infection among U.S. pregnant travelers - August 2015-February 2016. MMWR Morb Mortal Wkly Rep 2016;65(8):211–4.

77. Rasmussen SA, Jamieson DJ, Honein MA, et al. Zika virus and birth defects–reviewing the evidence for causality. N Engl J Med 2016;374(20):1981–7.

78. Adebanjo T, Godfred-Cato S, Viens L, et al. Update: interim guidance for the diagnosis, evaluation, and management of infants with possible congenital zika

virus infection - United States, October 2017. MMWR Morb Mortal Wkly Rep 2017;66(41):1089–99.

79. Centers for Disease Control and Prevention (CDC): zika virus. 2017. Available at: https://www.cdc.gov/zika/index.html. Accessed November 29, 2017.

80. Oduyebo T, Polen KD, Walke HT, et al. Update: interim guidance for health care providers caring for pregnant women with possible zika virus exposure - United States (Including U.S. Territories), July 2017. MMWR Morb Mortal Wkly Rep 2017; 66(29):781–93.

81. Woods CR. False-positive results for immunoglobulin m serologic results: explanations and examples. J Pediatric Infect Dis Soc 2013;2(1):87–90.

82. Pierson TC, Graham BS. Zika virus: immunity and vaccine development. Cell 2016;167(3):625–31.

83. National Institute of Allergy and Infectious Diseases (NIAID). Zika virus vaccines. 2017. Available at: https://www.niaid.nih.gov/diseases-conditions/zika-vaccines. Accessed September 17, 2017.

84. Larocca RA, Abbink P, Peron JP, et al. Vaccine protection against Zika virus from Brazil. Nature 2016;536(7617):474–8.

85. Verani JR, McGee L, Schrag SJ, Division of Bacterial Diseases, National Center for Immunization and Respiratory Diseases, Centers for Disease Control and Prevention (CDC). Prevention of perinatal group B streptococcal disease–revised guidelines from CDC, 2010. MMWR Recomm Rep 2010;59(RR-10):1–36.

86. Heath PT. Status of vaccine research and development of vaccines for GBS. Vaccine 2016;34(26):2876–9.

87. Centers for Disease Control and Prevention (CDC). Respiratory syncytial virus infection (RSV) for healthcare professionals. 2017. Available at: https://www.cdc.gov/rsv/clinical/index.html. Accessed June 1, 2017.

88. Safety study of respiratory syncytial virus (RSV)-fusion (F) protein particle vaccine. 2012. Available at: https://clinicaltrials.gov/ct2/show/NCT01290419. Accessed June 1, 2017.

89. Society for Maternal-Fetal Medicine (SMFM), Hughes BL, Gyamfi-Bannerman C. Diagnosis and antenatal management of congenital cytomegalovirus infection. Am J Obstet Gynecol 2016;214(6):B5–11.

90. Dollard SC, Grosse SD, Ross DS. New estimates of the prevalence of neurological and sensory sequelae and mortality associated with congenital cytomegalovirus infection. Rev Med Virol 2007;17(5):355–63.

91. Fowler KB, Stagno S, Pass RF, et al. The outcome of congenital cytomegalovirus infection in relation to maternal antibody status. N Engl J Med 1992;326(10):663–7.

92. Davis NL, King CC, Kourtis AP. Cytomegalovirus infection in pregnancy. Birth Defects Res 2017;109(5):336–46.

93. Boppana SB, Ross SA, Fowler KB. Congenital cytomegalovirus infection: clinical outcome. Clin Infect Dis 2013;57(Suppl 4):S178–81.

94. Arvin AM, Fast P, Myers M, et al, National Vaccine Advisory Committee. Vaccine development to prevent cytomegalovirus disease: report from the National Vaccine Advisory Committee. Clin Infect Dis 2004;39(2):233–9.

95. Schleiss MR. Cytomegalovirus vaccines under clinical development. J Virus Erad 2016;2(4):198–207.

96. Fu TM, An Z, Wang D. Progress on pursuit of human cytomegalovirus vaccines for prevention of congenital infection and disease. Vaccine 2014;32(22):2525–33.

97. Krause PR, Bialek SR, Boppana SB, et al. Priorities for CMV vaccine development. Vaccine 2013;32(1):4–10.

Thromboprophylaxis in Pregnancy

Diana Kolettis, MD, Sabrina Craigo, MD*

KEYWORDS

- Thromboembolism • Prophylaxis • Pregnancy • Thromboprophylaxis

KEY POINTS

- Venous thromboembolism is a significant contributor to maternal morbidity and mortality. Thromboprophylaxis for patients at highest risk of venous thromboembolism should be part of standard obstetric practice.
- Measures to mitigate the risk of venous thromboembolism after cesarean delivery should be used, including early ambulation and mechanical or pharmacologic thromboprophylaxis based on individual risk factors.
- Low-molecular-weight heparin and unfractionated heparin are safe and effective for use in pregnancy.
- Neither prophylactic nor intermediate dosing of low-molecular-weight heparin or unfractionated heparin requires monitoring of anti-Xa levels or activated partial thromboplastin time.
- Standard doses of low-molecular-weight heparin and unfractionated heparin may be inadequate in the obese population. Higher or weight-based dosing should be considered for severely obese patients.

BACKGROUND

Venous thromboembolism (VTE) is one of the leading causes of maternal death in the United States and the world. VTE includes deep vein thrombosis and pulmonary embolism (PE) as well as other more rare forms such as mesenteric vein thrombosis and intracranial venous thrombosis. The overall incidence is 2- to 4-fold higher than the rate in the nonpregnant population.[1] The risk is increased throughout pregnancy, but greatest in the postpartum period.[2] The incidence of VTE ranges from 1 to 2 per 1000 with up to 80% being DVTs in the antepartum period and 20% to 25% being PE.[3,4] In contrast, the incidence of PE is much higher postpartum, with 40% to 60% of all PEs occurring after delivery.[2] Recent efforts to address maternal mortality in the United States led to the development of strategies to help identify patients at

Disclosure Statement: None.
[a] Department of Obstetrics and Gynecology, Division of Maternal Fetal Medicine, Tufts Medical Center, 800 Washington Street, Box 360, Boston, MA 02111, USA
* Corresponding author.
E-mail address: scraigo@tuftsmedicalcenter.org

Obstet Gynecol Clin N Am 45 (2018) 389–402
https://doi.org/10.1016/j.ogc.2018.01.007
0889-8545/18/© 2018 Elsevier Inc. All rights reserved.

greatest risk of VTE, and to implement practices focused on prevention. The relatively low incidence of VTE makes prospective studies difficult. Recommendations for practice are, therefore, based largely on small retrospective studies, epidemiologic studies, and expert opinion.[5]

Pregnancy is considered a thrombogenic state, owing to venous stasis, an increase in coagulation factors, and relative immobility. Plasma levels of coagulation factors, fibrinogen, Von Willebrand factor, and other markers of thrombin generation are increased during pregnancy, theoretically to protect the mother from excessive bleeding during delivery.[5] Compression of the vena cava and pelvic vessels by the gravid uterus is another contributing factor. Universal prophylaxis is not recommended during pregnancy. Instead, efforts in prevention of VTE have focused on interventions for those patients with risk factors in addition to pregnancy.[6,7] Risk factors may be preexisting, such as a personal history of VTE or known thrombophilia, or may emerge during pregnancy, such as hospital admission or a need for surgery. In this article, we review the current recommendations for thromboprophylaxis in pregnancy, including outpatient antepartum, inpatient, perioperative, and postpartum thromboprophylaxis. We do not address therapeutic anticoagulation for VTE diagnosed in pregnancy, mechanical heart valve, atrial fibrillation, or other conditions requiring therapeutic anticoagulation.

DEFINITION, RISKS, AND GUIDING PRINCIPLES

Prophylaxis is an action taken to prevent disease, especially by specified means or against a specified disease. Thrombosis prevention can be achieved via mechanical or pharmacologic methods. The benefits of pharmacologic thromboprophylaxis in preventing the occurrence of VTE must be balanced by the increased risk of bleeding during pregnancy, delivery, and the postpartum period. There is wide variation among recommendations regarding indications, dosing, and duration of thromboprophylaxis for the pregnant patient.

Mechanical strategies to prevent VTE include early ambulation after surgery, graduated venous compression stockings, or sequential compression devices (SCD), all aimed at decreasing venous stasis. Several models of SCD have been developed. None are superior over the others in terms of preventing VTE[8]; however, all mechanical methods have been found to reduce the risk of deep vein thrombosis by two-thirds in general surgical patients.[9] There is little evidence for the efficacy of these methods in pregnancy because there are no large-scale studies. The American Congress of Obstetricians and Gynecologists (ACOG) recommends SCD for all women undergoing cesarean section who are not already on pharmacologic thromboprophylaxis.[6]

Pharmacologic thromboprophylaxis has been used for many decades to prevent VTE. The most common forms used include heparins and warfarin. Heparins act indirectly by binding to antithrombin, which then inhibits thrombin, and inactivates factor Xa.[10] Coumadin reduces the synthesis of active clotting factors by depleting the levels of functional vitamin K.[11] The use of any medication in pregnancy requires weighing the risks and benefits to the woman and her fetus. Anticoagulants are associated with an increased risk of bleeding, including placental abruption, postpartum hemorrhage, and perioperative bleeding.[11] The goal of thromboprophylaxis is to administer a dose of medication that reduces VTE risk while minimizing the risk of bleeding.

Warfarin has long been used in the nonpregnant population for prophylaxis against recurrent VTE. Warfarin crosses the placenta and has been associated with fetal anomalies, such as midface hypoplasia, stippled chondral calcification, scoliosis, and short proximal limbs when exposure occurs in the first trimester.

Use of warfarin later in gestation is associated with fetal intracranial hemorrhage and schizencephaly.[12–14]

Heparin medications, including unfractionated heparin (UFH) and low-molecular-weight heparin (LMWH) do not cross the placenta and thus are preferentially used during pregnancy.[15–19] LMWH has been modified from UFH by depolymerization, making the molecular size of the drug smaller. UFH can be associated with heparin-induced thrombocytopenia, and long-term use can be associated with bone loss. These risks are significantly lower with LMWH.[20] Advantages of UFH include lower cost and shorter half-life, which decreases the time required to reverse the anticoagulant effects. Advantages of LMWH include ease of administration and a more reliable anticoagulant effect.[15] LMWH is cleared completely through the renal system. Patients with severe renal insufficiency should receive UFH because its clearance is both hepatic and renal.[21] Rapid reversal of UFH and to some degree LMWH is possible with protamine sulfate. Neither prophylactic nor intermediate doses of LMWH or UFH require monitoring of anti-Xa levels or activated partial thromboplastin time.[21] If UFH is used, platelet counts should be checked before initiation. There is no standardized approach to monitoring platelets while on heparin in pregnancy.

Newer anticoagulation agents have been developed, although they have not been extensively studied in or approved for patients who are pregnant. Fondaparinux, which is a synthetic selective inhibitor of factor Xa, has been used in patients who develop adverse skin reactions with the use of heparin. A small observational study of 12 pregnancies in 10 women showed that fondaparinux did not cause hypersensitivity skin reactions and was not associated with bleeding complications to mother or fetus.[22] Apixaban (Eliquis) acts by inhibiting platelet activation and fibrin clot formation by inhibiting factor Xa. It is indicated for patients with atrial fibrillation, and to help prevent the recurrence of a deep vein thrombosis or PE after a proper treatment course. It can also be used for thromboprophylaxis in the postoperative period from hip and knee replacements. Apixaban is not recommended during pregnancy or breast feeding.[23] Clopidogrel (Plavix) is indicated for patients with acute coronary syndromes, recent myocardial infarctions, or recent stroke by reducing platelet aggregation. There have been case reports of successful pregnancies and deliveries for patients who were taking clopidogrel throughout their pregnancy for cardiac indications,[24] but it has not been used for VTE thromboprophylaxis.

The half-life of UFH is about 1.5 hours, whereas the half-life of LMWH is approximately 4 hours.[21] The risk of bleeding around the time of delivery and limitations in predicting the onset of labor make the use of anticoagulants in pregnancy challenging. Anticoagulation can also be associated with complications of regional anesthesia.[25] Obstetricians caring for patients on anticoagulants before delivery are required to anticipate these potential events and coordinate care around delivery. There are 2 common approaches to managing the use of thromboprophylaxis in this time period. One method involves transition from LMWH to UFH before delivery, with the patient being instructed to stop UFH when signs of labor occur. The other tactic involves stopping LWMH 24 hours before the scheduled induction of labor.[25]

Obstetricians face the challenge of assessing whether a patient is a candidate for thromboprophylaxis. Efforts initially focused on patients with a prior history of VTE. The approach has now broadened to identify those at risk based on several factors.[26] These additional risk factors include age greater than 35 years, obesity, cesarean delivery, black race, heart disease, sickle cell disease, diabetes, systemic lupus, tobacco use, and multiple pregnancy. Several screening strategies have been reported, but none have been uniformly adopted.[27] The Royal College of Obstetrics and Gynecology uses a scoring system to determine the level of risk and subsequent management of obstetric patients. A patient is assigned points based on their specific risk factors for VTE. A higher score is associated with a higher overall risk of VTE. For example, for a patient who is older than 35 years, is a smoker, and has a body mass index (BMI) of greater than 40 kg/m^2, it is recommended that thromboprophylaxis be considered from the first trimester.[7] The ACOG uses a screening strategy based on personal and family history of VTE, presence of low- or high-risk thrombophilia, and other risk factors (**Table 1**).[26] The American College of Chest Physicians (ACCP) categorizes risk factors into major and minor groups. If at least 1 major risk factor or at least 2 minor risk factors are present, the patient qualifies for prophylaxis (**Table 2**).[28]

By convention, recommendations for dosing regimens include prophylactic dosing, intermediate dosing, and therapeutic dosing.[6,28] The goal of prophylactic dosing is to decrease the risk of VTE without increasing bleeding complications. Prophylactic dosing of LMWH is 40 mg subcutaneously daily and UFH is 5000 U subcutaneously twice daily. Intermediate dosing is typically used to adjust prophylactic doses to account for weight gain or other changes over the course of pregnancy, or to address additional risk factors identified during the pregnancy. Current recommendations include increasing the dose of UFH as pregnancy advances to 7500 to 10,000 U twice daily in second trimester, and 10,000 twice daily in third trimester, although these recommendations are not definitive.[23] Regimens for intermediate dosing of LMWH include increasing the daily dose from 40 mg to 1 mg/kg/d or from 40 mg/d to 40 mg twice daily. Therapeutic dosing of anticoagulants is used to treat thromboembolic disease, but can, in some cases, be used prophylactically. For example, patients who have a history of 2 or more prior VTEs or patients taking life-long anticoagulation require therapeutic anticoagulation dosing during the antepartum period.[26]

Data on best dosing strategies are limited. The concept of intermediate dosing arose after pharmacokinetic studies suggested that a higher dose is needed later in pregnancy, owing to maternal weight gain.[11] In addition, a small retrospective study of women at high risk of VTE in pregnancy showed that, despite prophylactic LMWH, their incidence of VTE was still 7%, with 1.8% in the antepartum period. The investigators speculated that prophylactic doses of LMWH may not be as effective in the patients at highest risk. This finding suggests that intermediate or even therapeutic dosing may be needed in the patients at highest risk, but the authors note that further studies are needed to identify the most effective dosing regimen.[29]

ANTENATAL OUTPATIENT THROMBOPROPHYLAXIS

The ACCP and ACOG have released recommendations for thromboprophylaxis for those patients with conditions that increase their risk of VTE throughout pregnancy, including thrombophilias and a history of VTE.[26,28] These recommendations include the antepartum period, starting in the outpatient setting and in all cases continuing postpartum for at least 4 to 6 weeks. The ACOG recommends that patients who have a single previous episode of VTE associated with a transient risk factor outside pregnancy, such as major trauma or trauma to the lower extremity, and are otherwise considered low risk do not need antepartum prophylaxis. These recommendations are supported only by expert opinion. If an otherwise low-risk patient has a history of single VTE that was associated with either pregnancy or estrogen use, then antepartum prophylaxis is recommended. Patients with a history of multiple VTEs should receive prophylaxis, regardless of the cause. Patients who are already taking long-term anticoagulation require a therapeutic dose during the antepartum period. Those who have a low-risk thrombophilia (factor V Leiden heterozygous, prothrombin G20210A heterozygous, or protein C or protein S deficiency), but no personal or family history of VTE,

Table 1
Recommended thromboprophylaxis for pregnancies complicated by inherited thrombophilias

Clinical Scenario	Antepartum Management	Postpartum Management
Low-risk thrombophilia[a] without previous VTE	Surveillance without anticoagulation therapy	Surveillance without anticoagulation therapy or postpartum anticoagulation therapy if the patient has additional risks factors[b]
Low-risk thrombophilia with a family history (first-degree relative) of VTE	Surveillance without anticoagulation therapy	Postpartum anticoagulation therapy or intermediate-dose LMWH/UFH
Low-risk thrombophilia[a] with a single previous episode of VTE—Not receiving long-term anticoagulation therapy	Prophylactic or intermediate-dose LMWH/UFH or surveillance without anticoagulation therapy	Postpartum anticoagulation therapy or intermediate-dose LMWH/UFH
High-risk thrombophilia[c] without previous VTE	Surveillance without anticoagulation therapy, or prophylactic LMWH or UFH	Postpartum anticoagulation therapy
High-risk thrombophilia[c] with a single previous episode of VTE or an affected first-degree relative—Not receiving long-term anticoagulation therapy	Prophylactic, intermediate-dose, or adjusted-dose LMWH/UFH regimen	Postpartum anticoagulation therapy, or intermediate or adjusted-dose LMWH/UFH for 6 wk (therapy level should be at least as high as antepartum treatment)
No thrombophilia with previous single episode of VTE associated with transient risk factor that is no longer present—Excludes pregnancy- or estrogen-related risk factor	Surveillance without anticoagulation therapy	Postpartum anticoagulation therapy[d]
No thrombophilia with previous single episode of VTE associated with transient risk factor that was pregnancy- or estrogen-related	Prophylactic-dose LMWH or UFH[d]	Postpartum anticoagulation therapy
No thrombophilia with previous single episode of VTE without an associated risk factor (idiopathic)—Not receiving long-term anticoagulation therapy	Prophylactic-dose LMWH or UFH[d]	Postpartum anticoagulation therapy
Thrombophilia or no thrombophilia with two or more episodes of VTE—Not receiving long-term anticoagulation therapy	Prophylactic or therapeutic-dose LMWH Or Prophylactic or therapeutic-dose UFH	Postpartum anticoagulation therapy or Therapeutic-dose LMWH/UFH for 6 wk

(continued on next page)

Table 1 (continued)		
Clinical Scenario	**Antepartum Management**	**Postpartum Management**
Thrombophilia or no thrombophilia with two or more episodes of VTE— Receiving long-term anticoagulation therapy	Therapeutic-dose LMWH or UFH	Resumption of long-term anticoagulation therapy

Postpartum treatment levels should be greater or equal to antepartum treatment. Treatment of acute VTE and management of antiphospholipid syndrome are addressed in other Practice Bulletins.

Abbreviations: LMWH, low molecular weight heparin; UFH, unfractionated heparin; VTE, venous thromboembolism.

[a] Low-risk thrombophilia: factor V Leiden heterozygous; prothrombin *G20210A* heterozygous; protein C or protein S deficiency.

[b] First-degree relative with a history of a thrombotic episode before age 50 years, or other major thrombotic risk factors (eg, obesity or prolonged immobility).

[c] High-risk thrombophilia: antithrombin deficiency; double heterozygous for prothrombin *G20210A* mutation and factor V Leiden; factor V Leiden homozygous or prothrombin *G20210A* mutation homozygous.

[d] Surveillance without anticoagulation therapy is supported as an alternative approach by some experts.

Table 2 ACOG, ACCP, and RCOG thromboprophylaxis risk assessment and management recommendations after cesarean delivery		
	Degree of Risk	**Management**
ACOG	Low	Sequential compression devices
	Additional risk factors	Perform an individual risk assessment, as some patients may require prophylaxis with sequential pneumatic compression devices and UFH or LMWH.
ACCP	Presence of ≥1 major or ≥2 minor risk factors (see **Table 3**)	Prophylactic LMWH, or mechanical prophylaxis (for those with contraindications to anticoagulants) while in the hospital after delivery
	Considered very high risk (multiple additional risk factors that persist in puerperium)	Prophylactic LMWH with elastic stockings and/or intermittent pneumatic compression
	High-risk patients with risk factors that persist after delivery	Extended prophylaxis for ≤6 wk after delivery
RCOG	All women who have had an unscheduled cesarean delivery	Consider LMWH for 10 d after delivery
	Those having an elective cesarean delivery with additional risk factors (see **Table 4**)	
	Intermediate, high and very high risk	Prophylactic LMWH for 6 wk postpartum

Abbreviations: ACCP, American College of Chest Physicians; ACOG, American Congress of Obstetricians and Gynecologists; LMWH, low-molecular-weight heparin; RCOG, Royal College of Obstetrics and Gynecology; UFH, unfractionated heparin.

do not require antepartum thromboprophylaxis. Patients with high-risk thrombophilias (antithrombin deficiency, double heterozygous for factor V Leiden mutation, and prothrombin G20210A mutation or homozygous prothrombin gene mutation) but no history of VTE can be followed without thromboprophylaxis during the antepartum period, or prophylactic dosing can be considered. Prophylactic or intermediate-dose LMWH or UFH is also indicated for patients who have a high-risk thrombophilia with single prior VTE or have a family history of VTE (see **Table 1**).[26]

For those women who are candidates for antepartum thromboprophylaxis, LMWH or UFH should be started in the first trimester and continued throughout pregnancy. If additional risk factors are identified during pregnancy, such as immobility, or if hospital admission is required, adjustment from prophylactic dosing to intermediate dosing should be considered. Thromboprophylaxis is used for women considered at increased risk of VTE events, but does not prevent all thromboembolisms, so patients should be educated regarding the signs and symptoms of VTE. Likewise, patients should be counseled regarding the potential for bleeding complications, and should be instructed to report any concerning symptoms to their obstetric provider.

As a pregnancy nears term, UFH is often preferred owing to the ease of reversal. Regional anesthesia, including labor epidurals and spinal anesthesia for cesarean delivery, is contraindicated if a patient is receiving LMWH.[22] Our ability to predict the onset of labor is limited, so transitioning prophylactic LMWH to prophylactic UFH around 36 to 37 weeks of gestation is a reasonable approach. Patients should be instructed to discontinue any thromboprophylactic medication with onset of symptoms of labor.[6] If delivery (vaginal or cesarean) occurs after more than 4 hours have elapsed since administration of prophylactic UFH, the risk of hemorrhage is not significantly increased. Spinal anesthesia can be administered 12 hours after UFH or 24 hours after LMWH.[6,25] Some practitioners prefer to continue LMWH until 24 hours before a scheduled induction of labor or a scheduled cesarean delivery. There are no data to suggest that 1 method is superior, and providers may individualize their approach to patients based on other clinical information, such as desire for regional anesthesia or likelihood of delivering before 39 weeks of gestation.

The continuation of pharmacologic thromboprophylaxis is not recommended during labor and delivery, but patients treated with thromboprophylaxis antenatally will require continuation through the postpartum period. LMWH can be restarted 6 hours after vaginal delivery and 6 to 12 hours after cesarean delivery.[26]

POSTPARTUM THROMBOPROPHYLAXIS

Likely owing to the physiologic changes and relative immobility that can occur after delivery, the risk of VTE is greatest in the postpartum period, and extends for at least 6 weeks.[4] In a large study using claims data from hospitalizations in California from 2005 to 2010, investigators evaluated the risk of thrombotic events (including VTE, myocardial infarction, and stroke). As expected, the highest risk was in the first 6 weeks postpartum, but from 7 to 12 weeks postpartum the risk was still increased over the risk of these outcomes 1 year later. The absolute risk during the 7- to 12-week postpartum period was low, but the investigators recommended further study into the optimal duration of thromboprophylaxis for high-risk patients. They also recommended that clinicians evaluating patients for possible thrombotic events should recognize that the risk remains increased for at least 3 months postpartum.[30]

Guidelines from the ACCP and ACOG recommend postpartum thromboprophylaxis for all patients with any personal history of VTE, all patients with high-risk thrombophilia, and patients with low-risk thrombophilias and a family history of VTE.

Thromboprophylaxis is also recommended during the immediate postoperative period for those with low-risk thrombophilias and no personal or family history of VTE with additional risk factors such as obesity or immobility.[26,28]

THROMBOPROPHYLAXIS FOR OTHER SIGNIFICANT EVENTS
Hospital Admission

Hospitalization is associated with an increased risk of VTE in the general nonpregnant population. The ACCP guidelines recommend LMWH thromboprophylaxis for any acutely ill or immobilized patient.[28] A Cochrane Review showed the benefit of UFH thromboprophylaxis in reducing VTE in nonpregnant medical patients with acute medical illness.[31] Analysis of a national database of more than 200,000 women hospitalized during pregnancy for nondelivery indications from 1997 to 2000 showed the VTE risk was 18-fold higher during hospitalization than during time outside the hospital.[32] The risk remained 6-fold higher for the 28 days after discharge, compared with time outside the hospital. The highest rates were observed in women with a BMI of greater than 30 kg/m^2, age of greater than 35 years, admitted during third trimester, and with hospital stays of greater than 3 days.[32] Although there is general agreement that hospitalization, or the reason for hospitalization, places a pregnant woman at increased risk for VTE, there are no data to demonstrate which method of thromboprophylaxis should be used, or if any method is effective in preventing VTE in hospitalized pregnant women.

Women who are already being treated with pharmacologic thromboprophylaxis as an outpatient should have it continued while hospitalized, unless there is a high risk of bleeding. Consideration should be given to beginning thromboprophylaxis during the inpatient stay for women admitted with medical or surgical complications, with orthopedic injuries, who are immobilized or on prolonged bed rest, or who have multiple other risk factors for VTE such as obesity or age greater than 35 years.[5]

Prophylactic anticoagulation increases the risk of bleeding complications related and unrelated to pregnancy, so caution should be used when considering pharmacologic thromboprophylaxis for patients with these conditions (ie, placenta previa). Mechanical methods of thromboprophylaxis could be considered as an alternative to pharmacologic prophylaxis in this group. Pharmacologic thromboprophylaxis is a reasonable option for many patients admitted without bleeding concerns, and if used should be continued until the patient is fully ambulatory.[26]

Cesarean Delivery

More than 80% of maternal deaths related to PE occur after cesarean delivery, but the benefit of thromboprophylaxis for cesarean delivery has not been well-studied.[33] A case-control study demonstrated the overall risk of VTE was 6-fold higher among those undergoing cesarean delivery compared with those with a vaginal delivery (0.18% vs 0.3%).[4] Still, the individual risk for a VTE after cesarean delivery in a low-risk woman is similar to the risk seen in low-risk nonobstetric surgical patients, for whom routine thromboprophylaxis is not recommended.[23] Guidelines for prophylaxis after cesarean delivery, therefore, vary widely, owing to the difficulty in determining who will benefit from thromboprophylaxis and the lack of information on optimal duration of therapy (see **Table 2**).[7,26,28] Early ambulation after surgery has multiple known benefits.[8,9] It is thought to decrease venous stasis and is recommended after cesarean delivery. The ACOG also recommends use of SCD on all patients undergoing cesarean delivery who are not already receiving pharmacologic thromboprophylaxis.[6] Observational studies of a large cohort of patients with universal use of SCD at the time of cesarean delivery showed a significant lowering of VTE risk.[34] Continuing the SCD until the patient is fully ambulatory is a reasonable approach. The ACOG guidelines also recommend considering a combination of SCD and pharmacologic thromboprophylaxis for women considered at high risk of VTE, including those with a BMI of greater than 35 kg/m², a prior history of VTE, any thrombophilia, or multiple additional factors.[6] Because of concerns of hemorrhage immediately after surgery, pharmacologic thromboprophylaxis is started 6 to 12 hours postoperatively and is continued until the patient is fully ambulatory, or throughout the postpartum period, depending on risk factors. For example, a patient who is greater than 35 years of age and obese but has no other risk factors for VTE might be given thromboprophylaxis until ambulatory or until discharged, whereas a patient with a history of VTE will receive thromboprophylaxis for 6 weeks. Dosing for postcesarean delivery prophylaxis is 40 mg of LWMH daily or UFH 5000 units twice daily. For morbidly obese women with a BMI of greater than 40 kg/m², a weight-based LMWH dosing regimen should be considered.

The AACP recommends early ambulation for all patients undergoing cesarean delivery, and pharmacologic prophylaxis for those with risk factors for VTE, recommending the addition of graduated compression stockings or SCD for women at very high risk of VTE (multiple additional risk factors; **Table 3**).[28] In contrast, the Royal College of Obstetrics and Gynecology recommends considering thromboprophylaxis with LMWH for 10 days after elective cesarean delivery if any risk factors are identified, and for 10 days in all patients undergoing nonelective cesarean delivery. Some risk factors that are identified include parity greater than 3, smoker, age greater than 35 years, gross varicose veins, multiple pregnancy, preterm birth, prolonged labor, and postpartum hemorrhage with more than 1 L blood loss or requiring blood transfusion. They also recommend continuing LMWH for 10 days for women at intermediate risk and 6 weeks for high-risk women, using a risk assessment scoring system (**Table 4**).[7] No prospective trial of this approach has been reported, and it is estimated that these guidelines would lead to more than 1 million patients in the United States each year receiving thromboprophylaxis.[33] The universal adoption of this type of recommendation in the United States will require more evidence regarding safety and efficacy of such an approach.

Table 3
American College of Chest Physicians guidelines: risk factors for VTE resulting in a baseline risk of postpartum VTE of greater than 3%; after a Cesarean section

Major Risk Factors (OR >6)	Minor Risk Factors (OR >6 When Combined)
Presence of ≥1 risk factor suggests a risk of postpartum VTE >3%	Presence of ≥2 risk factors or 1 risk factor in the setting of emergency cesarean section suggests a risk of postpartum, VTE of >3%
Immobility (strict bed rest for ≥1 wk in the antepartum period)	BMI >30 kg/m²
Postpartum hemorrhage ≥1000 mL with surgery	Multiple pregnancy
Previous VTE	Postpartum hemorrhage >1 L
Preeclampsia with fetal growth restriction	Smoking >10 cigarettes/d
Thrombophilia (antithrombin deficiency, factor V Leiden, prothrombin G20210A)	Fetal growth restriction (gestational age + sex-adjusted birth weight <25th percentile
Medical conditions: SLE, heart disease, sickle cell	Thrombophilia (protein C or S)
Blood transfusion	Preeclampsia
Postpartum infection	

Abbreviations: BMI, body mass index; OR, odds ratio; SLE, systemic lupus erythematosus; VTE, venous thromboembolism.

Table 4
Royal College of Obstetrics and Gynecology Risk Assessment for VTE

Total score ≥4 antenatally, consider thromboprophylaxis from the first trimester

Total score ≥3 antenatally, consider thromboprophylaxis from 28 wk

Total score ≥2 postnatally, consider thromboprophylaxis for ≥10 d

If admitted to the hospital antenatally, consider thromboprophylaxis

If prolonged admission (≥3 d) or readmission to hospital within the puerperium consider thromboprophylaxis.

	Score
Preexisting risk factors	
Previous VTE (except a single event related to major surgery)	4
Previous VTE provoked by major surgery	3
Known high-risk thrombophilia	3
Medical comorbidities: for example, cancer, heart failure, active SLE, inflammatory polyarthropathy or inflammatory bowel disease; nephrotic syndrome; type 1 diabetes mellitus with nephropathy; sickle cell disease; current intravenous drug use	3
Family history of unprovoked or estrogen-related VTE in a first-degree relative	1
Known low-risk thrombophilia (no VTE)	1
Age (>35 y)	1
Obesity	1 or 2
Parity ≥3	1
Smoker	1
Gross varicose veins	1
Obstetric risk factors	
Preeclampsia in current pregnancy	1
ART/IVF (antenatal only)	1
Multiple pregnancy	1
Cesarean section in labor	2
Elective cesarean section	1
Midcavity or rotational operative delivery	1
Prolonged labor (>24 h)	1
PPH (>1 L or transfusion)	1
Preterm birth <37 wk in current pregnancy	1
Stillbirth in current pregnancy	1
Transient risk factors	
Any surgical procedure in pregnancy or puerperium except immediate repair of the perineum, for example, appendectomy, postpartum sterilization	3
Hyperemesis	3
OHSS (first trimester only)	4
Current systemic infection	1
Immobility, dehydration	1

Abbreviations: ART, assistive reproductive technology; IVF, in vitro fertilization; OHSS, ovarian hyperstimulation syndrome; PPH, postpartum hemorrhage; SLE, systemic lupus erythematosus; VTE, venous thromboembolism.

Adapted from Royal College of Obstetricians and Gynaecologists. Reducing the Risk of Venous Thromboembolism during Pregnancy and the Puerperium. Green-Top Guideline No. 37a 2015. © Royal College of Obstetricians and Gynaecologists; reproduced with permission.

ADDITIONAL CONSIDERATIONS
Obesity

Obesity, as defined by the Centers of Disease Control and Prevention as a BMI of 30.0 kg/m^2 or greater,[35,36] is an independent risk factor for VTE. Obesity is considered a chronic inflammatory state with upregulation of inflammatory markers, which stimulate the liver to produce coagulation factors. Tissue factor may also be upregulated with obesity. Obesity and the postpartum period together pose a significant risk for VTE, particularly in the setting of immobilization.[37,38] The Royal College of Obstetrics and Gynecology guidelines published in 2015 recommended postpartum prophylaxis with LMWH in obese women regardless of mode of delivery and the ACCP guidelines suggest pharmacologic thromboprophylaxis for obese patients after cesarean delivery.[14,28] The ACCP guidelines are largely extrapolated from data from nonpregnant populations. The ACOG recommends SCD for all patients after a cesarean delivery and suggests that pharmacologic thromboprophylaxis should be considered based on individual risk factors, including obesity.[6]

The approach to the obese pregnant population is further complicated by the lack of consensus on the optimal dosing regimen for pharmacologic therapy. The standard doses of LMWH for thromboprophylaxis are thought to be ineffective with severe obesity, possibly owing to the increased volume of distribution of the drug.[16] Alternatively, patients who are obese have a lower proportion of lean body mass as a percentage of total body weight. Thus, dosing based on total body weight could lead to supratherapeutic anticoagulation. One prospective trial demonstrated that weight based dosing (0.5 mg/kg of LMWH every 12 hours) led to adequate anti-Xa levels more often than a BMI-stratified standard dosing regimen (40 mg twice daily for a BMI of 40–59 60 kg/m^2 and 60 mg twice daily for BMI >60 kg/m^2). Weight-based dosing led to adequate prophylactic anti-Xa levels in 86% of cases versus 21% of those in the stratified dosing regimen.[37]

Immobilization

Immobilization is a recognized risk factor for VTE and likely contributes to the risk of VTE observed in patients admitted to the hospital, and observed with long flights. Data on LMWH prophylaxis for nonpregnant patients with immobilization of the lower extremities showed a significant reduction of VTE.[37] There are no specific guidelines for pregnancy, suggesting VTE thromboprophylaxis for immobilization only, but it is considered a minor risk factor in several guidelines.[6,7] When possible, early ambulation after surgery is recommended, with the intent of reducing venous stasis. Likewise, ambulation during hospital admission should be encouraged when possible. Recent studies showing adverse effects related to activity restriction for obstetric conditions have led to recommendations to avoid prescribing bed rest.[39–41]

Breastfeeding

The commonly used anticoagulants, including LMWH, UFH, and even warfarin, do not accumulate in breast milk and thus are considered safe to use during lactation.[42] In cases in which another class or type of anticoagulant is used, specific information regarding safety during breastfeeding should be reviewed in detail before making recommendations.

SUMMARY

VTE is a significant contributor to maternal morbidity and mortality. Strategies to decrease the incidence of VTE in pregnancy include using mechanical and pharmacologic thromboprophylaxis for women at highest risk. Identifying patients who may benefit from thromboprophylaxis involves thinking critically about each patient's risk factors in the antepartum period, during hospital admission, at the time of cesarean delivery, and in the postpartum period. Current guidelines rely on clinicians individualizing use of thromboprophylaxis based on risk factors. Large-scale prospective trials are needed to determine how thromboprophylaxis can best be used to minimize VTE-related complications.

REFERENCES

1. Ginsberg JS, Bates SM. Management of venous thromboembolism during pregnancy. J Thromb Haemost 2003;1:1435–42.
2. Heit JA, Kobbervig CE, James AH, et al. Trends in the incidence of venous thromboembolism during pregnancy or postpartum: a 30-year population-based study. Ann Intern Med 2005;143(10):697–706.
3. James AH, Jamison MG, Brancazio LR. Venous thromboembolism during pregnancy and the postpartum period: incidence, risk factors, and mortality. Am J Obstet Gynecol 2006;194:1311–5.
4. Simpson EL, Lawrenson RA, Nightingale AL, et al. Venous thromboembolism in pregnancy and the puerperium: incidence and additional risk factors from a London perinatal database. Br J Obstet Gynaecol 2001;108(1):56–60.
5. Bain E, Wilson A, Tooher R, et al. Prophylaxis for venous thromboembolic disease in pregnancy and the early postnatal period. Cochrane Database Syst Rev 2014;(2):CD001689.
6. The American Congress of Obstetricians and Gynecologists (ACOG) Committee on Practice Bulletins-Obstetrics. Practice bulletin no. 123: thromboembolism in pregnancy. Obstet Gynecol 2011;118:718–29.
7. Thrombosis and embolism during pregnancy and the puerperium, reducing the risk. Green-top guideline no. 37a. London: The Royal College of Obstetricians and Gynaecologists (RCOG); 2015.
8. Morris R. Evidence- based compression: prevention of stasis and deep vein thrombosis. Ann Surg 2004;239(2):162–71.
9. Amaragiri SV, Lees TA. Elastic compression stockings for prevention of deep vein thrombosis. Cochrane Database Syst Rev 2000;(3):CD001484.
10. Muñoz EM, Linhardt RJ. Heparin-binding domains in vascular biology. Arterioscler Thromb Vasc Biol 2004;24(9):1549–57.
11. Clark NP. Unfractionated heparin dose requirements targeting intermediate intensity antifactor Xa concentration during pregnancy. Pharmacotherapy 2010;30(4): 369–74.
12. Wesseling J, van Driel D, Heymans HS, et al. Coumarins during pregnancy: long-term effects on growth and development of school-age children. Thromb Haemost 2001;85:609–13.
13. Lee HC, Cho SY, Lee HJ, et al. Warfarin-associated fetal intracranial hemorrhage: a case report. J Korean Med Sci 2003;18:764–7.
14. Pati S, Helmbrecht GD. Congenital schizencephaly associated with in utero warfarin exposure. Reprod Toxicol 1994;8:115–20.
15. Marik PE, Plante LA. Venous thromboembolic disease and pregnancy. N Engl J Med 2008;359:2025–33.
16. Forestier F, Daffos F, Rainaut M, et al. Low molecular weight heparin (CY 216) does not cross the placenta during the third trimester of pregnancy. Thromb Haemost 1987;57(2):234.

17. Ginsberg JS, Kowalchuk G, Hirsh J, et al. Heparin therapy during pregnancy. Risks to the fetus and mother. Arch Intern Med 1989;149(10):2233.
18. Greer IA, Nelson-Piercy C. Low-molecular-weight heparins for thromboprophylaxis and treatment of venous thromboembolism in pregnancy: a systematic review of safety and efficacy. Blood 2005;106(2):401.
19. Weitz JI. Low-molecular-weight heparins. N Engl J Med 1997;337(10):688.
20. Blann AD, Landray MJ, Lip GYH. An overview of antithrombotic therapy. BMJ 2002;325(7367):762–5.
21. Iturbe-Alessio I, Fonseca MC, Mutchinik O, et al. Risks of anticoagulant therapy in pregnant women with artificial heart valves. N Engl J Med 1986;315(22):1390.
22. Knol HM. Fondaparinux as an alternative anticoagulant therapy during pregnancy. J Thromb Haemost 2010;8(8):1876–9.
23. Agnelli G. Apixaban for extended treatment of venous thromboembolism. N Engl J Med 2013;368(8):699–708.
24. Reilly CR. Successful gestation and delivery using clopidogrel for secondary stroke prophylaxis; a case report and literature review. Arch Gynecol Obstet 2014;290(3):591–4.
25. Horlocker TT, Wedel DJ, Rowlingson JC, et al. Regional anesthesia in the patient receiving antithrombotic or thrombolytic therapy: American Society of Regional Anesthesia and Pain Medicine evidence-based guidelines (third edition). Reg Anesth Pain Med 2010;35(1):64–101.
26. The American Congress of Obstetricians and Gynecologists (ACOG) Committee of Practice Bulletins: obstetrics practice bulletin #138 inherited thrombophilias in pregnancy. Obstet Gynecol 2013;122(3):706–17.
27. Dargaud Y, Rugeri L, Vergnes MC, et al. A risk score for the management of pregnant women with increased risk of venous thromboembolism: a multicenter prospective study. Br J Haematol 2009;145:825–35.
28. Bates SM, Greer IA, Middeldorp S, et al. VTE, thrombophilia, antithrombotic therapy, and pregnancy: antithrombotic therapy and prevention of thrombosis, 9th ed: American College of Chest Physicians evidence-based clinical practice guidelines. Chest 2012;141(2 Suppl):e691S.
29. Roeters van Lennep JE, Meijer E, Klumper FJ, et al. Prophylaxis with low-dose low-molecular-weight heparin during pregnancy and postpartum: is it effective? J Thromb Haemost 2011;9(3):473.
30. Kamel H, Navi BB, Sriram N, et al. Risk of a thrombotic event after the 6-week postpartum period. N Engl J Med 2014;370:1307–15.
31. Alikhan R, Cohen AT. Heparin for the prevention of venous thromboembolism in general medical patients (excluding stroke and myocardial infarction). Cochrane Database Syst Rev 2009;(3):CD003747.
32. Sultan A, West J, Tata LJ, et al. Risk of first venous thromboembolism in pregnant women in hospital: population based cohort study from England. BMJ 2013;347:f6099.
33. Sibai BM, Rouse DJ. Pharmacologic thromboprophylaxis in obstetrics: broader use demands better data. Obstet Gynecol 2016;128:681.
34. Clark SL, Christmas JT, Frye DR, et al. Maternal mortality in the United States: predictability and the impact of protocols on fatal postcesarean pulmonary embolism and hypertension-related intracranial hemorrhage. Am J Obstet Gynecol 2014;211:32.e1-9.
35. Centers for Disease Control and Prevention (CDC). Defining adult overweight and obesity. Available at: www.cdc.gov/obesity/adult/defining.html. Accessed November 25, 2017.

36. Morgan ES, Wilson E, Watkins T, et al. Maternal obesity and venous thromboembolism. Int J Obstet Anesth 2012;21:253–63.

37. Overcash RT, Somers AT, LaCoursiere DY. Enoxaparin dosing after cesarean delivery in morbidly obese women. Obstet Gynecol 2015;125:1371–7.

38. Ettema HB, Kollen BJ, Verheyen CPM, et al. Prevention of venous thromboembolism in patients with immobilization of the lower extremities: a meta-analysis of randomized controlled trials. J Thromb Haemost 2008;6:1093–8.

39. Grobman WA, Gilbert SA, Iams JD, et al. Activity restriction among women with a short cervix. Obstet Gynecol 2013;121(6):1181–6.

40. da Silva Lopes K, Takemoto Y, Ota E, et al. Bed rest with and without hospitalization in multiple pregnancy for improving perinatal outcome. Cochrane Database Syst Rev 2017;(3):CD012031.

41. MCarty-Singleton S, Scissione AC. Maternal activity restriction in pregnancy and the prevention of preterm birth: an evidence-based review. Clin Obstet Gynecol 2014;57(3):616–27.

42. Richter C, Sitzmann J, Lang P, et al. Excretion of low molecular weight heparin in human milk. Br J Clin Pharmacol 2001;52(6):708–10.

Moving?

Make sure your subscription moves with you!

To notify us of your new address, find your **Clinics Account Number** (located on your mailing label above your name), and contact customer service at:

Email: journalscustomerservice-usa@elsevier.com

800-654-2452 (subscribers in the U.S. & Canada)
314-447-8871 (subscribers outside of the U.S. & Canada)

Fax number: 314-447-8029

Elsevier Health Sciences Division
Subscription Customer Service
3251 Riverport Lane
Maryland Heights, MO 63043

*To ensure uninterrupted delivery of your subscription, please notify us at least 4 weeks in advance of move.